DOWN THE COVID-19 RABBIT HOLE

DOWN THE COVID-19 RABBIT HOLE

INDEPENDENT SCIENTISTS AND PHYSICIANS UNMASK THE PANDEMIC

EDITED BY STEVEN PELECH
AND CHRISTOPHER A. SHAW

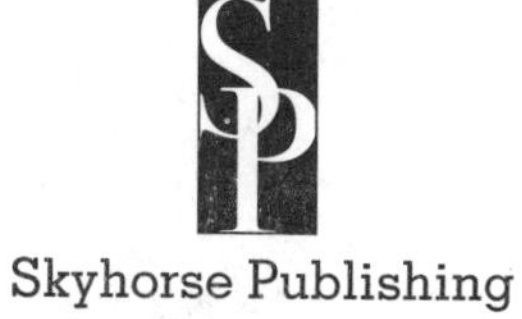

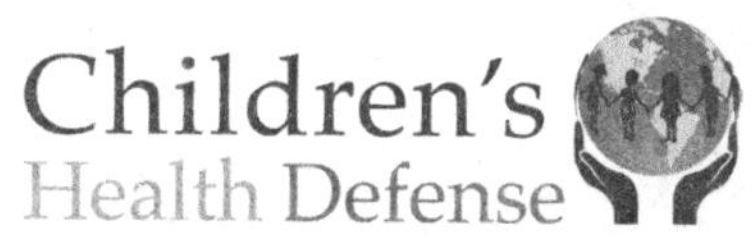

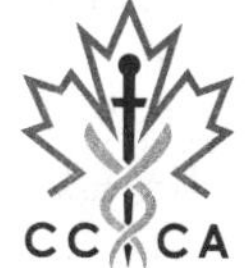

Skyhorse Publishing books may be purchased in bulk at special discounts for sales promotion, corporate gifts, fund-raising, or educational purposes. Special editions can also be created to specifications. For details, contact the Special Sales Department, Skyhorse Publishing, 307 West 36th Street, 11th Floor, New York, NY 10018 or info@skyhorsepublishing.com.

10 9 8 7 6 5 4 3 2 1

Library of Congress Cataloging-in-Publication Data is available on file.

Cover image by Getty Images

Print ISBN: 978-1-5107-7959-4
Ebook ISBN: 978-1-5107-7960-0

Printed in the United States of America

Contents

This book is dedicated to all the people who lost their lives or who suffered greatly from the consequences of the actions taken by those in positions of power. There were millions of victims. We hope that somehow lessons can be learned from the COVID-19 pandemic to avoid similar future situations. All proceeds from the book are donated to the work of the Canadian Citizens Care Alliance (CCCA).

Acknowledgments

Many people contributed to this book, prominently members of the Scientific and Medical Advisory Committee of the Canadian Citizens Care Alliance (CCCA). In particular, we would like to acknowledge the extensive contributions of Drs. John Hardie, Kanji Nakatsu, York Hsiang, Philip Oldfield, and Mariko Uda, as well as their work, including their corrections and suggestions, which have vastly improved this book. Almost all author contributions are acknowledged in the chapters and in the biographies at the end. However, some authors have chosen to remain anonymous for fear of reprisals in view of their sensitive positions. We thank Anne Champagne, MES (Green Words Writing and Editing) for her work formatting the extensive list of references, and further editing provided by Catherine Sutter. We are grateful for the contributions and advice from Alan Cassels, Mariane Klowak, and Rodney Palmer, and Professors John Oller, Russell Blaylock, and David Wiseman. We also acknowledge those at Skyhorse who helped us through all the stages of book writing and preparation for publishing. These include Tony Lyons, Nicole Mele, Zoey O'Toole, Caroline Russomanno, and many others who worked behind the scenes. Our thanks also to Mary Holland who kindly provided the Foreword to this book.

Foreword

Mary Holland
Children's Health Defense

The authors of this groundbreaking book deserve our immense gratitude. They have pulled together many scientific strands from the COVID-19 pandemic—the disease, tests, masks, vaccines, therapeutics—and have started putting together this "massive jigsaw puzzle."[1] While governments and mainstream media continue to cower from any truthful analysis of the COVID-19 fiasco, this courageous group of twenty-four-plus scientists and physicians banded together to rigorously analyze what happened and produce this book. They dedicate the book to all the people who lost their lives or who suffered greatly from the consequences; the victims are in the millions. They also dedicate the book to the proposition that we may still overcome our ignorance and fear to prevent this from ever happening again. It's not too late to turn around the pandemic prevention and response complex that is being institutionalized as we go to print.

This group of highly credentialed authors comes out of the Canadian Citizens Care Alliance, to which all book proceeds will be donated. The authors have provided a critical stepping stone in what they rightly call the "herculean task of repairing the damage." They have given us well-founded knowledge, so that we have the possibility to chart a better course. They opine that we are either at the beginning of a resurgence of our democracies—or at the threshold of a rapid descent into dystopia. The choice is ours.

Among the book's greatest virtues is that it remains grounded in well-cited fact throughout. It leaves for another day speculation about why all this happened. And although the book treats in depth the science behind infectious disease, the pathology of SARS-CoV-2, the safety and efficacy of COVID-19 vaccines and masks, and the therapeutics for the disease, the book is meant for the intelligent lay reader, not just scientists. It is well-written, well-organized, and well-cited, with over 1,070 primary sources. It is essential reading for anyone who wants to understand what co-editor Steven Pelech calls ones of "the greatest whodunnit mysteries" of all time.

The book points out how astonishingly unscientific the whole COVID-19 phenomenon was—from the official narratives to the measures employed to allegedly combat COVID-19. In chapter 2 on "truth," we learn that science only progresses through constant challenge to existing dogma: "Debate is a critical component of the scientific endeavor." And yet during COVID-19, debate was shut down, with dissenting views from the official narrative branded "disinformation" or "malinformation," typically with no justification except that the views differed from orthodoxy.

While the book focuses on the North American experience, it is relevant to anyone who lived through the last five years, regardless of location. And it is comprehensive—starting with the basics of the scientific method, epidemiology and immunology, giving the reader everything needed to better assess the tools employed—and not employed—to respond to the declared COVID-19 public health emergency.

The authors' credentials are impressive—with degrees in a wide variety of scientific fields—biochemistry, medicine, pharmacy, pathology, surgery, epidemiology, toxicology, genetics, immunology, bioinformatics, virology, microbiology, and neuroscience to name a few. This is hardly a rogue group of outsiders. On the contrary, the authors were or are in positions at prestigious universities throughout Canada, renowned in their fields. No doubt many suffered extreme professional hardships because of their willingness to step out of the COVID-19 lockstep dogma.

The tone of the book is also welcome—no spin or rhetoric—just a sober, detailed account of the many scientific dimensions of what occurred. Because of its extraordinarily well-documented nature and clear presentation, the book will be especially valuable to policymakers, scientists, and physicians as a reference as we continue to peel back the layers of what really happened since 2020. It also contains a useful glossary of scientific and other terms necessary for this discourse.

Although the focus of the book is undoubtedly science, the authors do not shy away from pointing out other important features of the COVID-19 years: (1) that 1 percent of the global population vastly increased its financial fortunes while the other 99 percent became poorer; (2) that "the unvaccinated" and "unmasked" experienced "levels of inconceivable discrimination" in this ironic era of diversity, equity, and inclusion, setting dangerous precedents for future government action; and (3) that governments in the United States, Canada, and elsewhere told their citizens the same "outright lies" with the same timing as elsewhere, suggesting that there may have been a "higher level of control" than simply at official government levels.

The authors do not shrink from forceful conclusions. They argue that the COVID-19 vaccines, which stop neither infection nor transmission, are not logically vaccines but rather gene therapies of limited use to suppress symptoms. They state that "authorization of these products should be suspended until the concerns raised [in the book] have been resolved and publicly verified by the regulatory authorities." In other words, they join the millions of laypeople and scientists around the world calling for the mRNA COVID injections to be pulled off the market immediately.

Chapter 3, putting COVID-19 in the context of infectious disease transmission, clarifies that infectious diseases have not been the major causes of morbidity and mortality in Canada for many years. In fact, from 2001 to 2016, infectious diseases accounted for 1.4 to 1.6 deaths per hundred thousand Canadians annually, which increased to about 2.4 deaths per hundred thousand in 2019 and 2020. Furthermore, the authors conclude that government COVID-19 measures adopted in 2020 were not the reason for the same mortality rate in both years. Based on these morbidity and mortality numbers, governments created entirely unjustifiable panic.

The book dissects the myth of "asymptomatic transmission," which led to the massive PCR testing for COVID-19 worldwide. The book disabuses the reader of any notion that the PCR test should have been the "standalone 'gold standard'" test for defining COVID-19: "A positive result with a PCR test does not mean a person has COVID-19 and is able to transmit the disease." And yet as this book goes to press, the PCR test is again being catapulted to prominence as the gold standard test for bird flu and any other possible Disease X.

In the chapter on masks, weighing their effectiveness against risk, the authors point out a little discussed dimension: that 52 billion disposable masks were produced in 2022, with about 1.6 billion ending up in the oceans in just that year. Mask pollution in the ocean, as elsewhere, was significant and will endure for a very long time.

Chapter 13, on the safety of COVID-19 vaccines, is striking. Table 13.2 from the World Health Organization's VigiAccess on vaccine adverse events is simply shocking. It points out that the rate of adverse events from COVID-19 shots is 31,822 times greater than the rate of adverse events from the diphtheria vaccine, whose adverse events have been tracked since 1979. Thankfully, people have caught on to the extraordinary injuriousness and failure of COVID-19 vaccine shots. By the end of 2024's first quarter, Pfizer and Moderna COVID-19 vaccine sales plummeted by 88 percent and 92 percent respectively, compared to 2023.

Chapter 14 discusses many therapies used—and not used—to treat COVID-19. The chapter examines particularly suppressed treatments, including ivermectin, hydroxychloroquine, cannabinoids, and specific nutraceuticals. There were several well-established treatment options that would likely have been effective for treating viral infections before the release of the Emergency Use Authorization in the United States or the Interim Order in Canada. The authors argue that these treatments were not pursued because of the "obsession on the part of the medical establishment, government, and media that only vaccines would return the world to 'normal.' Such pronouncements were seemingly the result of some fixed agenda that may have had little to do with health." The dismissal of these well-established viral treatments by public health officials was "unconscionable."

Chapter 15 touches on some of the future unknown consequences of the COVID-19 shots. The manufacturers of the experimental mRNA COVID-19 vaccines knew from *in vivo* animal biodistribution studies that the mRNA in the lipid nanoparticle coating would be distributed to multiple organ systems, including the central nervous system. This too could be a grave concern for the future "as the short- or long-term consequences of these molecules passing into neural cells are still unknown." And despite this lack of knowledge, manufacturers are barreling ahead with all kinds of mRNA injections for humans and livestock.

Chapter 15 further warns about the potential effects of the mRNA injections on human reproduction. "Given their accumulation in reproductive organs and the already apparent decrease in birth rates, these lipid nanoparticle-enclosed genetic materials may be capable of further accelerating the forecasted world population decline." The authors point out that citizens and governments may have to contemplate how to continue to function as societies when a significant fraction of the population is chronically ill. The post-COVID-19 future may look very distinct from the past.

The book explains the intangible "loss of trust" in all the entities that foisted draconian COVID-19 measures on the world "as more people and their friends and relatives are harmed by the medical measures imposed during the pandemic, the backlash will grow." Trust in all our major institutions—political, financial, medical, legal, and media—are "the inevitable long-term casualties of the pandemic response, arguably vastly more severe in both short- and long-term consequences than the pandemic itself."

I am delighted that the authors have already embarked on a next book—about the "regulatory capture" of mainstream medicine and media and the role of governments that exaggerated the pandemic, leading to needless deaths. If the next book is as strong as this one, it too will be on the must-read list.

This book is truly a monumental achievement. For anyone curious about what we just lived through during the last five years, it is essential reading. While it doesn't answer all the questions we may have about COVID-19, it certainly answers many of the most important ones. And it illuminates how to act—and not act—scientifically to prevent future assaults on our rights and freedoms.

Preface

Christopher A. Shaw

"Nothing in life is to be feared; it is only to be understood. Now is the time to understand more, so that we may fear less."[1]

—Marie Curie

The responses to COVID-19 over the past four and a half years have illustrated how clearly society has failed to put the recent pandemic into anything approaching a clear perspective. We have collectively permitted our ignorance of the disease to allow those who seek to use it for their own ends to flourish. From this ignorance, and the incessant drum beat of fear from government, the media, and, not least, the medical profession, we have collectively become a terrified and manipulated population across the planet.

Whose fault was this? The aforementioned are some of the culprits who brought us to this state. But who is really to blame? We are.

One of the major scenes in the movie *V for Vendetta* is when the protagonist V takes over a television station and tells the audience that they are to blame for the dystopian fascistic country they now live in. The population was lazy and cared more about their creature comforts than their freedom. Those who wanted power even used a manufactured pandemic and vaccine to silence any dissent.

V for Vendetta was, of course, science fiction. However, in the last few years we have seen that just as art imitates life, sometimes, as now, life imitates art. The lockdowns, the mandates, the COVID-19 vaccine hysteria to get one, then two, then an annual shot into every arm, and the demonization of those who refused have led us to where we are today.

We now face the herculean task of repairing the damage done to people and institutions in Canada, the United States, and in many other countries. The first step is to provide a truly scientific evaluation of the pandemic. We need to understand the pathophysiology of COVID-19, the measures taken by government, and the damage done by the experimental COVID-19 vaccines to see just how we were collectively misled by false assumptions about the nature of the disease and its potential cures. This book is our collective response as members of the Canadian Citizens Care Alliance (CCCA), formerly known as the Canadian COVID Care Alliance, in recognition of the broader challenges our society is facing.

As a society, we are at the beginning of either a resurgence of our democracy or a rapid descent into a *V for Vendetta*-like world. Knowledge is key to the former; the lack of it propels us toward the latter.

Read this book, challenge our facts and conclusions, and then decide for yourself.

The choice is still ours to make, and it is not too late.

CHAPTER 1

Why This Book?

Steven Pelech

"You take the blue pill, the story ends, you wake up in your bed and believe whatever you want to believe. You take the red pill, you stay in wonderland, and I show you how deep the rabbit hole goes."

—Morpheus (from the 1999 film *The Matrix*)

The COronaVIrus Disease 2019 (COVID-19) pandemic qualifies as one of the greatest whodunit mysteries of the last century. Over seven million victims worldwide have been officially reported to have died from this respiratory disease, with the total death tally claimed to be much higher. The pathogenic agent was officially identified early on in January 2020 as a novel betacoronavirus of still debatable origin, but most likely a genetically-engineered bat virus. On February 11, 2020, the International Committee on Taxonomy of Viruses (ICTV) named the causative pathogen for COVID-19 as Severe Acute Respiratory Syndrome CoronaVirus 2 (SARS-CoV-2).[1] Nearly five years have transpired since the first official reports of the emergence of this mysterious and severe respiratory disease in Wuhan, China. Even now, the whole muddled affair remains clouded in controversy, starting with the mysterious origin of SARS-CoV-2, through to the ineffectiveness of the various measures that our institutions and societies used to fight this virus and counteract its effects.

Much has been written and said about SARS-CoV-2 and the effectiveness of strategies to mitigate its threat. Much more will surely be documented and discussed by historians in the decades to come. This book serves to record many of the observations made during the COVID-19 pandemic. Google Scholar already lists over 5.3 million publications concerning COVID-19 alone. The tsunami of data regarding the virus and its disease has been overwhelming, often contradictory and inconsistent. Even among the medical and scientific community, there remain more unanswered questions than clear answers. Apparently, a large majority of scientists and medical doctors have been just as confused and misguided as the public about what transpired during the COVID-19 pandemic.

Now that the COVID-19 pandemic has been declared "over," most people just want to move on with their lives and put the whole COVID-19 affair behind them.[2] Others want answers, especially those families that have suffered greatly from either COVID-19 itself or government mishandling of the pandemic. Many people were reduced to second class citizens for resisting COVID-19 vaccine mandates. It is critical to look back with hindsight and evaluate honestly what happened, whether best practices were applied, and what improvements are still needed. This is what government commissions are called for, and what in the military is known as an "After Action Report." Even as this book is being written, public health authorities in Canada and elsewhere are still calling for continued masking and updated COVID-19 vaccinations.

The way our major institutions dealt with the COVID-19 threat has exposed significant inadequacies in these institutions that are supposed to maintain the integrity, cohesion, and health of our societies. These include not just the incompetency and insensitivity within our health care and research systems, but also our governance, legal system, and news media outlets. Many, especially those within these organizations, insist these institutions are to be celebrated for their success in the face of a new adversary, where the projected casualties could have been ten times greater were it not for their decisiveness and resolve to enforce measures not exercised since wartime. Others, however, are bitterly disappointed with the performance of these institutions and their apparent indifference and even outright hostility to those who chose not to go along and take the novel experimental vaccines for COVID-19.

On the one hand, the world largely, particularly in the West, united in confronting a common threat, which resulted in an unprecedented sharing of information and resources. Scientific publications that would previously have been behind paywalls were made freely available if they related to COVID-19. Strategies to curtail the spread of the SARS-CoV-2 virus were quickly shared, although many potential solutions were not endorsed nor promoted by government and mainstream media. Our populations largely embraced the demanded sacrifices of individual freedoms in the name of the greater good to protect the lives of others as well as themselves. They were patriotic in exercising their civic duties in response to the rallying calls that proclaimed that "we are all in this together." Fear and coercion were also driving factors for mass compliance.

On the other hand, to confront the COVID-19 threat, clear abuses in human rights were consistently practiced by countries around the globe, with Canada being one of the worst. The net result was ultimately highly divisive for society at large. These divides, carved primarily by fear and ignorance, even separated friends and family members from each other. Rather than uniting the public, people were divided into those that were vaccinated and those that were not. COVID-19 vaccination was rapidly adopted as the ultimate panacea for confronting the disease. Legitimate concerns were voiced early on that the public health measures taken were not only poorly effective, but they were often more harmful than the disease they were supposed to protect us from. In the frenzy and chaos of the early days of the COVID-19 pandemic, governments implemented solutions with little regard for the overall impacts on society and particularly the most vulnerable.

To combat SARS-CoV-2, promising existing therapeutics already known to be safe were repressed or ignored in favor of more expensive and poorly tested drugs. Novel genetic vaccines were rushed through development and unleashed on the public with minimal testing and available efficacy and safety data. Those who had concerns about these vaccines were subjected to ridicule and even the loss of their jobs with levels of discrimination that are inconceivable in a time when equity, diversity, and inclusion have become fashionable and top priorities for many Western governments and academic institutions. Many people were victims and died from the very measures that were supposed to protect them. Some have even argued based on recent data for all-cause mortality that COVID-19 vaccines have already caused more deaths than the SARS-CoV-2 virus.[3] Very dangerous precedents were clearly established during the COVID-19 pandemic. The abuses exercised during the COVID-19 pandemic are poised to happen again when the next global threat comes along if measures are not put into place to limit the impact on natural and civil rights.

The lessons learned from this global pandemic experience need to be highlighted so that the most effective measures are identified, and mistakes are not repeated in the future. This book aims to contribute to our understanding of what got us to this point and what needs to change so that such disruptions of our societies from the threat of an infectious disease, which frankly was never as deadly as portrayed by government health officials and mainstream media, never happen again.

More than twenty-four of the authors and contributors to this book are research scientists who assembled early on during the COVID-19 crisis to critically evaluate the threat of the virus, the effectiveness of the products offered by the pharmaceutical industry, and the measures instigated by public health authorities. Most of the authors are members of the Scientific and Medical Advisory Committee (SMAC) of what was formerly the Canadian COVID Care Alliance (CCCA) and is now known as the Canadian Citizens Care Alliance.

The CCCA was established in early 2021 as a volunteer, non-profit coalition of researchers, physicians, other health-care practitioners, and legal and ethical professionals dedicated to educating Canadians and people from other nations about the local and international responses to COVID-19. The organization's objective has been to provide top-quality, balanced, evidence-based information that is free of conflicts of interest such as funding from industry or government. The SMAC is one of several committees of the CCCA that has met weekly by Zoom and communicated daily by email for more than three years. The SMAC includes over thirty research professors from major universities across Canada, as well as medical practitioners with diverse expertises in immunology, virology, vaccinology, biotechnology, biochemistry, statistics, and public health. The SMAC reviews the scientific literature, clinical trials, and public health agency data on matters related to COVID-19 with an unbiased view, and what the CCCA publishes in articles and videos are produced with the consensus of the SMAC. While we hope that our findings will be helpful to ongoing discussions with our scientific and medical colleagues, we also recognize that the public needs some guidance in view of the distorted perspectives that have dominated the mainstream legacy media, which has simply parroted the changing and conflicting pronouncements from public health agencies.

Much of the information in this book reflects the Canadian experience with respect to government handling of the COVID-19 pandemic. Canada had one of the highest rates of COVID-19 vaccine adoption, and federal and provincial governments in the country enacted some of the most sweeping restrictions in the world. Canada also saw some of the most vociferous grassroots protests against these restrictions, which was epitomized by the Trucker Freedom Convoy in 2021, with one of the largest protests in Canadian history occurring in Ottawa, the capital city of Canada. The largest public inquiry in the world into a country's government's response to the COVID-19 pandemic, the National Citizens Inquiry, was also undertaken in Canada. Those from other countries will easily recognize that many of our observations are generally applicable globally. The messaging from public health officials and government leaders worldwide has been remarkably consistent, almost verbatim, and uncannily delivered with precision timing in unison.

For some examples, we uniformly heard during the pandemic that quarantining for two weeks was going to flatten the curve of the increase in COVID-19 disease incidence and prevent overwhelming our hospitals; that COVID-19 was very deadly with lethality rates that exceeded the worst flus; that the COVID-19 vaccines were well tested and highly effective in preventing infection and were very safe or at least that these vaccines prevented illness with COVID-19 and stopped its transmission. When all of that turned out to be false, health authorities claimed these vaccines significantly reduced symptoms of COVID-19 and prevented serious disease. As will become apparent from this book, the consistent espousing of unsupported statements ultimately undermined the credibility of health authorities and our health-care systems.

Also, the consistency and timing of the various public health/government pronouncements hints at a higher level of control that transcends nations. Present proposals to further empower the World Health Organization during its future declared pandemics certainly support such notions.

COVID-19 has resulted in a pandemic of misinformation and, according to some, disinformation. This has prompted the establishment of alliances such as the Trusted News Initiative (TNI), which involved government-funded news outlets and social media giants censoring almost all contrarian or dissenting views on matters such as COVID-19 prevention and treatment measures. Self-labeled facts-checkers worked diligently to discredit those who offered statements conflicting with the approved narrative. But who checked the fact-checkers? What were their credentials, and how were they funded? Mainstream and social media avoidance of balanced presentation of the full facts and unbiased critical review of controversial issues surrounding the COVID-19 response represented a colossal failure of these legacy news outlets and the dominant social media giants. A dearth of reliable information from such sources has steered many to seek alternative media outlets that offered more critical presentations of news and views such as the *Epoch Times*, *Rebel News*, *TrialSite News*, *True North*, and the *Western Standard* in Canada and the United States. At times, however, alternative social media information sources misunderstood the "facts" and caused further confusion and distraction from what is true, relevant, and significant.

At the CCCA, we do not entertain or support extreme conspiracy theories, although we can understand why some people might hold such views in the face of some of the available evidence over the last four and a half years. We are certainly not against vaccination in general as a medical prophylactic strategy, although from our investigations we have come to have major misgivings regarding some vaccines, in particular the COVID-19 genetic vaccines. We recognize that to some, *any* criticism of *any* vaccine by *any* author will be characterized as "anti-vax." The word is a "suitcase" word that acts like a dog whistle to imply that those with any concerns whatsoever are scientifically and medically ignorant, as well as selfish and uncaring about the well-being of others.

We recognize that misinformation abounds in legacy media, social media, and other types of alternative media. We believe that the Canadian public and the rest of the world need to be well informed about the evidence that informs public health policy. People should be able to make their own decisions about interventions that jeopardize bodily autonomy and the doctor-patient relationship and statements of "fact" that are not warranted by the available evidence. Our goal is to alert the public where there is controversy and help ferret out the truth, regardless of how inconvenient it might be. Effective solutions to society's problems must be grounded in truth and not influenced by the pursuit of profit or political power.

To really understand the threat posed by SARS-CoV-2, it is necessary to know about this virus and other pathogenic viruses as well as our immune responses to them. Consequently, some of the chapters of this book will be somewhat technical for the lay person. This is unavoidable due to the complex nature of the subject matter. However, because much of what we have uncovered seriously challenges the mainstream narrative, it is critical to scrutinize the scientific underpinnings of the pronouncements of health authorities. To weigh the available evidence, we need to understand that evidence.

To assist the reader, in this book we have included chapters that introduce the scientific method, genes and proteins, viruses, the immune system, and vaccines. Now, nearly five years into the COVID-19 pandemic, we expect that many readers will already possess some knowledge about these matters. Nevertheless, there are people that still question whether SARS-CoV-2 and other viruses even exist. There is a wealth of information available about this virus that is unprecedented in detail. Much is also known about our immune system, which is our best defense against viruses and other infectious pathogens. In fact, immunological systems in animals have effectively dealt with viruses for eons before the existence of humans. There is little doubt that preventative intervention with vaccines has been a powerful strategy to reduce infectious disease spread, which contributed to the elimination of smallpox. Prior to smallpox's eradication, it wreaked havoc and devastation on humanity. However, improvements in sanitation, nutrition, access to clean water, and better living conditions have had the largest impacts on controlling infectious diseases. This book will provide some basic primer information on these topics so that readers are better equipped to understand the science and mythology surrounding the SARS-CoV-2 virus and countermeasures against it.

The identification of the villains and heroes in this war on COVID-19, as in other human conflicts, is often dependent on the eye of the beholder. Powerful individuals, organizations, and governments have seized the opportunity to promote their own agendas, which frequently include the accumulation of power and wealth. During the first two years of the COVID-19 pandemic, the richest 1 percent of the population amassed close to two-thirds of all new global wealth.[4] At the same time, the incomes of 99 percent of the world's population declined due to lockdowns, business closures, lower international trade, less international tourism, and other factors.[5]

However, it is counterproductive and irrational to assume an organized nefarious intent to unleash a deadly virus—or even COVID-19 genetic vaccines—to reduce the human population. The researchers who manipulated the genetic structure of the SARS-CoV-2 virus or developed dubious SARS-CoV-2 vaccines, as well as public health officials, may have had the best of intentions. Certainly, very dedicated health-care workers made herculean efforts to stop and treat COVID-19 cases, and often did so at the risk of their own health and lives. Ironically, many of the health-care workers who were celebrated for this service in the first year of the pandemic were later persecuted when they refused to be subjected to newly available COVID-19 vaccinations.

It is important to analyze the accepted beliefs related to the prevention and treatment of COVID-19 and the impacts of public health policy measures, and to determine whether the data truly supported the claims made throughout the pandemic. We cite over 1070 primary sources throughout this book from peer-reviewed scientific literature, public health data websites, and information provided directly from drug and vaccine manufacturers. These clues have been assembled like pieces of a massive jigsaw puzzle to form a picture and a reasonable sense of what happened during the COVID-19 saga, at least from the scientific angle.

In the first movie of the Matrix film series released in 1999, the character Morpheus asks the protagonist Neo whether he wants to take a blue pill that will allow him to remain contented with naivety and with a false representation of reality or take a red pill to learn unsettling and life-changing truths. The same choice is now yours. You are encouraged to read this book and learn how deep the rabbit hole goes. Do not be afraid, as illumination will be provided throughout this deep and twisting tunnel of COVID-19 pandemonium toward an egress of enlightenment.

CHAPTER 2

COVID-19 and Science—Information, Misinformation, and the "Truth"

John Hardie & Steven Pelech

"And you will know the truth, and the truth will set you free."
—New Testament, John 8:32

2.1. Defining Science and "Truth"

During the COVID-19 pandemic, political and public health leaders have repeatedly stated in all manner of contexts that they are "following the science." Dr. Anthony Fauci, the former head of the US National Institute of Allergy and Infectious Diseases even declared at one point "I am the Science."[1] These have become mantras, as they are just repeated words. But do these officials even comprehend what "science" embodies, or are these words intended simply to make their audiences feel better, trust them, and follow their directives without challenge? Another mantra heard often during the last three years is "the science is settled," an assertion more akin to a statement of religious faith than an illustration of how science works.[2] Some authors have even called such pronouncements cult-like.[3] To begin with, a clear understanding of science and how it is practiced by scientists is necessary.

The definition of "science" according to the Encyclopedia Britannica is "any system of knowledge that is concerned with the physical world and its phenomena and that entails unbiased observations and systematic experimentation." Merriam-Webster defines science as "knowledge or a system of knowledge covering general truths or the operation of general laws especially as obtained and tested through scientific method." The Cambridge dictionary describes science as "(knowledge from) the careful study of the structure and behavior of the physical world, especially by watching, measuring, and doing experiments, and the development of theories to describe the results of these activities."

The power of science has been its success in tracking complex phenomena and the formulation of hypotheses to explain the underlying mechanisms that might account for these observations. The understanding that comes with the application of science allows outcomes to be predicted if certain courses of actions are exercised.

True "scientists" are those who engage in or have expert knowledge of the study of one or more of the natural sciences such as geology, biology, chemistry, physics, and astronomy. They are learned individuals who systematically research and gather data and other evidence to generate hypotheses and test them to gain and share understanding and knowledge. Effective scientists have been described as having attributes such as curiosity, patience, persistence, courage, creativity, attentiveness to detail, open mindedness, lack of bias, critical thinking, and problem-solving ability.[4] The art of scientific enquiry has been so successful because its practitioners have emulated these characteristics in the past and been willing to follow the data and evidence, even when the new hypotheses that result might challenge prevailing opinion at the time. This is why courage and persistence are such important attributes in a scientist.

Science only progresses thanks to constant challenges to the existing dogma by those who seek to test and re-evaluate existing notions and, upon finding flaws, speak out and inform others of their concerns and the need to formulate better hypotheses and explanations of observed phenomena. Debate is a critical component of the scientific endeavor.[5] Without it, science cannot progress to better understand nature and to guide and inform public policy when called upon to do so.

Nevertheless, since the beginning of the COVID-19 crisis, words such as "consensus," "misinformation," and "disinformation" have been repeatedly used to describe reports and articles that either support or challenge the prevailing narratives. This has led to much confusion within the published scientific and general literature. The confusion rests with how the practice of scientific work has been misguidedly transformed. While debate is a fundamental aspect of scientific progress, in the last four years, it has often not been practiced.

According to the Merriam-Webster dictionary, the definition of "misinformation" is "incorrect or misleading information," and "disinformation" is "false information deliberately and often covertly spread (as by the planting of rumors) in order to influence public opinion or obscure the truth." Those who are uncomfortable with critical and contrarian viewpoints are quick to claim that the purveyors of these views are spreaders of misinformation and disinformation. Such challenges to the prevailing narratives are presently seen as a major threat to the integrity of science and the trust of the public in scientific institutions.[6] There is little doubt that many public health officials and scientists will consider this book as a dangerous source of misinformation and disinformation. However, the views of those unwilling to debate contrarian views on these matters are only opinions that are not as well supported as proclaimed.

Truth is an elusive concept in science. Therefore, scientists rarely talk about the pursuit of *truth*. Instead, they talk about the pursuit of *knowledge*, which is generated by application of standardized principles and approaches, known as the scientific method. While the public may interpret the most current, accepted, and publicized scientific knowledge (i.e., information) as "the truth," scientists know very well (or at least they ought to know well enough) that this is not the case. That information (i.e., knowledge) is only the most current interpretation of data produced by scientists applying the scientific method to the best of their abilities.

2.2. Application of the Scientific Method

During the pandemic, scientists from different backgrounds, including physical scientists, social scientists, medical scientists, basic scientists, epidemiologists, and statisticians, have been widely cited. Although these scientists work in their own areas, the structure of their work—the scientific method—is remarkably similar. Its structure can be seen in the way that scientific articles are usually written.

2.2.1. Step 1: Defining the Problem

The first step in the scientific method consists of defining a question to investigate. Classically, scientific questions have come from observation and data collection of a phenomenon that has captured a scientist's attention, or a phenomenon perceived as problematic, as is the case for a disease. Here, relevant information is organized as it applies to the topic at hand. This involves starting with established concepts or ideas that are widely accepted as being correct and applicable to those working in the field in question (e.g., the once widely held idea that the world is flat). Then information that challenges some part of the accepted truth is introduced, often in the articulation of an alternative hypothesis (e.g., the world is spherical). This can be in the form of a statement or a question. For instance, if the accepted position is that Vitamin D is ineffective against COVID-19, then based on additional new information an alternative hypothesis that "Vitamin D is effective in treating COVID-19" can be proposed.

2.2.2. Step 2: Methods and Materials

This step involves identification of the nature and sources of materials used in the study that are relevant to other laboratories should they attempt to replicate a given experiment. A component as simple as water might make a difference in results. For example, tap water in Vancouver, British Columbia, Canada contains only small amounts of dissolved minerals, whereas tap water in the American Midwest might contain a significant quantity of calcium. If the subject of the study is calcium-activated, different results could be observed between laboratories in the different locations if calcium levels were not controlled.

The methods and procedures are also carefully described in this step. In the context of COVID-19, much research from laboratory-only experiments to large-scale human clinical trials were undertaken. For example, the hypothesis "Vitamin D reduces deaths caused by COVID-19" could be studied in a laboratory setting or in a clinical trial. For the laboratory setting, the variables could be standardized so that the only difference between the experimental condition and its control is the presence of Vitamin D. Cultures of cells infected with SARS-CoV-2 plus Vitamin D or no Vitamin D could be studied to determine what proportion of cells supplemented with Vitamin D died compared to those cells that did not receive Vitamin D.

Testing the same hypothesis in a clinical trial might be more challenging due to variability among human subjects. These variables might include sex, age, weight, general health, diet, genetics, the complement of enzymes affecting Vitamin D metabolism, and even the microbiome of participants, which includes their resident microflora of bacteria, viruses, and fungi. Done correctly, both types of studies are very valuable, as positive results from laboratory experiment—often with animals—may lead to later testing in human subjects.

Eliminating bias is key to verifying that the observed findings are a close representative of the "truth." In laboratory experiments, the use of "positive" controls (gives the answer wanted for comparative purposes) and "negative" controls (does not give the answer wanted for comparative purposes) should ideally be done. In the example of Vitamin D and the virus that causes COVID-19, in the laboratory with cultured cells, the test cells would be those that receive Vitamin D and SARS-CoV-2, whereas the control would be cells that received only the virus. In addition, a positive control would be a group of cells that receive only Vitamin D but are not exposed to the virus, whereas a negative control would be a group of cells that have no exposure to Vitamin D or the virus. As will be discussed later in Chapter 14, although controversial, Vitamin D does appear effective in reducing progression to severe COVID-19.

2.2.3. Step 3: Results

This step describes the observations made by the researchers. These could be as simple as counting the numbers of people in the various study groups who have exhibited improvement in disease symptoms with a drug treatment or a demonstrated reduction in incidence of an infectious disease after vaccination. Generally, this section contains much data, which may be effectively presented as tables or figures, as well as appropriate statistical analyses to determine whether the results are significant or not.

2.2.4. Step 4: Discussion and Conclusions

This is the last step where the authors offer their interpretation of the data or observations. Often the data are discussed in terms of whether they disprove or are consistent with the hypothesis. To revisit the hypothesis that "Vitamin D is effective in treating COVID-19," the researchers might observe that in the treated group only two of twenty-six people died compared with thirteen of twenty-five in the untreated control group. These observations are consistent with the stated hypothesis and might be interpreted as supporting the hypothesis, but they *do not prove* that the hypothesis is true. This is because there could be extenuating circumstances that contributed to the difference in results. For example, the untreated controls might have had an underlying condition that renders them more likely to die. Science cannot provide proof, such as can be produced in a discipline such as mathematics; it can only increase (or decrease) the probability that a particular hypothesis is correct. Sometimes a theory can work extremely well to explain phenomena until further application demonstrates that it is deficient. For example, Newtonian physics was highly predictive of the behaviors of macroscopic objects, including the motions of the planets and their moons in our solar system. However, it failed with subatomic particles, necessitating new theories, including those associated with quantum mechanics.

It may be helpful here to distinguish between a theory and a hypothesis. A useful definition of a theory is that it is a structured explanation about a group of facts or phenomena in usually the natural world.[7] In comparison, a hypothesis is a short statement or proposition that attempts to explain a phenomena or facts based on limited evidence that serves as a starting point for further investigation.[8] Thus, a theory might be widely accepted, whereas a hypothesis is a statement that might or might not be correct. Accordingly, a hypothesis should be written so that it can be proven incorrect by testing. The most productive approach is to design experiments that disprove the hypothesis, i.e., a hypothesis should be falsifiable. Scientific mentors expound the concept that "you can never prove a hypothesis, you can only disprove it." However, when a hypothesis has been tested extensively and not disproven, it has the potential to become a trusted part of a specific body of information or knowledge.

One last thing to note is that while various hypotheses can be advanced to explain any observation, experience tends to favor the simplest hypothesis that effectively explains the observation. This is termed Occam's Razor or the Law of Parsimony.

Chapter 9 will further discuss the application of the scientific method in the context of the formulation and execution of clinical trials for drugs and vaccines.

CHAPTER 3

Agents and Transmission of Infectious Diseases

John Hardie, J. M. & Steven Pelech

"In times of stress and danger such as come about as the result of an epidemic, many tragic and cruel phases of human nature are brought out, as well as many brave and unselfish ones."

—William Crawford Gorgas

"Gentlemen, the microbes will have the last word."

—Louis Pasteur

3.1. Deaths from Infectious and Other Diseases in Canada

While infectious diseases have taken a significant toll in Canada, they are not the major causes of morbidity and mortality in this country. From 2001 to 2016, infectious diseases accounted for 1.4 to 1.6 deaths per 100,000 Canadians annually, which increased to about 2.4 deaths per 100,000 in 2019. In 2020, the first official year of the COVID-19 pandemic and in the absence of any suitable vaccines for SARS-CoV-2, this number remained unchanged from 2019.[1] It may be tempting to suggest that drastic measures by public health officials to confront COVID-19, including shutting of international borders, quarantining the healthy, the closures of schools, businesses, and entertainment venues, social distancing, universal masking, and increased handwashing, kept the SARS-CoV-2 virus in check. However, as will be discussed later, this was clearly not the case.

With a population of around thirty-eight million at the time, the total number of deaths from all causes in Canada was 285,270 in 2019, and 307,205 in 2020.[2] Infectious diseases accounted for only 8.6 percent of these deaths in 2019 and 12.6 percent of deaths in 2020, whereas cancer and cardiovascular diseases (including strokes) accounted for 27.0 percent and 23.2 percent of all deaths in

Canada, respectively. In 2020, the total number of deaths with COVID-19 was 16,151 (of which about half were due to a co-morbidity or contributing medical conditions), which accounted for 5.25 percent of all deaths.[2] Most of these COVID-19 deaths were ultimately from (secondary and) terminal bacterial pneumonia ("the old man's friend") and could likely have been better averted by treatment with antibiotics and reduced overuse of ventilators.

In some of the Canadian provinces such as British Columbia, Alberta, and Ontario, daily deaths by illicit drug overdose approached or surpassed those from COVID-19 during the pandemic. Presently, drug overdose is the leading cause of death in these provinces for those under sixty years of age. Since the onset of COVID-19, the rate of accidental apparent opioid toxicity deaths has doubled from pre-COVID-19 rates, worsening the opioid crisis that first started significantly rising in 2016.[3] The vast majority of these deaths were from fentanyl overdoses, and usually in those in the twenty-to fifty-nine-year-old age bracket. Since most COVID-19 deaths in Canada and elsewhere in the last four years have been in the very elderly, drug overdose has resulted in more years of life lost than COVID-19.

3.2. Infectious Diseases Caused by Bacteria and Viruses

Infectious diseases are caused by pathogens that replicate in living organisms or cells. Such pathogens include helminths (parasitic worms), protozoa, fungi, bacteria, viruses, and even proteins like the prion proteins that cause mad cow disease, scrapie in sheep, and Creutzfeldt-Jakob disease in humans. These pathogens are unable to reproduce and spread without the assistance of a host. Large parasites and bacteria flourish in the gut, blood stream, skin, or in certain organs of a host. In fact, most successful parasites are benign to their hosts and do not induce disease. As will be discussed later in chapter 14, one of the most successful drugs for treating parasitic infections is ivermectin, which has also been demonstrated to be very promising in the treatment of COVID-19.

In humans, over a thousand different species of bacteria can co-exist with each other and with the body, especially in the intestines, and constitute what is known as the resident flora or microbiota. In total, some forty trillion bacteria co-exist with the approximately fifty trillion human cells in an adult human body.[4] A thriving gut flora helps maintain body weight[5] and reduces the risk of inflammatory bowel disease such as ulcerative colitis.[6] These bacteria aid in digestion, produce vitamin K, and help fight off pathogenic bacteria that can cause disease. There are only around a hundred different bacterial species that are known to be pathogenic to humans, despite the existence of over ten thousand documented bacterial species and more likely tens of millions of bacterial species on the planet.[7]

There are some two hundred species of viruses that are known to cause disease in humans,[8] even though about three hundred thousand species of viruses are thought to co-exist in mammals alone, nevermind in other animals and plants.[9] There are also viruses, called bacteriophages, which infect bacteria. There are even viruses, called virophages, that are genetic parasites of giant viruses.[10] Moreover, there are also viroids, which consist of only naked ribonucleic acid (RNA) without a protective protein and/or lipid (fat) coat, and obelisks, which are also comprised of RNA that can encode proteins known as "oblins." The total number of viruses that reside in a healthy human body has been estimated to be close to 380 trillion, the vast majority of which simply co-exist without causing disease.[11] Some of these have integrated into the human genome as proviruses or endogenous viral elements.[12] Every person appears to have a unique virome and microbiome.

The reason why so few viruses or bacteria can infect and cause disease in humans and other species is because they must co-evolve with those or highly related species. To enter a host cell, viruses and bacteria need to have evolved proteins on their surfaces that can tightly bind to specific proteins or sugars that are on the surface of the host's cells. Then they must traverse through the cell's outer membrane, known as the plasma membrane, which is a lipid and protein barrier that keeps the contents of the host cell in and the undesirable substances and microbes out. Once inside a cell, a virus must hijack the cell's biosynthetic enzymes to produce proteins, nucleic acids, sugars (saccharides), and lipids that are the building blocks for forming new, infectious viral particles. This requires precision production of viral proteins that can efficiently interact with the cell's own enzymes. It might take thousands of years before a virus can evolve to infect a new host species, but the process can be much faster if the virus has already been adapted to a highly related host species. When this happens, it is known as cross-species transmission. If the virus is transferred from a non-human species to humans and results in disease, this is called zoonosis. Just a few complementary mutations in the structure of the genome of the virus might be sufficient to allow the leap between species in a matter of months.

This incredible requirement for co-evolution of a virus and its host is the main reason why the three-week quarantine of the first Apollo mission astronauts that returned from the Moon was absurd. The Moon with no atmosphere and continuous radiation bombardment from the Sun was likely to be a sterile environment to begin with. Moreover, there would have been no chance for any microbes on the Moon to co-evolve with life forms on the Earth. Similarly, the scenario offered in H. G. Well's *War of the Worlds* novel, which was later adapted into two Hollywood films, is also highly unlikely. In this fictional story, humanity is defeated by superior, technically advanced, and morally depraved aliens, but ultimately saved by the lowly microbes on Earth. The alien physiology would likely be too different to permit Earth bacteria and certainly viruses to easily infect their cells.

Ideally, for a virus or bacteria to flourish in a population, it must be very durable, highly infectious, and should not harm its host. A host that is unaware of its active infection with a virus or bacteria is more likely to live as normal and interact with other potential hosts, which more readily spreads the infecting pathogen. During transit from host to host, the virus or bacteria must also be able to survive the changing environment. Some viruses have tough protein shells that assume geodesic polyhedron shapes to withstand the elements. However, other viruses have lipid membranes that can easily dry out and become destroyed. To be infectious, the virus must have proteins on its own surface that can recognize with high affinity a protein or polysaccharide on the surface of a host cell to which it can attach for entry. But the real challenge is to subvert the cell's own enzymes to replicate the genome and proteins of the virus.

To understand how difficult this really is, it is necessary to have some understanding of basic biochemistry and molecular biology.

3.3. DNA Makes RNA Makes Proteins

The chromosomes of animals, plants, and microbes are comprised of long polymers of deoxyribonucleic acid (DNA) and structural proteins called histones. Known as the genome, the DNA component contains the stored genetic information for the construction of all RNA and proteins in cells and, ultimately, their functionalities. DNA features nucleotide bases that are interlinked like beads in incredibly long chains. Each bead is built from one of four possible types: Adenine (A); Thymine (T); Cytosine (C); and Guanine (G). These building blocks, called bases, are joined in combinations that store information on how to construct ribonucleic acids (RNA) and functional proteins. Just as computer code written in binary (base two) with zeroes and ones allows for storing information, the genetic code operates in quaternary (base four) in living organisms for the same purpose.

DNA is found in chromosomes, and humans usually have two sets of twenty-three separate chromosomes in most cells of the body. In each cell, the length of the genome (genetic material) in each set of chromosomes is about 3.2 billion base pairs long,[13] which when unraveled and put end to end is about two meters in length. If all the DNA packed in all the cells of a single adult human body were attached and stretched out, it would go from here to the sun and back over three hundred times. This illustrates how incredibly long and thin DNA can be.

The human genome features just over twenty thousand genes that encode proteins as well as over a thousand other genes that specify RNA molecules that play structural roles (e.g., transfer-RNAs and ribosomal-RNAs) and regulatory roles (e.g., micro-RNAs).[14] Remarkably, less than 4 percent of the human genome DNA harbors genes for proteins or RNA. Another 4 percent encodes the remnants of past viral integrations into the human genome of our ancestors. A large portion of the human genome appears to be non-essential baggage described as "junk" or "dark" DNA, although it also encodes various obscure regulatory or non-coding elements.

To make proteins, the DNA sequence of nucleotide bases in a gene needs to be re-written—i.e., transcribed—by enzymes called RNA polymerases into RNA copies. RNA uses similar building blocks to DNA, including A, C, and G bases, but T is replaced with Uracil (U). The sequence of nucleotides in RNA is dictated by the DNA template by base-pairing, in which an A selectively binds to a U, and a G specifically binds to a C. Consequently, a short strand of DNA with the sequence AAATTTCCCGGG will be transcribed by RNA polymerases into the RNA sequence UUUAAAGGGCCC. Actually, genes can be thousands of nucleotide bases long, as will be their RNA copies. These resultant RNA copies are known as messenger-RNA (mRNA) molecules. These mRNAs are positive, single-stranded RNA polymers of nucleotides that are directly readable by protein synthesis factories known as ribosomes. Whereas DNA is very stable and found deep inside the nucleus of cells, mRNA is transient and rapidly degraded. However, this mRNA can last long enough to leave the nucleus of cells and encounter ribosomes that are found in the cytoplasm of cells.

Proteins are long beaded chains of interconnected amino acids. Thermodynamic forces and weak chemical bonds help fold the protein chain into distinct functional three-dimensional structures. There are twenty types of common amino acids found in proteins. In humans, nine of these amino acids must be acquired in the food we eat; whereas, we can produce the other eleven by biosynthetic enzymes that operate within the metabolic pathways in cells. These enzymes are themselves proteins. Like molecular robots, proteins can build and degrade other proteins, nucleic acids, sugars, lipids, and other small molecules, acting as biological catalysts of the biochemical reactions that allow cells to live, reproduce, and even die when required. Each of the approximately twenty thousand proteins encoded by the human genome has a specialized function that is dictated by the sequence of possible amino acids in each protein. The primary amino acid sequence of proteins ultimately determines their three-dimensional structures, which permits them to carry out their diverse activities, including their interactions with other proteins and other molecules. In addition to acting as biological catalysts of biochemical reactions, proteins can also play structural roles to maintain the shape and mobility of cells.

The ribosomes are large complexes of proteins and ribosomal-RNA that together function as protein synthesis factories. They read the sequence of nucleotide bases in the messenger-RNA to find and assemble the corresponding amino acids into a growing protein that is specified by the RNA nucleotide sequence. Essentially, the ribosomes are translators of specific RNA sequences to generate the corresponding protein sequences. In these molecular assembly plants, each new amino acid is affixed to the previously selected amino acid by the binding of transfer-RNA molecules that are also specifically attached to one of the twenty possible amino acids and ferries them to the ribosomes.

Sequential triplets of the nucleotides specify each amino acid in what is known as the Genetic Code. Sixty-one possible nucleotide triplets select one or more of the twenty possible amino acids. This redundancy in the genetic code means that certain amino acids can be specified by up to six triplet combinations of the four possible nucleotides. For example, the amino acid arginine is selected when the RNA sequence of a triplet is CGU, CGC, CGA, CGG, AGA, or AGG. Other amino acids like methionine and tryptophan are uniquely specified by AUG and UGG, respectively. As a consequence, the portion of the RNA sequence UUUAAAGGGCCC described earlier would be translated by ribosomes to yield a segment of a protein with the sequence phenylalanine-lysine-glycine-proline.

All life forms on the Earth and viruses use the same genetic code for the triplets of nucleotides in transfer-RNAs that select each amino acid. Thus, all living organisms use the same nucleotides and amino acids and have very similar biochemistry in what has been referred to as central metabolism. This shared biochemistry is why invading viruses can be parasitic to their hosts. This common biochemistry is also why many scientists believe that life on Earth first arose from a common ancestor. In a theory known as *panspermia*, some scientists believe such a microbe came with ice asteroid fragments from another living world that hit Earth billions of years ago.[15] Through the process of evolution, a diversity of life-forms on our planet eventually flourished to populate the entire surface of the globe and create our biomes. Of course, evolution and panspermia are theories that can never be proven, despite their high probability. Panspermia can be viewed as a sleight of hand to explain away the origin of life on Earth as it shifts it to an elusive world elsewhere, leaving still the mystery of how life started in the first place. However, it affords another ten billion years for its beginning in the known universe.

The bottom line is that many steps are required for a virus to be able to successfully replicate itself in a host. Because viruses have very small genomes relative to those found in host cells, they must take advantage of, and be compatible with, the proteins and other molecules of host cells. Without the ability to divert the normal functions of the host proteins toward their own ends, these parasitic entities would be unable to replicate and propagate in new hosts. Viruses appear to have evolved from cells during evolution of life, in part from the loss of most genes that are found in cells and in part from the development of novel genes that encode proteins that are specialized to allow viruses to enter and hijack host cells to optimize their replication.[16]

The simpler the structure of the virus, the more durable it may be, the faster it can be produced, and the quicker it can evolve from random mutations. Such mutation can arise from the low rate of fidelity in the reproduction of genomes by enzymes or by chemical mutagens or radiation in the environment. Most mutations are inconsequential or even deleterious to infectious pathogens, but occasionally these mutations might improve their ability to infect and replicate in a host. Bacteria can replicate quickly in a matter of minutes, although not as fast as viruses. By contrast, animal and plant cells typically take a few days to reproduce. After birth, most multicellular organisms require months or years to reach a mature, reproductive stage. As a consequence, viruses can mutate and adapt much more rapidly than their hosts. However, hosts have developed counter-defenses to resist new infectious disease-causing pathogens, which will be discussed in chapter 7. Before the immune systems of hosts are considered, it is necessary to discuss how infectious diseases spread.

3.4. Transmission of Infectious Diseases

Many deadly infectious diseases like the bubonic plague (also known as the "Black Death" and caused by the bacterium *Yersinia pestis*) and disfiguring diseases like leprosy (caused by *Mycobacterium leprae*) have been known for thousands of years. The pathogenic bacteria that are responsible for these and many other infectious diseases only became visible and identifiable through magnification with the advent of light microscopes. Other infectious diseases like smallpox, chickenpox, measles, and polio, all caused by viruses, have also been known for thousands of years. Over a hundred years ago, many other diseases were recognized as being caused by very tiny pathogens that easily penetrated very fine filters that normally trapped bacterial cells and larger microbes. They only became recognizable with the development of more powerful electron microscopes in the 1930s. Over the centuries, knowledge has continued to accumulate about these tiny contagions that inflict humans, other animals and plants, such as how they propagate, and most recently their further identification by genomic sequencing. Following the completion of the Human Genome project, the tremendous advancements in the efficiencies of DNA sequencing technologies with dramatic reductions in costs have resulted in the identifications of thousands of new microbial and viral species in the twenty-first century.

For transmission of an infectious disease to occur, a chain of independent events must be linked together in the proper order. Six of these links are described as follows:

3.4.1. Link 1—Sufficient Dose of an Infectious Pathogen

In the controlled environment of a laboratory, it is possible to calculate the infective or lethal dose of a pathogen. It is, however, impossible to determine a precise infective dose for human pathogens out in the real world. Although different species of pathogens vary widely in their ability to cause disease (e.g., a single *Rickettsia tsutsugamushi* microbe can cause a symptomatic infection as opposed to a million or more of the organism *Salmonella typhi*),[17] the level of the infective dose varies with the competency of a new host's defense mechanisms.

Two factors are essential if a potential pathogen is to cause disease. Firstly, it must establish itself in or on the host tissue. This necessitates that at a location within the host there is an environment with appropriate pH and oxygen tension levels, temperature, and nutrients that are suitable for the survival and growth of the pathogen. This is referred to as "the fertile soil" of the pathogen.[18] Due to this necessity, pathogens tend to favor specific anatomic locations. For example, the unique environment of the skin is conducive to the growth and infectivity of the bacteria, *Staphylococcus aureus* and *Streptococcus pyogenes* (staph and strep), whereas the completely different acidic nature of the gastrointestinal tract is better suited to infection by *Escherichia coli* and *Salmonella enterica* (E. coli and salmonella).

Secondly, apart from locating in fertile soil, a pathogen must overcome the defense system of the potential host to attain a critical mass that, for that pathogen in that host, produces overt evidence of an infection.

3.4.2. Link 2—Existence of a Viable Infectious Pathogen

To induce infection, not only must there be a critical mass of a pathogen, but that mass must remain viable. A potentially infectious mass of a pathogen relocated from its fertile soil to a hostile environment loses its viability and its infectivity. Viruses are intracellular parasites and must be so located if their viability is to be retained. A door handle often does not provide that environment. Viruses from the handle might have their viability resuscitated through sophisticated laboratory techniques, but that does not imply that the door handle is a fomite, i.e., a source of viable infectious pathogens. Notably, the fear of COVID-19 viruses on fomites was an early, and mistaken, concern propagated by many health authorities.

3.4.3. Link 3—A Portal of Escape

A pathogen prior to its invasion of a new host must escape from its primary source. The portal of escape is usually related to where the pathogen is located on the body. Human pathogens leave the body from the respiratory tract, in fecal material, and in body fluids such as blood, semen, vaginal secretions, urine, saliva, sweat, and breast milk.

3.4.4. Link 4—A Mode of Transmission

Once a sufficient dose of a viable pathogen leaves its primary source, it must be transmitted to its new host before the potential for infection exists. Sneezing and coughing produce a spray of respiratory pathogens that might be inhaled by potential new hosts. COVID-19, tuberculosis, and streptococcal pharyngitis are spread by this route. Direct person-to-person contact spreads infectious mononucleosis by kissing and sexually transmitted disease by intimate sexual behavior. A less direct route of transmission occurs when a food handler shedding *shigella* or *salmonella* pathogens or the hepatitis A virus contaminates food because of inappropriate hand washing.[19] The sharing of syringes containing contaminated blood is a common method of transmitting the hepatitis B virus among intravenous drug abusers. Microorganisms pathogenic to humans can also be transmitted by bites from insects such as mosquitoes, fleas, and ticks.

In summary, the common routes of transmission are respiratory via inhalation, fecal-oral from ingestion of contaminated fecal material, sexual from direct contact with mucous membranes, body fluids from infected blood, semen, sweat and urine, and via vectors such as insects and animals that bite.

3.4.5. Link 5—A Portal of Entry

The potential for infection does not exist unless the transmitted critical mass of a viable pathogen accesses the fertile soil of host tissues. The usual portals of entry are the same as the portals of escape. They include the respiratory, gastrointestinal, and genitourinary tracts plus skin and mucous membrane surfaces that are broken or otherwise compromised.

3.4.6. Link 6—A Susceptible Host

The ability of a sufficient dose of an invading viable pathogen to elicit disease is dependent on the susceptibility of the potential new host to that pathogen. Factors that contribute to susceptibility include general malaise, poor socio-economic and living conditions, malnutrition, chronic disease, obesity, increasing age, stress, and the frequency of previous infectious diseases.[20] More significantly, the resistance to susceptibility is enhanced by a healthy lifestyle, a balanced diet, a functioning immune system, low stress, and sufficient sleep.[21] Thus, a young, physically fit individual would be much more tolerant of high numbers of a particular pathogen than would an older, infirm person with diabetes mellitus.

An important factor governing susceptibility is the capacity to develop an immune response in time to prevent the multiplying pathogen from reaching a critical mass. For example, a robust immune system might not resist a low dose of a highly virulent, rapidly multiplying pathogen. Similarly, a large mass of a low virulent pathogen could overcome a delayed and weakened immune response.

3.4.7. Analyzing the Links

Critical to the development of an infection, the six links constituting the Chain of Infection must be joined in the order of: Sufficient Dose of an Infectious Pathogen, Existence of a Viable Infectious Pathogen, A Portal of Escape, A Mode of Transmission, A Portal of Entry, and A Susceptible Host. Breaking this chain by removing or incapacitating one of the links prevents the transmission of an infectious disease. Although each link is critical, the most significant one regarding the transmission of an infectious disease is host susceptibility.

The clinical importance of this conclusion is more readily appreciated by focusing on host resistance rather than host susceptibility. This allows the probability of an infectious disease occurring to be represented by the following equation.[22]

$$\text{Infection} = \frac{\text{Virulence of the Pathogen x Dose of the Pathogen}}{\text{Host Resistance}}$$

This equation illustrates two factors relevant to the transmission of all infectious diseases. First, infection is not an inevitable outcome of exposure to a pathogen but depends on an interrelated series of events constituting the Chain of Infection. Second, host resistance is more pertinent to the development of an infectious disease than are the specific characteristics of a potential pathogen.[23] The significance of this factor is appreciated when the heterogeneous nature of a population is considered.

The factors that decrease host resistance (increase susceptibility) not only accumulate with advancing age but have an increasing variability within each successive decade of life. For example, two young cousins ages five and eight years are likely to share similar health and socio-economic circumstances resulting in both having a similar resistance to infection no matter the potency of the pathogen. However, their respective grandparents ranging in age from sixty-five to seventy-five years could have a wide spectrum of life and health experiences resulting in each of them having vastly different co-morbidities and consequently various levels of resistance and susceptibility to a potential pathogen. Public health programs to prevent the spread of an infectious disease will be of questionable utility if they ignore the diversity of susceptibility to infection that exists within all populations. However, this is precisely what happens with broad vaccine mandates.

Noted medical historian Dr. Mary Dobson of Cambridge University emphasized this fundamental concept in her 2007 book, *Disease: The Extraordinary Stories behind History's Deadliest Killers,* when she said, "there is always a complex set of inter-related biological, genetic, environmental and social factors meaning that some people succumb, while others survive or remain untouched by the circulating pathogen or potentially fatal disorder."[24]

Apart from appreciating the significant roles of host resistance and susceptibility in disease transmission, disease prevention programs must address what constitutes the diagnosis of an infectious disease and recognize the concept of asymptomatic transmission as both relate to the identification and understanding of infectious disease transmission.

3.5. Diagnosis of an Infectious Disease

A confirmed case of an infectious disease is dependent on the co-existence of two essential factors. One is the presence of its characteristic symptoms and the other is the identification of the causative pathogen.[25] For example, an individual might have the typical signs and symptoms of a flu from influenza. However, unless laboratory tests reveal the presence of one of the flu viruses, a confirmed diagnosis of flu cannot be made. Similarly, an appreciation for the Chain of Infection indicates that a noncritical mass of *Streptococcus pyogenes* could be present on a throat swab, but without the appropriate symptoms, a diagnosis of strep throat is questionable.

The methods and criteria associated with testing for SARS-CoV-2 will be discussed later in chapter 8. However, their complexities combined with the non-specific nature of COVID-19 symptoms (cough, fever, chills, fatigue) have likely led to an overestimation of the number of COVID-19 cases, hospitalizations, and deaths during times of high testing (during times of low testing, underestimations were likely produced). The SARS-CoV-2 tests based on PCR detection also had excessively high rates of false-positive identifications, as will be discussed in chapter 8.

3.6. Asymptomatic Transmission

The concept of asymptomatic transmission is that an individual who has no symptoms of an infectious disease can still transmit it. But in health care, a patient who no longer has symptoms is considered *well.* Therefore, the question is, "Can a well patient transmit an infection?" In addition, can a person at the early stages of an infectious disease be transmitting that disease? The idea of asymptomatic transmission has been a major driver of policies, procedures, and mandates associated with infections and has been a feature in many of the public health policies during the COVID-19 pandemic.

The Chain of Infection dictates that for infection to become established, a sufficient dose of viable respiratory virus like influenza must be transmitted through the air from an infectious carrier to a potentially susceptible new host. It is the force associated with the symptoms of coughs and sneezes that expels infectious doses of a respiratory virus from the respiratory tract of the primary host with sufficient velocity to be transmitted as aerosols through the air and be inhaled by a new host, where they must overcome that person's natural defenses (intact mucous membranes) and immunological responses. Without coughs and sneezes the potential for a respiratory virus transmission is very low and effectively nonexistent.

The Chain of Infection reveals that an individual might harbor a virus and have nonexistent-to-mild non-specific symptoms, but unless the viable virus is expelled in sufficient amounts by sneezing or coughing and overcomes the resistance of a new host, the potential for transmission remains relatively insignificant. Nevertheless, the promotion by government and media sources that a healthy, well, symptom-free person could transmit a respiratory virus enhanced the levels of public fear and paranoia and facilitated the introduction of mandated procedures such as societal lockdowns, travel restrictions, and school closures. If it does occur, the concept of asymptomatic transmission through the air is a rare phenomenon and should never be used to justify public health policies and procedures.

In January 2020, before the onset of the pandemic, Dr. Anthony Fauci, the director of the US National Institute of Allergy and Infectious Diseases at that time, supported this concept when he said, "In all the history of respiratory borne viruses of any type, asymptomatic transmission has never been the driver of outbreaks. The driver of outbreaks is always a symptomatic person."[26] Further evidence on the low level of asymptomatic transmission for SARS-CoV-2 was provided by Dr. Maria Van Kerkhove, head of WHO's emerging diseases and zoonosis unit, on June 8, 2020, when she said that, "from the data we have, it still seems to be rare that an asymptomatic person actually transmits onward to a secondary individual." She continued to say that "We have a number of reports from countries who are doing very detailed contact tracing. They're following asymptomatic cases. They're following contacts. And they're not finding secondary transmission onward. It's very rare."[27]

The role of asymptomatic transmission in spreading a respiratory virus like SARS-CoV-2 appears to be inconsequential compared to the way in which the Chain of Infection governs the transmission of this and other pathogens. Recent studies have shown that only about 9 percent of 242 asymptomatic patients at a tertiary care facility had detectable minus strand SARS-CoV-2 RNA, which is a measure of active virus.[28] (The minus strand of RNA is an intermediate opposite copy of the positive, sense strand of RNA and is required to make more copies of the RNA for packaging into new virus particles. It cannot be used by ribosomes to make proteins.) This demonstrated that the vast majority of asymptomatic patients who had tested positive by traditional PCR methods were not particularly infectious, contrary to earlier assumptions.

3.7. Application of the Chain of Infection to COVID-19

The principles governing the transmission of infectious diseases are multidisciplinary. The following chapters will discuss the role these specialties have in unravelling the numerous contradictions and dilemmas associated with SARS-CoV-2 and COVID-19. By defining certain terms and assembling the Chain of Infection, this chapter provides a primer on the basic elements controlling the transmission of an infectious disease.

These factors reveal that a one-size-fits-all approach to combatting a respiratory disease pandemic fails to account for the diverse range of susceptibility to the disease. An understanding of the Chain of Infection would have directed targeted preventive measures to the least resistant rather than assume that everyone was equally susceptible. Similarly, public health efforts to increase resistance to infection within all strata of society should have recognized the fundamental concepts inherent in the Chain of Infection.

The diagnosis of an infectious disease requires that its symptoms be present, and its causative pathogen identified. As shall be seen in upcoming chapters, the spectrum of symptoms associated with COVID-19 and the laboratory manipulations required to identify viable SARS-CoV-2 should have tempered the enthusiasm for readily confirming cases of COVID-19. The specter of SARS-CoV-2 being transmitted by healthy individuals incited public fear and paranoia. An elementary knowledge of the Chain of Infection would have revealed the implausibility of such an occurrence. The concepts inherent in the Chain of Infection are time tested and easy to understand. Ensuring that it was intact and operational when dealing with COVID-19 would have reduced much of the misunderstanding associated with this infectious respiratory disease.

CHAPTER 4

Pre-COVID-19 Coronaviruses and Other Respiratory Disease Viruses

Steven Pelech

"Viruses have not failed to follow the general law. They are strict parasites which, born of disorder, have created a very remarkable new order to ensure their own perpetuation."

—André Lwoof

"Our species has co-evolved alongside many others to which we were in contact, especially through scavenging, hunting, and then animal husbandry, all of which would have exposed us to novel pathogens and zoonotic diseases. As a species, we had to adapt to these new pathogens without the benefits of modern medicine. The newly emerging diseases of recent decades, while novel in themselves, are but a repeat of patterns which humans have survived over several millennia."

—Kimberly A. Plomp

4.1. Viral Respiratory Diseases

Many human infectious diseases are caused by airborne viruses. Notably, these include respiratory syncytial virus, influenza, and coronaviruses. These viruses are highly contagious and are mainly transmitted in aerosols received through the mouths and noses of victims. They produce very similar symptoms, which include runny nose, coughing, sneezing, wheezing, fever, and decreases in appetite. The symptoms are largely consequences of the body's counter-reactions to a respiratory infection. These viruses infect humans largely through inhalation of virus-laden air. As such, their first opportunity to infect the human body occurs in the larger passages of the upper respiratory tract—the nose, pharynx, larynx, trachea, and bronchi.

Once these viruses invade cells of the upper airways, they hijack the human intracellular machinery to replicate and often cause cell damage in the process by lysing the infected cells. If the human body responds well, the immune system will prevent these viruses from spreading beyond the upper airways and will quickly terminate any illnesses induced by these viruses. If the immune response is insufficient, the infection might spread into the lower airways (alveoli) and develop into a much more serious systemic infection (including secondary infections such as bacterial pneumonia). The immune response to respiratory viruses in airway spaces is rather different when compared to an infection of the bloodstream from a skin wound or even an injection of a vaccine.

4.2. Respiratory Syncytial Virus (RSV)

RSV generally induces mild, cold-like symptoms, and most people recover within two weeks or less. It produces a seasonal disease that occurs mostly early in the fall. RSV, however, can also cause serious lung infections in some infants and older adults, especially those with pre-existing serious medical problems. One study noted that 42 percent of adults infected with RSV are asymptomatic and transmit the virus at a very much lower rate than those who were symptomatic.[1] RSV normally infects about 97 percent of children before the end of their second year of life. It kills fewer than one in 2,500 for children under five, and those that succumb usually have significant co-morbidities.[2] The actual RSV case fatality rates (deaths due to RSV divided by all patients who develop RSV infection) are difficult to estimate. The reported numbers vary dramatically from zero deaths in smaller studies, to between one in 714 to one in 7,805 in a few of the larger US studies. With about twenty-three million children under the age of five in the United States, and the number of RSV deaths annually ranging from one hundred to three hundred per year, rates of closer to one death per 77,000 RSV infections annually in this age group can be calculated.

In 2019 (pre–COVID-19), there were almost nineteen thousand RSV cases reported in Canada. From August 2020 until May 2021, there were just 239 cases. This remarkable 98.5 percent decrease was attributed to masking, distancing, handwashing, and closure of day-care and schools. However, it is likely that many RSV cases were incorrectly counted as COVID-19 cases. By late October 2022, RSV cases had "surged" to 486 according to one mainstream article.[3] This increase of over 100 percent compared to the previous period, however, was a mere 2.5 percent of the 2019 count, which was itself consistent with previous years. A 2019 investigation noted that in Canada during 2003–2013, a total of seventy-nine RSV-associated infant deaths were recorded, with thirty-two of these being attributable solely to an RSV infection.[4]

Until recently, a vaccine for RSV has been elusive. Previous attempts were largely thwarted by safety concerns.[5] By October 2021, at least four companies (Pfizer, Moderna, GSK, and Johnson & Johnson) had been testing candidate RSV vaccines in Phase 3 trials. On May 23, 2023, Pfizer received US Food and Drug Administration (FDA) approval for Abrysvo as a bivalent vaccine to prevent RSV infection in adults sixty years and older[6] based on positive clinical trial data.[7]

Abrysvo is composed of two RSV proteins (known as Pre-Fusion proteins) that were selected to optimize protection against RSV A and B strains. In another clinical Phase 3 trial study for Abrysvo that was described in the *New England Journal of Medicine*,[8] pregnant women (twenty-four- through thirty-six-weeks gestation) received a single intramuscular injection of 120 micrograms (⊠g) of the Abrysvo vaccine or placebo. (A microgram is one millionth of a gram.) Less than 1.7 percent of both the vaccinated (3,682 participants) and placebo-treated (3,676 participants) mothers had babies who had medically treated severe RSV-associated lower respiratory tract infections up to 180 days after birth, with nineteen cases in the vaccinated cohort and sixty-two cases in the placebo cohort. With such low numbers of recorded infections, there are issues with the statistical confidence and the real effect size of the benefit from the vaccine could have been lower than 50 percent. In addition, the vaccine protection was found to wane rapidly in the infants after their birth and did not last beyond a year.

Along with the rarity of severe RSV in babies, it is easily treatable. There are currently two drugs approved for RSV disease: palivizumab and ribavirin, which can be used prophylactically. Palivizumab (Synagis) is a humanized monoclonal antibody that targets the fusion (F) glycoprotein on RSV and blocks the fusion of the virus with membranes of host cells, aborting its entry into cells.[9] Ribavirin is a more generic antiviral nucleoside drug that prevents the synthesis of the genomes of RSV, hepatitis C, and Lassa fever by multiple mechanisms following its further modification and activation inside of cells. It acts as an inhibitor of the enzyme inosine-5′-phosphate dehydrogenase and reduces the levels of guanosine-triphosphate (GTP), which is necessary to support DNA and RNA synthesis. Ribavirin also directly inhibits certain viral RNA polymerases that are necessary for viral genome replication.[10]

In the fall of 2022, there were increased incidences of RSV, COVID-19, and influenza infections. As a result, Canadian public health authorities expressed concern that pediatric units in hospitals could be overwhelmed by a surge in those infections.[11] It was evident that the median age of RSV cases in hospitalized infants was higher in 2022 than typically observed prior to the onset of COVID-19 in Canada.[12] Thus, the guidelines and efforts to "flatten the curve" for reducing hospital cases of COVID-19 in the early years of the pandemic ultimately delayed and then concentrated the cases of RSV and influenza in hospitals in 2022, thus "sharpening" their curves.

4.3. Influenza

Influenza has been recognized as a seasonal illness for over a century with annual variations in prevalence and severity. Adults can become infectious about a day before they manifest any symptoms, and they can remain infectious for five to seven days after the appearance of flu symptoms. These symptoms can include fever, cough, runny nose, body aches, nausea, vomiting, and diarrhea. The symptoms can be very mild to severe, with full recovery occurring in usually one to two weeks.

From the Orthomyxoviridae family, the influenza viruses occur in four types, A, B, C, and D. The A and B types are mainly responsible for seasonal epidemics of the flu, whereas the C type produces mild illness, and the D type primarily infects cattle.[13] Their genomes consist of eight segments of negative-sense stranded RNA. Co-infection of the same cell with two different influenza viruses allows the mixing of these segments to generate new variants, especially if one of the influenza strains is from another animal species.

The Influenza A viruses are divided into subtypes based on two proteins, i.e., hemagglutinin (H) and neuraminidase (N), which are located on the surface of the virus. There are eighteen different hemagglutinin subtypes (H1 though H18) and eleven different neuraminidase subtypes (N1 through N11). More than 130 influenza A subtype combinations have been identified in nature, mainly from wild birds, but there are likely additional influenza A subtype combinations given the propensity for virus "reassortment" of the eight RNA segments. The H1N1 and H3N2 subtypes have been responsible for the more recent influenza pandemics.

The most devastating influenza pandemic on record is the 1918 "Spanish" flu, which was caused by the H1N1 influenza virus A. It has been estimated to have produced disease in at least five hundred million people, about a third of the world's population at the time, and resulted in around fifty million deaths.[14] There were four waves of the Spanish flu, with the first occurring between February 15 and June 1, 1918, and the last wave occurring from December 1, 1919 to April 30, 1920.[15] Some fifty thousand Canadians and 675,000 Americans appear to have succumbed to this H1N1 influenza A virus between 1919 and 1920. It had an estimated mortality rate of 2.5 percent and primarily affected twenty-five- to forty-year-olds. The deaths were primarily due to subsequent secondary bacterial pneumonia. The epidemic is likely to have originated in Haskell County, Kansas, home to Ft. Riley of the US 7th Cavalry,[16] although it may have started elsewhere in the United States, Spain, or France. The Spanish flu was probably one of the major factors that led to the end of World War

I. The high lethality rate of the Spanish flu was likely a reflection in part of the high rates of war injuries, including damage to the airways and lungs by gas warfare, poor nutrition and inadequate sanitation, and high stress levels during the end and aftermath of World War I. On the termination of the war, the spread of the flu was exacerbated by the return of soldiers to their home countries.

H1N1 influenza subtypes were prevalent in the 1950s and then largely disappeared until 1977 when they reappeared, causing a pandemic that originated in the former USSR.[17] The 1977 H1N1 subtype had a fatality rate of less than 0.005 percent and was fairly mild; it primarily affected people twenty-six years of age or younger. The gene sequence of the 1977 H1N1 was almost identical to the N1H1 subtype from 1950,[18] leading scientists to believe it was likely to have "escaped" from a lab that was developing a vaccine against influenza.[19] People older than twenty-six in 1977 probably already had lasting immunity against the H1N1 strain due to prior exposure. However, influenza A viruses tend to mutate faster than influenza B type viruses, and so evasion of pre-existing immunity is more likely with influenza A viruses. The H1N1 subtype that emerged during the 2009–2010 flu season (called "swine flu" in the media) was caused by a combination of influenza A viruses that infected pigs, birds, and humans.

Vaccines against influenza are usually developed for North America based on a mix of the subtypes that appear to be prevalent during the prior flu season in the Southern Hemisphere. Often, these predictions fail, and new influenza vaccines prove to be less effective than desired for the new flu season. For example, in a meta-analysis study of vaccine effectiveness from the 2009–2010 influenza pandemic, it was estimated that in the Northern Hemisphere it was only 22 percent effective.[20] But when most circulating flu viruses are well-matched to those used to make flu vaccines, a reduction of flu illness between 40 and 60 percent can typically be observed.[21]

In the 2019–2020 flu season from November 17, 2019, to March 28, 2020, there were higher than usual levels of influenza detections (55,379 cases) and hospitalizations (2,493 cases) in Canada, but the flu season ended about eight weeks sooner than the average end of flu season, which resulted in a lower annual total than usual.[22] The abrupt drop in influenza cases after the end of March 2020 was attributed to instigation of public health measures to limit the spread of COVID-19.

One of the mysteries during the COVID-19 pandemic was why the incidence of influenza cases in Canada and worldwide so dramatically declined. In the 2020–2021 flu season, there was essentially no community spread of influenza, with only sixty-nine confirmed detections of the influenza virus in Canada, usually occurring in people under twenty years of age, and none were hospitalized.[23] Despite double the average annual testing rates in Canada, influenza percent positivity did not exceed 0.01 percent of tested cases. Like RSV, the number of influenza cases was historically low when compared to the previous six years. The same trends were also observed in the United States, and in most countries in both the northern and southern hemispheres. Depending on the country, the historical average rates of influenza positivity ranged from 0.8 to 25.1 percent of those tested.[24]

About 45 percent of the recorded influenza cases in Canada in the 2020–2021 season were in people who were recently vaccinated against the virus.[25] Since the influenza viruses in most vaccines tend to be attenuated, i.e., weaker strains of influenza A viruses, there is a risk that some individuals who have weak immune systems that are unable to mount a sufficiently protective immune response might contract the disease. Some inactive influenza vaccines use heat-killed virus or some of its proteins rather than the whole virus, but these tend to be less effective. The very low rates of influenza cases in Canada continued in the 2021–2022 flu season, which began on August 29, 2021. There was a resurgence of influenza cases in the 2022–2023 flu season in Canada, but the total was still lower than typically seen in the flu seasons that preceded COVID-19. From August 28 to December 31, 2022, there were only 59,459 influenza cases reported nationally.[26] In the United States in the 2022–2023 flu season, the H3N2 influenza viruses predominated, vaccine effectiveness was moderate at about 35 percent for preventing hospitalization, and of the hospitalization for influenza, 52.8 percent had been fully vaccinated beforehand for the flu.[27]

It should be noted that most people who die with influenza actually die from secondary bacterial pneumonia. For that reason, Statistics Canada usually reports deaths from both influenza and pneumonia together. In the 2019–2020 flu season, there were 306 ICU admissions and 120 deaths with influenza in Canada, and over 70 percent were from influenza A. Over 90 percent of the deaths were associated with at least one comorbidity, usually hypertension or another heart disorder. Typically, about 3,500 deaths with influenza occur annually in Canada.[28] It should be appreciated that the risk of death for children less than fifteen years of age is about ten- to a hundred-times higher from influenza than from COVID-19.[29]

It seems reasonable that the reduction of flu-like illnesses in Canada during 2020–2021 and 2021–2022 was partly due to misdiagnosis as COVID-19 cases. But why would the incidence of COVID-19 in the first two years of the pandemic result in almost complete suppression of the spread of influenza? It has been estimated that over 430,000 people arrived in the United States from China during the early phase of the COVID-19 pandemic before the Trump administration imposed travel restrictions.[30] Consequently, there was still ample opportunity for the latest influenza variants from China to travel to North America in January through to mid-March of 2022. One possible explanation for the reduction in influenza cases in the 2020–2021 and 2021–2022 flu seasons is the widespread infection with the novel SARS-CoV-2 virus. Apart from stimulating an adaptive immune response to SARS-CoV-2, there might have been a general upregulation of the innate immune response at the same time. While this is less specific, the innate immune response would confer protection against infections in general. For example, it is reported that people who received the bacillus Calmette–Guérin (BCG) vaccine for tuberculosis, which stimulates an innate immune response, were much less prone to getting severe COVID-19.[31] However, this BCG-vaccine effect on COVID-19 incidence has been controversial.[32]

Even without prior immune protection from previous infection or vaccination, influenza can be successfully treated in most cases with antiviral drugs. Influenza A and influenza B viruses are sensitive to the recent antivirals oseltamivir (Tamiflu) from Roche and zanamivir (Relenza) from GalaxoSmithKline. These are inhibitors of the neuraminidase enzyme on the surface of the influenza particles, which is needed to permit budding and release of the virus from infected host cells.

4.4. Common Cold Coronaviruses

The first time a coronavirus was identified as being responsible for a respiratory infection was back in 1937, when this virus produced a devastating effect on the poultry industry. By 1965, it was demonstrated that coronaviruses were responsible for approximately 15 to 30 percent of common colds in humans.[33] Coronaviruses appear to have infected humans as far back as at least twenty thousand years ago.[34] Among the most common human coronaviruses are the alphacoronaviruses 229E and NL63 and the betacoronaviruses HKU1 and OC43. All of these coronaviruses produce relatively mild, but inconvenient, symptoms that rarely require hospitalization.[35] The symptoms include runny nose, sore throat, headache, fever, cough, and a general feeling of malaise. A lower-respiratory tract illness, such as bronchitis or pneumonia, may develop, particularly in people with heart and lung (cardiopulmonary) disease, those that are immune-compromised, young infants, and the elderly. In addition to the discussed coronaviruses, there are several types of viruses that can potentially cause the common cold, including rhinoviruses, enteroviruses, and human metapneumovirus.

The OC43 coronavirus shares 51 percent nucleotide identity in its whole genome with SARS-CoV-2, and the encoded spike proteins share 28 percent amino acid identity.[36] The more similar the nucleotide sequences of two genes, the more likely it is that they have a common origin. Likewise, the more similar the amino acid sequences of two proteins, the more likely that they arise from the same or related genes and have similar functionality. *Nucleotide identity* means exactly the same nucleotide base types (out of four possible types) appear in precisely the same aligned position in the two gene sequences being compared. *Amino acid identity* means exactly the same amino acid type (out of twenty possible amino acids) is located in the same aligned position in the two protein sequences being compared. *Amino acid similarity* comparisons make allowances for highly related amino acids being substituted with each other in making such comparisons (e.g., a negatively charged amino acid replacing another negatively charged amino acid, or a positively charged amino acid replacing another positively charged amino acid). Thus, two proteins can have lower amino acid identity, but more amino acid similarity. OC43's 51 percent nucleotide identity to SARS-CoV-2 indicates that both viruses emerged from a common ancestor in the distant past. However, they will not necessarily behave the same way regarding virulence and host infectivity.

As with other coronaviruses, these particular common-cold viruses are characterized by their "crown-like" appearance in electron microscopic images. The projections correspond to bundles of three interwoven copies of the large spike protein that is encoded by the S gene in the genomes of this family of single-stranded RNA viruses, which are embedded in a lipid membrane that envelopes the virus. The interaction of the spike protein trimer with a receptor that is normally present on the surface of a suitable host cell is critical in permitting entry, by first allowing the virus to latch on to it. In the cases of OC43 and HKU1, their spike proteins interact with 9-O-acetylsialic acid to invade host cells.[37] The 229E spike protein exploits amino-peptidase N (ANPEP) as its host cell receptor to mediate viral infection,[38] whereas the NL63 spike protein utilizes angiotensin-converting enzyme 2 (ACE2) as its host receptor.[39] As will be discussed later in chapter 5, ACE2 is an important enzyme in the regulation of blood pressure. In addition to NL63, the spike proteins of SARS-CoV-1 and SARS-CoV-2 utilize ACE2 as a receptor for viral attachment to host cells.

In one study of serum antibody samples collected from 251 people between August 2013 and March 2020, 2.2 percent had cross-reactive antibodies against full-length SARS-CoV-2 spike protein, 0.6 percent had antibodies against its receptor-binding portion, and 23.9 percent had antibodies against its nucleocapsid protein.[40] In the same study, the authors reported that SARS-CoV-2 infection increased the detection of antibodies against the OC43 spike protein. However, the presence of these antibodies against OC43 spike protein did not correlate with a reduced risk of acquiring a SARS-CoV-2 infection as demonstrated with a PCR test performed with a nasal swab sample when the 251 people that were positive for SARS-CoV-2 RNA were compared to 251 people that did not test positive for the virus. Another study showed that those individuals with an infection between 2015 and 2020 with the endemic 229E, NL63, HKU1, or OC43 (eCoV-positive) had a similar rate of SARS-CoV-2 infections as measured by PCR tests when compared to those without previous recent infection with these cold coronaviruses (eCoV-negative). However, prior exposure to endemic 229E, NL63, HKU1, or OC43 was associated with 90 percent reductions in intensive care unit (ICU) admissions and a trend toward lower odds of mechanical ventilation compared to those without (eCoV-).[41] The percentage of hospitalized patients who eventually died over follow-up was also lower in the eCoV-positive (4.8 percent) group as compared with the eCoV-negative (17.7 percent) group. Thus, antibodies against the common-cold coronaviruses might not have prevented SARS-CoV-2 infection, but they might have reduced the severity of COVID-19 illness and death. This likely accounts for the low rates of COVID-19 deaths in international refugee camps and the Downtown Eastside of Vancouver, BC, a zone with disproportionately high levels of drug use, homelessness, poverty, crime, mental illness, and sex work.

4.5. SARS-CoV-1

The first report of a SARS-CoV-1 (originally called SARS-CoV) case with more severe pneumonia-like symptoms was in late 2002 in Guangdong province in southern China.[42] The new disease was named severe acute respiratory syndrome (SARS) and appeared to have a high mortality rate of about 3 percent.[43] Earlier estimates placed the mortality rate as high as 11 percent, but this underestimated the number of people who were actually infected and was based largely on total hospitalized cases of SARS.

The SARS-CoV-1 virus spread to over twenty-eight countries, but was predominantly in five countries, including Canada, during its short course. It caused over eight thousand hospitalizations and resulted in over eight hundred deaths worldwide, although 83 percent of all SARS deaths were in Mainland China and Hong Kong. Canada's main SARS outbreak was in Toronto, Ontario, starting in February 2003, and resulted in about 438 recorded hospital cases and forty-four deaths in the country.[44]

Within a month of its detection, the complete genome structure of the SARS-CoV-1 virus was first elucidated at the Genome Sciences Centre in Vancouver, British Columbia, in collaboration with the National Microbiology Laboratory in Winnipeg, Manitoba,[45] and a week later it was also reported by the US Centers for Disease Control and Prevention (CDC).[46]

The successful containment of SARS-CoV-1 has been attributed to most infections occurring in hospital settings during the late and symptomatic phase of the disease.[47] However, it is remarkable that the SARS-CoV-1 virus apparently disappeared from the human scene within two years of its emergence, without the use of preventive measures such as vaccines or specific antiviral treatments.[48] The last probable SARS-CoV-1 cases were reported in China in April 2004.[49]

Masked palm civets (*Paguma larvata*, a member of the mongoose family), which are known to be sold in the animal markets of the Chinese city of Guangzhou, were initially hypothesized to be the source of SARS-CoV-1 infection in humans.[50] It should be appreciated that there were two SARS-CoV-1 outbreaks in 2002–2004, each arising from separate palm civet-to-human transmission events. The first emerged in late 2002 and ended in August 2003, and the second arose in late 2003 from a lingering population of SARS-CoV progenitors in civets.

A decade and a half later, the origin of SARS-CoV-1 was eventually traced back to a remote cave in Yunnan province in China, to a single population of horseshoe bats of the *Rhinophidae* family, which harbors various virus strains that have high genetic similarity to SARS-CoV-1.[51] Among the bat coronaviruses isolated from the Yunnan cave, the Rs3367, RsSHC014, WIV1, and WIV16 strains were the closest matches to SARS-CoV-1 with respect to their overall genetic sequences. This included the regions encompassing the S1 (spike), ORF3, and ORF8 genes, which are known to be more variable between coronaviruses. ORF's are open-reading frames in genome sequences that are known or suspected to encode proteins. Furthermore, many of the proteins produced from the genomes of these bat coronavirus shared greater than 98 percent amino acid sequence identities with the human/civet SARS-CoVs.

It remains a puzzle as to how a virus from bats in Yunnan could travel to infect animals and humans about a 1100 kilometers away in Guangdong without causing any suspected cases in the Yunnan area itself. This reduces the likelihood that a bat from Yunnan directly transmitted SARS-CoV-1 to a human. It is feasible that the masked palm civets were infected by a bat SARS coronavirus that was the direct progenitor of SARS-CoV-1. This progenitor was generated from a series of recombination events with highly related bat coronaviruses. However, the closest civet SARS coronavirus lacks portions of the S1 spike protein gene that permits optimal binding of the virus to human ACE2 protein, which is the primary host receptor for SARS-CoV-1.[52] Of note, the SARS-CoV-1 virus itself shows 79 percent nucleotide identity in the whole genome with SARS-CoV-2, and their spike proteins share 76 percent amino acid identity.[53] SARS-CoV-1 was less infectious than SARS-CoV-2, but it caused more severe illness with greater lethality.

4.6. MERS-CoV

In 2012, at least eight years after SARS mysteriously disappeared, another pandemic outbreak with a SARS coronavirus erupted in the Middle East, with a small number of imported cases in Europe, North Africa, Asia, and North

America. The virus was designated Middle East Respiratory Syndrome coronavirus (MERS-CoV) and ultimately infected around 2,500 people, primarily in Saudi Arabia.[54]

MERS's mortality rate appeared to be much higher than that of SARS-CoV-1, since approximately 35 percent of the MERS patients who were reported to the World Health Organization (WHO) died. The disease is manifested by severe respiratory infection, often with kidney (renal) and other multi-organ failure.

About 80 percent of cases of MERS-CoV infections in humans were the result of direct or indirect contact with camels or infected individuals, with the latter largely being health-care workers. The dromedaries were the principal host for the virus and the only known zoonotic source. For MERS-CoV transmission, direct close contact with an infected individual was necessary. MERS-CoV binds to host cells by attachment to dipeptidyl peptidase 4 (DPP4), which is expressed in the upper respiratory tract of epithelial cells of camels, but much less so in humans. DDP4 is an example of a protease, which is a class of enzymes that cleave other proteins into smaller segments. The lack of DDP4 receptors in the human upper respiratory tract likely accounts for the restricted transmission of MERS-CoV in humans.[55] DPP4 receptors are known to be expressed in human kidney cells, small intestine cells, and immune T cells.[56]

The MERS-CoV virus displays 53 percent nucleotide identity in its whole genome with SARS-CoV-2, and the respective spike proteins share 26 percent amino acid identity.[57] The lower rate of spike protein amino acid identity with SARS-CoV-1 and SARS-CoV-2 likely accounts in part for the differences in their spike protein recognition of host cell proteins. The interaction of MERS-CoV with DPP4 is mediated via its spike protein.

The spike proteins of coronaviruses are not only important for host cell receptor recognition, but they facilitate the fusion of the host cell surface membrane with the coronavirus lipid membrane as well. This provides for the delivery of the genetic material, i.e., the RNA genome of the virus into the cell. The cell and virus membrane fusion mediated by the spike protein is improved following its cleavage at subunits by the protease furin for certain coronaviruses like MERS-CoV.[58] Proteases, also known as proteinases, are enzymes that cut other proteins between specific amino acid sequences. This can lead to their target protein's activation, inactivation, or ultimate degradation. The furin recognition sequence motif in MERS-CoV, which results in the formation of the S1 and S2 subunits of the spike protein and increases the infectivity of MERS-CoV also occurs in SARS-CoV-2, but not in common-cold coronaviruses, SARS-CoV-1, or the closest bat and civet coronaviruses related to SARS-CoV. MERS-CoV also features an additional furin cleavage site in the S2 subunit that is not found in SARS-CoV-2. In the human body, furin is widely expressed in different tissues and cell types.[59] MERS-CoV is also able to enter cells using an alternative pathway at the cell surface with activation by the transmembrane protease serine 2 (TMPRSS2) and by TMPRSS4, which can also target SARS-CoV-2 at the S1/S2 furin cleavage site.[60] Once the viral load is high enough to establish a MERS-CoV infection, the increased affinity for DPP4 by the furin cleavage might contribute to the higher rate of multiple system failure and death caused by MERS.[61]

There are many different respiratory viruses that produce very similar symptoms. Some of these are seasonal like RSV, influenza, and the cold coronaviruses. However, SARS-CoV-1 and MERS-CoV had very limited runs, ultimately fizzling out as viruses of concern with relatively little imposition of public health measures to curtail their spread. For the coronaviruses, the spike protein is central to their ability to infect host cells, and while ACE2 was a common target for many of them, other host cell proteins were exploited by some of the coronaviruses. The next chapter will offer a detailed description of the SARS-CoV-2 virus, which is responsible for COVID-19.

CHAPTER 5

The SARS-CoV-2 Virus

Steven Pelech & Wendi Roscoe

"Only one form of contagion travels faster than a virus. And that's fear."
—Dan Brown

"Know thy enemy and know yourself; in a hundred battles, you will never be defeated. When you are ignorant of the enemy but know yourself, your chances of winning or losing are equal. If ignorant both of your enemy and of yourself, you are sure to be defeated in every battle."
—Ancient Chinese General Sun Tze

To become better acquainted with the SARS-CoV-2 virus, a little more introduction to heavy-duty biochemistry and cell biology may be necessary. The level of detail provided in this chapter may exceed the interest and patience of many of the readers of this book. However, for those that desire a closer look at the tiny enemy virus that spurred the COVID-19 pandemic, this chapter is for them. Likewise, in chapter 7, the body's elegant immune defenses against infectious pathogens like the SARS-CoV-2 virus are detailed. Such knowledge of the enemy and the strength of our own defenses will provide for ultimate victory over this recent scourge of humanity.

5.1. The Structure of SARS-CoV-2 Genome and Proteins

SARS-CoV-2 is the seventh major coronavirus to affect humans in recent times, after HKU1, NL63, OC43 and 229E, SARS-CoV, and MERS-CoV.[1] It is taxonomically placed in the order *Nidovirales*, subfamily *Orthocoronavirinae*, which has four genera, namely *Alphacoronavirus*, *Betacoronavirus*, *Gammacoronovirus*, and *Deltacoronoavirus*. Like SARS-CoV-1 and MERS-CoV, SARS-CoV-2 is a betacoronavirus.[2]

Characteristic of coronaviruses, SARS-CoV-2 is a ribonucleic acid (RNA) containing virus that has a single, positive-stranded genome around 29,903 nucleotides long. Its genome encodes the information for construction of at least twenty-eight different viral proteins that permit the reproduction of the infectious viral particle. The locations of the genes that encode the SARS-CoV-2 structural and non-structural (NSP) proteins are illustrated in Figure 5.1 in the insert. Non-structural proteins are generally considered those proteins that are not found in the completed infectious viral particle. NSP, along with accessory proteins, are critical for replication of viruses inside of cells, but they are not necessary to be assembled in the final infectious virus and are usually absent due to packing limitations.

Each protein has an amino acid composition and sequence that is dictated by the sequences of the nucleotides in the SARS-CoV-2 virus genes. Like other viruses in the coronavirus family, SARS-CoV-2 is characterized by a crown-like appearance under an electron microscope, which arises from the location of multiple large spike protein complexes on the viral particle surface. The spike protein, which is made initially as a 1273- to 1278-amino-acid-long precursor protein, is clipped into S1 and S2 subunits that remain tightly interlinked (Figure 5.2 in the insert). When presented on the surface of a virus or cell, the spike protein is located in trimeric complexes of three S1 subunits and three S2 subunits that are intertwined. The S1 subunit features a region called the receptor binding domain (RBD) through which the virus can attach to receptors on host cells, including particularly the angiotensin converting enzyme 2 (ACE2) protein, thus gaining access to cells where it has the potential to replicate.

Apart from copies of the membrane and envelope proteins that are also exposed on the outside of the virus, any of the other viral proteins that are present in the fully formed viral particle are buried in its interior. The other SARS-CoV-2 genome-encoded proteins are not likely to be commonly present in the viral particle, except for the nucleocapsid protein, which interacts with the RNA genome to facilitate its packing. Internal viral proteins are less useful for immune cell recognition of the intact virus particle for its removal. However, antibodies that are produced against the nucleocapsid can be useful to indicate a past infection with SARS-CoV-2 long after recovery from COVID-19 or after an asymptomatic infection.

In view of the virus surface accessibility and large size of the spike protein complex, it has been specifically targeted for the production of vaccines that can evoke the adaptive immune system in people to produce two main classes of lymphocytes, i.e., T cells and B cells, which will recognize the spike protein on the virus particle and infected cells. The bivalent COVID-19 vaccines produced mixed versions of the spike protein gene from both the original Wuhan strain and Omicron BA.4/5 strains that predominated in mid-2022, all of which were essentially extinct and supplanted by the Omicron XBB strains by early 2023. The bivalent COVID-19 vaccines allow for the formation of four possible combinations of triplets, two of which are not found naturally in any virus strains. X-ray crystallographic structures of the spike protein complexes isolated from cells that have been treated with bivalent vaccines have not been described in the scientific literature. The effects of the mixed, heterogeneous versions of the spike protein complexes that result from the new bivalent vaccines are unclear.

5.2. Receptors for the SARS-CoV-2 Spike Protein

As mentioned, the spike protein through its RBD is able to attach to the ACE2 protein, which is expressed on the surface of diverse human cell types. Attachment to ACE2 is possible when the RBD is accessible following flipping to the open position in the S1 subunit. When the spike protein is finally presented on the surface of the SARS-CoV-2 virus or on the surface of host cells following the uptake of COVID-19 genetic vaccines, it can exist in both open and closed conformations.

It should be appreciated that ACE2 is not the only host cell protein that SARS-CoV-2 can bind via its spike protein. Neuropilin (NRP1) is another target receptor for the spike protein.[3] NRP1 binds to vascular endothelial growth factor-A (VEGF-A), which mediates pain reception and growth of blood vessels.[4] Like ACE2, NRP1 is highly present in the endothelial and epithelial cells of the nose and lungs. Moreover, a wide range of immune cell receptors (CCR9, CD2, CD4, CD7, CD26, CD50, CD56, CD106, CD150, and XCR1)[5] and the nicotinic acetylcholine receptor have been implicated as other targets for the spike protein by molecular modeling studies.[6]

Finally, spike protein can bind more loosely to sialylated glycans that are generally expressed on the surface of cells, and which are extremely prevalent on red blood cells, platelets, and the endothelial cells that line blood vessels.[7] While these particular cells express low levels of ACE2, spike protein can induce the clumping of red blood cells, and this may contribute to blood clotting and other cardiovascular issues known to be associated with COVID-19 and the COVID-19 vaccines.

ACE2 is one of the main enzymes of the renin-angiotensin system (RAS), which is central to the regulation of blood pressure, fluid, and salt balance.[8, 9] As a protease, ACE2 clips the eight-amino-acid-long hormone angiotensin 2 to a slightly shorter seven-amino-acid-long peptide called Ang (1–7), which then mediates vasodilation and increases blood flow.[10]

Angiotensin 2 promotes vasoconstriction of blood vessels, inflammation, and subsequent thickening and scarring of tissues. By binding to its receptor ACE1, angiotensin 2 turns on signaling pathways inside of cells to ultimately increase blood pressure, directly by causing constriction of small arteries and indirectly by causing the release of the hormones aldosterone, from the adrenal glands above the kidneys, and vasopressin, from the pituitary gland at the base of the brain. The binding of SARS-CoV-2 to cells appears to inhibit the enzymatic activity of ACE2 and permit accumulation of angiotensin 2.

ACE2 is widely and differentially expressed in diverse human tissues. Among the thirty-one tested human tissues in one study, ACE2 gene expression was highest in cells of the testes, small intestine, kidneys, heart, thyroid, and adipose tissue, and lowest in blood, spleen, brain, and skeletal muscle.[11] Similarly, the Human Protein Atlas (HPA)[12]database shows that ACE2 has relatively high protein expression levels in the duodenum, small intestine, gallbladder, kidneys, testes, seminal vesicles, colon, rectum, and adrenal glands.

As often observed with diverse viruses, SARS-CoV-2 spike protein can interact with multiple cell receptors leading to pathophysiological consequences linked to the perturbation of the normal activity of the cells expressing those receptors. Among the myriad of symptoms associated with COVID-19, immune-related complications—such as over production of immune lymphocytes (lymphocytopenia) and immune mediators (cytokine storms)—are common in severe diseases. One possible path for such pathologies is the recent finding that SARS-CoV-2 spike protein can also bind to CD4 receptor and mediate its entry in T helper cells, thereby affecting its normal function and leading to viral persistence and disease severity.[13] More about how the immune system fights viral infection will be provided in chapter 7.

5.3. Demographics of SARS-CoV-2 Hosts

The structure of the ACE2 in different species largely dictates whether SARS-CoV-2 can infect them. Initially in the COVID-19 pandemic, the Wuhan strain of SARS-CoV-2 poorly infected rats and mice. The inability to evoke responses in these rodents compromised early pre-clinical safety studies of vaccines and necessitated the production of transgenic mice that expressed the human version of ACE2 in their tissues to study drugs that might potentially block infection of the virus and its replication. However, as SARS-CoV-2 mutated within the human population, it was able to expand its range of potential host species. For example, wild rats in the sewers of New York City ultimately became susceptible to infection with the Alpha, Delta, and Omicron variants of SARS-CoV-2.[14]

SARS-CoV-2 has also been shown to infect a wide range of other wild, domestic, and captive animals since its early identification in pangolins and civets. An ever-expanding list of infected animals includes ferrets, minks, Syrian golden hamsters, bushy-tailed woodrats, striped skunks, domestic cats, lions and tigers, wild deer, and gorillas.[15, 16, 17, 18, 19, 20, 21, 22] For example, about 36 percent of 360 nasal swab samples collected between January and March 2021 from the free-ranging white-tailed deer in northeastern Ohio in the United States were infected with SARS-CoV-2.[23] In another study conducted in Ohio between December 2020 and January 2021, more than 80 percent of the tested deer were determined to be SARS-CoV-2 infected.[24] So far, cottontail rabbits, fox squirrels, Wyoming ground squirrels, black-tailed prairie dogs, house mice, and raccoons have been resistant to SARS-CoV-2 infection.[25] This ability of SARS-CoV-2 to infect and propagate in so many diverse species means that even if the human population could temporarily eliminate the virus, it will be able to re-infect humans in the future from animal reservoirs.

5.4. Roles of SARS-CoV-2 Viral Proteins

Binding of SARS-CoV-2 to the ACE2 protein on a suitable host cell triggers a cascade of events that lead to internalization of the virus into the cell, as shown in Figure 5.3. Loose binding of the virus with sialylated glycans (polysaccharide sugar side-chains) on proteins in host cells may facilitate initial interactions, which is followed by high affinity binding to ACE2 and other receptors.[26] After the attachment of SARS-CoV-2 to ACE2 via its RBD, the transmembrane protease serine 2 (TMPRSS2), which is present on the surface of the host cells, clips the spike protein to generate its S1 and S2 subunits. The conformational change in the S2 subunit facilitates fusion of the outer membrane of the virus particle with the plasma membrane on the surface of the host cells. This results in the release of the viral ribonucleoprotein complex into the cytoplasm of the host cell. The ribonucleoprotein component is the positive, single strand of RNA decorated with nucleocapsid proteins.

While this is the main means of entry into most host cells, there are other routes, including the capture of the viral particle by a process known as endocytosis. In this case, the S1 and S2 subunits of the spike protein are generated by cleavage by proteases in the cathepsin family.[27, 28, 29] As mentioned, there are other known receptors such as NRP1 and other potential candidates. Proteases that might also cleave the S1 and S2 subunits include cathepsin L, TMPRSS11D, and TMPRSS13.[30, 31]

Once inside the host-cell, the viral RNA genome is released and later replicated through viral proteins that are encoded by the SARS-CoV-2 genome. The RNA sequence is the template that allows for the production of the viral proteins. It is unclear how many intact virus particles are produced that can be assembled and then spread to nearby cells. A large portion of the packaged viral particles contain mRNA that is missing the back end and is defective for producing new virus.[32] Such defective viral genomes are commonly produced with other single-stranded RNA viruses, including RSV, measles, influenza, Ebola, and dengue viruses.

Through a series of subsequent steps for which the details remain sketchy, different genes are translated by ribosomes into viral proteins with the aid of existing host proteins that further facilitate the production of negative-sense

RNA copies of the positive-sense RNA genome. These negative-sense RNA copies in turn serve as templates to make several more positive-sense RNA genomes, which are eventually packaged into new infectious virus particles. The non-structural protein and accessory proteins encoded by the viral genome ultimately provide for the synthesis of viral spike (S), envelope (E), membrane (M), and nucleocapsid (N) proteins, which are required components in the completed virus particle.

The spike protein is a type I transmembrane protein that is 1273 to 1279 amino acids long with several polysaccharide attachments (i.e., it is N-linked and O-linked glycosylated with polymers of various sugars). Some of these N-glycans are thought to be important in modulating the conformation of the RBDs. Glycosylation of foreign proteins can also reduce their recognition by host antibodies. About three-quarters of the surface of the spike protein trimer complex is shielded by the glycan chains.

The viral membrane protein is 223-amino-acids-long, occurs in a dimeric form, and is also glycosylated (i.e., it is O-linked glycosylated). Although it is found in the lipid membrane of the virus particle, it binds the nucleocapsid protein, which in turn is also associated with the viral RNA genome. This plays an important role in the final assembly of the virus particle so that it contains the genetic payload.

The viral envelope protein is seventy-five amino acids long, and it plays a role in the assembly and release of the viral particle. Like the spike and membrane proteins, the envelope protein features a trafficking signal sequence that enables its integration into the endoplasmic reticulum (ER) membranes of the cell.

The viral nucleocapsid protein is 420 amino acid long, and it has three highly evolutionary conserved domains: an N-terminus domain, an RNA-binding domain, and a C-terminus domain. The RNA-binding domain undergoes heavy modification by a process known as protein phosphorylation, which appears to be essential for the ability of the nucleocapsid protein to bind RNA and in the replication of the virus. This appears to be performed by an enzyme known as glycogen synthase kinase-3, and inhibitors of this kinase block SARS-CoV-2 replication in cells in culture.[33] Multiple nucleocapsid proteins work together to facilitate the packaging of RNA in the viral particle. This protein also enhances virus transcriptional efficiency.

Upon entry into the host cell, the ORF-1a and ORF-1ab genes found near the beginning of the genome are translated by the ribosomes to produce two large polyproteins, pp1a and pp1ab, which undergo proteolytic cleavage to form several smaller proteins (NSPs 1 to 16). Some of these reassemble into a functional viral RNA polymerase that is sometimes referred to as a replicase. The pp1a non-structural protein is processed by proteolysis into NSP1 to

NSP11 and the pp1ab non-structural protein is similarly processed to produce NSP12 to NSP16. The second half of the viral genome encodes the remainder of the viral proteins, including the spike, envelope, membrane, nucleocapsid, and NSPs specified by the ORF3a, ORF3d, ORF6, ORF7a, ORF7b, ORF8, ORF9b, ORF14, and ORF10 genes. These latter proteins are generated by a carefully orchestrated sequence of replication-transcription events that lead to the synthesis of subgenomic RNAs from the negative-sense RNA strand that was produced by the replicase complex. These shorter positive-sense RNAs are translated to produce several of the other structural and accessory proteins that participate in the assembly and encapsulation of the genomic RNA into the final virus particle.

The roles of many of the other twenty-five proteins encoded by the SARS-CoV-2 have been elucidated, in part due to their similarity with other coronavirus proteins.[34] For example, the NSP9 proteins of SARS-CoV-1 and SARS-CoV-2 share about 97 percent amino acid sequence similarity.[35] Many of these viral proteins are RNA polymerases, which are enzymes that act to replicate the RNA genome and produce mRNAs that encode for the viral proteins that are required at the later stages of the assembly and export of the final virus particles. Several of the other viral proteins are proteases that cleave the viral proteins into intermediate and mature functional proteins. Some of these viral RNA polymerases and proteases have been targeted for development of antiviral drugs against SARS-CoV-2. Many of the other viral proteins target the production of immune cell mediators known as cytokines, which are released from infected host cells to recruit immune cells to the site of the infection. Interferon regulatory transcription factor-3 (IRF3) is often affected in the infected host cells, which results in reduced or enhanced production of interferons (IFNs). Many of the actions of the NSP and the accessory ORF proteins appear to be in conflict with inhibiting or activating the immune system, although there is a trend toward early suppressions of host cell efforts to recruit the immune system.

The process of viral replication with RNA viruses necessitates the creation of a double-stranded RNA molecule intermediate. This can trigger a cascade of events leading to antiviral effects by the host cell. Double-stranded RNA is not normally found in host cells, and there are sensory proteins, such as double-stranded RNA-dependent protein kinase, which can activate countermeasures, such as the production of IFNs. SARS-CoV-2 is able, through several of the NSPs and some of the ORF viral proteins, to suppress IFN production as well as general cellular mRNA translation to support viral mRNA translation. For example, NSP5 and the nucleocapsid protein have been found to suppress the formation of stress granules in host cells, which are important as the cellular protective responses to viral infection, including type I and type III IFN responses.[36]

The production of the structural proteins by ribosomes is near the membranous endoplasmic reticulum (ER) of cells. The ER is an extensive network of membranes in cells from which the Golgi apparatus derives. The Golgi apparatus allows for the transport of membrane lipid and proteins throughout the cell. In the case of the spike protein, most of it is driven into the luminal side (as opposed to the cytoplasmic side) of the ER following its biosynthesis, but it remains anchored in the ER membrane by its transmembrane domain and by covalent attachment of copies of the fatty acid palmitate at multiple sites. The spike, membrane, envelope, and nucleocapsid proteins and genomic RNA remain in close proximity within the ER following their production, and eventually get trafficked together via the Golgi apparatus in vesicles to the cell surface, where the virus particles in these vesicles are released following fusion of the lipid bilayers of the vesicles with the lipid bilayer of the plasma membrane.

The traditional explanation of viral replication involves the production of new virus particles that infect more cells and continue to make new virus particles in a logarithmic fashion until the immune system turns the tide to control the infection. However, as will be discussed in chapter 7, if the immune system initially fails to contain the virus and prevent the early spread of SARS-CoV-2, a loss of control of immune cell activation can result in a devastating "cytokine storm," with the overproduction of immune modulatory proteins such as interleukins and interferons, which can make the clinical situation far worse.

5.5. SARS-CoV-2 Mutation to "Variants of Concern"

Canada-wide, since the first recorded wave of COVID-19 cases that peaked around May 6, 2020 (seven-day daily average = 45.6 per million people (pmp)), there have been at least nine more waves. These nine additional peaks occurred around January 13, 2021 (**Wave Two**: seven-day daily average = 210.9 pmp), April 19, 2021 (**Wave Three**: seven-day daily average = 227.0 pmp), September 22, 2021 (**Wave Four**: seven-day daily average = 221.6 pmp), January 9, 2022 (**Wave Five**: seven-day daily average = 1091.6 pmp), April 15, 2022 (**Wave Six**: seven-day average = 263.8 pmp), August 1, 2022 (**Wave Seven**: seven-day daily average = 123.8 pmp), October 22, 2022 (**Wave Eight**: seven-day daily average = 79.7 pmp), and December 26, 2022 (**Wave Nine**: seven-day daily average = 64.6 pmp).[37] There was a steady decline of COVID-19 cases since the beginning of 2023, and starting in September there was a slight uptick in COVID-19 cases with the onset of the flu season, which started to decline again in January 2024. In this last peak, the number of COVID-19 cases remained lower in incidence than any of the earlier waves.

In Canada, as elsewhere, major initiatives to sequence the genomes of SARS-CoV-2 variants as well as human hosts were undertaken. With the CDN$40 million CanCOGeN project funded particularly by Genome Canada, over 433,475 viral samples and 7,171 human samples were fully sequenced at the genome level by April 2022.[38] Such sequencing studies in Canada and many other countries have revealed just how quickly SARS-CoV-2 mutates; over ten thousand mutant forms of the SARS-CoV-2 virus have been sequenced and identified. However, interest has focused on what have been called variants of concern (VOC) or variants of interest, which have mutations that appear to increase the infectivity of SARS-CoV-2, and in doing so have allowed these VOC to out-compete other variants and predominate for a time, until they are displaced by other VOC. Typically, SARS-CoV-2 mutants have lifetimes of about four months before they begin to fade from their previous prevalence.[39]

In Canada, each of these subsequent COVID-19 waves after the original Wuhan strain were largely defined as being dominated by one or more new VOCs: January 2021 **Wave Two** by B.1.160, B.1.438.1, B.1.2, B.1.1.176; April 19, 2021 **Wave Three** by B.1.1.7 (Alpha) and P.1.14 (Gamma); September 2021 **Wave Four** by AY.25.1 and AY.27 (Delta); January 2022 **Wave Five** by BA.1 (Omicron); April 2022 **Wave Six** by BA.2 variants including BA.2 (Omicron); August 2022 **Wave Seven** by BA.5 variants including BA.5.2 and BA.5.2.1 (Omicron); October 2022 **Wave Eight** also by BA.5 variants including BA.5.2 and BA.5.2.1 (Omicron); December 2022 **Wave Nine** by other BA.5 variants, BQ1, and BQ.1.1 (Omicron); mid-September 2023 by EG.5 (Eris), EG.5.1, XBB.1 and XBB.2 (Omicron) variants, and by April 2024 by JN.1.[40]

Early in the COVID-19 pandemic, certain VOC accounted for most cases within a wave. However, as the pandemic has progressed, there has been a greater diversity of competing VOCs. This phenomenon is likely due to an optimization of the mutations to increase the affinity of the SARS-CoV-2 spike protein for the ACE2 protein on host cells to improve entry, reduce its virulence so the host is less likely to be sick, and more readily go out and transmit the virus, and better avoidance of immune cell defenses so the propagation of the virus can be extended. Ultimately, those variants that maximize these properties out-compete earlier variants. It should be appreciated that all of the VOC are still extremely similar in structure to the original Wuhan strain. For example, all of their spike proteins are at least 96 percent identical in amino acid sequence. Some of the mutations in the spike protein associated with VOC are shown in Figure 5.3 in the insert. Interestingly, the Wuhan SARS-CoV-2 spike protein has about a ten- to twenty-fold greater affinity for ACE2 than SARS-CoV-1.[41, 42]

By January 7, 2022, 84.2 percent of Canadians twelve years and older had been vaccinated for COVID-19 at least once, 77.9 percent at least twice, and 31 percent three times. However, this did not prevent the largest wave of COVID-19 cases, which at the time were dominated by the Omicron BA.1 and BA.2

VOCs. In November 2021, it was the Delta VOC that predominated. Within a month, Omicron BA.1 effectively out-competed the Delta variant. Studies have indicated that Omicron BA.1 was three- to six-times more infectious than previous SARS-CoV-2 variants.[43] Despite almost an 850 percent increase in the total number of COVID-19 cases between the peaks of the fourth and fifth waves, there was only a 221 percent increase in total hospitalizations, a 29 percent increase in total ICU admissions, and a 53 percent increase in total deaths. These data clearly demonstrate that Omicron BA.1 and BA.2 variants were much less severe than the Delta variant. The duration of the illness for those with COVID-19 was also about half the length of time. The same relatively low rates of hospitalization, ICU admissions, and deaths have been observed with the subsequent VOCs.

The Omicron BA.1 VOC was first identified in South Africa (although it appears to have originated in Europe), and there were very few deaths per capita in South Africa from this variant. Only about 40 percent of the South African population was vaccinated at least once by the end of 2021, and in 2023 about 50 percent were double or more vaccinated.[44] At the peak of the Omicron BA.1 wave in South Africa with 2.93 deaths per million people per day (seven day average), there were 4.29 deaths per million people per day (seven day average) in Canada in the same wave.[45] This might be partly explained by a lower average age in South Africa (median age is 27.6 years compared to forty-one years in Canada). Typical life expectancy in Canada is 81.75 years, compared to 65.25 years in South Africa. The average age of death from COVID-19 in Canada in 2020, pre-vaccination, was 83.8 years, whereas in 2019, the average age of death from all causes was 76.5 years.[46]

Since the first emergence of the Omicron VOCs, the incidence of COVID-19, hospitalization, and deaths have remained low in Canada for over two years. This is despite the multitude of over thirty other Omicron variants of SARS-CoV-2 (including BA.1, BA.2, BA.5.1.27, BA.5.2.34, BA.5.5.1, BE.1.1.1, BE1.2, BE.9, BF.11, BF.7, BN.1.3, BN.1.3.1, BQ.1, BQ.1.1, BQ.1.2, BQ.1.3, BQ.1.5, BQ.1.8.2, BR.2.1, BW.1.1, CH.1.1, CK.1, CM.8.1, CV.1, DJ.1.1, BF7, XBB.1, XBB1.5, XBB1.16, XBB.2, EG.5 (Eris), EG.5.1, FL1.5.1, HV.1, HK.3, and JN.1) that accounted for COVID-19 cases in September 2023. By the end of the third week of August 2023, EG.5 was responsible for 20.6 percent of all US cases of COVID-19, and the FL15.1 strain accounted for about 13.3 percent of US COVID-19 cases.[47] The substantially reduced progression to severe COVID-19 outcomes seen with the early Omicron variants as compared to the Delta variant was also described in a meta-analysis of the large, integrated healthcare system in Southern California.[48] The SARS-CoV-2 virus has continued to evolve to be as infectious and benign as it can be, such that none of the new variants really predominated in 2023 in Canada. However, since January 2024, the JN.1 variant and its derivatives have predominated after its first emergence in August 2023, and while this variant remains relatively benign, it has been more immune evasive. The new L455S mutation in the JN.1 variant is believed to contribute to its immune evasiveness and increased competiveness versus other SARS-CoV-2 variants despite its reduced affinity for ACE2.[49]

The high rate of mutation of SARS-CoV-2 is in part due to the poor fidelity of its RNA-dependent RNA polymerase to faithfully reproduce the complete genome of the virus without introducing mistakes. There is also a phenomena of RNA recombination whereby simultaneous infection of the same host cells by two or more related SARS-CoV-2 virus variants can produce new hybrid variants.[50] Many different RNA viruses can undergo mutation by recombination. The mechanism involves the viral RNA-dependent RNA polymerase detaching from one RNA template strand with the partially completed nascent RNA strand intact. It then attaches to another RNA template strand at the identical or a similar position and resumes elongation of the nascent RNA strand. Such jumping on and off different RNA templates can occur multiple times before the nascent RNA strand is fully completed.

Genome sequencing studies have revealed that about 2.7 percent of the SARS-CoV-2 genomes investigated have evidence of a recombination ancestry.[51] The highest rates of recombination in an RNA virus, as much as 25 percent, has been reported for mouse hepatitis virus.[52] The SARS-CoV-1[53] and MERS-CoV[54] viruses are believed to have emerged from RNA recombination events. Such a mechanism can provide for zoonotic transmission of coronaviruses and contribute to the species jump with other RNA viruses.

It has been suggested by Tanaka and Miyazawa on *Zenodo* (2023) that the extra mutations in the Omicron BA.1 variant are too many to be accounted for by natural mutation, and that Omicron variants were already present in 2020.[55] Compared to the original Wuhan strain designated 614G, there were at least fifty mutations identified in Omicron BA.1 variant, with thirty-two of these causing amino acid substitutions in the spike protein, and half of these were in its receptor binding domain. There are twice as many mutations in the BA.1 variant of the spike protein than any of the previous variants. BA.1 also features three mutations in the membrane protein and six mutations in the nucleocapsid protein compared to the Wuhan proteins.[56] Moreover, BA.2 has eight additional unique mutations not found in BA.1 and is missing thirteen mutations that are found in BA.1. In fact, all of the BA.1, BA.2, and BA.3 lineages appear to have arisen at about the same time, with additional Omicron variants later arising from different lineages. Thus, these newer Omicron variants did not simply come from a few additional mutations in earlier VOCs. Of the fifty mutations in Omicron variants, twent-six were unique to Omicron, ten were shared with Delta, and six were found in the Beta VOC.

Tanaka and Miyazawa (2023) carefully tracked the occurrence of the spike mutations in the BA.1 and BA.2 strains, and these authors came to the conclusion that these were genetically engineered.[57] Alternative hypotheses have been proposed that these variants first emerged by: 1) cryptic spread and were already present earlier on but not picked up by the standard viral surveillance and sequencing; 2) evolving in a chronically infected COVID-19 patient, who was probably immunocompromised; and 3) zoonosis where Omicron accumulated in a nonhuman host, such as a mouse, and then jumped into humans.[58] The detection of very similar sequences of the spike protein isolated from places like Puerto Rico in 2020 supports the first explanation,[59] although the question arises: Why did Omicron variants not spread much sooner globally, since they are so infectious?

The second hypothesis is partly supported by the high rate of immunosuppression from HIV-infection in as much as 20 percent of the South African population.[60] But this also begs the question that if Omicron came to South Africa from elsewhere, why did it not spread quickly in Puerto Rico or Europe, where it had been detected previously?

The third hypothesis of a zoonosis origin such as from a mouse is also problematic[61] since the mutations in the spike protein of Omicron would have optimized for a nonhuman species in which the ACE2 receptor for the spike protein is likely to be slightly different from humans.

The possibility still remains that the early Omicron variants may have resulted from genetic engineering and a release from a laboratory. Whether intentional or not, this release may have resulted in the development of a self-replicating vaccine that permitted "natural" immunity with more infectious and benign SARS-CoV-2 variants.

Although not discussed more fully in this book, one of the leading hypotheses among scientists is that the original Wuhan strain of SARS-CoV-2 was the result of genetic engineering in the Wuhan Institute of Virology and its accidental release in late 2019 rather from zoonosis.[62] When the genome structure of the Wuhan SARS-CoV-2 strain was initially sequenced, it was first identified as most closely related to that of a horseshoe bat (*Rhinolophus affinis*) SARS-like betacoronavirus designated RaBtCoV/4991 (renamed RaTG13). The genome nucleotide sequence of RaTG13 is 96.2 percent identical to that of SARS-CoV-2. The Wuhan-Hu-1 strain of the SARS-CoV-2 virus, which is the first sequenced genome of this virus, has 153 amino acid variations in total (thirty-three in the spike gene) when compared to RaTG13. More recently, Temmam et al. (2022) discovered bat coronaviruses in northern Laos (Southeast Asia) including BANAL-52 (*Rhinolophus malayanus*) that had an even higher nucleotide identity (96.8 percent) with the whole SARS-CoV-2 genome than RaTG13, but the RaTG13 spike protein amino acid sequence more closely resembles that of SARS-CoV-2.[63]

SARS-CoV-2 is more related in its viral protein sequences to RaTG13 than it is to SARS-CoV-1, but it does feature some portions that are more similar to SARS-CoV-1 than RaTG13.[64] In addition, the furin cleavage sites in the SARS-CoV-2 spike protein, which makes the virus more infectious, are not present in SARS-CoV-1, RaTG13, or BANAL-52.[65,66] Ambati et al. (2022) recognized that this furin cleavage site was 100 percent identical to a reverse complement of a nineteen-nucleotide long portion of the mRNA that encodes the totally unrelated human DNA repair protein mut S homolog 3 (MSH3), making this highly unlikely to be a random coincidence.[67, 68] Finally, the genome of SARS-CoV-2 features sites that are commonly used in genetic engineering.[69] Research into bat coronaviruses was ongoing in the Wuhan Institute of Virology for almost a decade before COVID-19, so the laboratory leak hypothesis seems most plausible.

CHAPTER 6

The Pathology of COVID-19

York N. Hsiang, Steven Pelech, Glenn Chan, & Christopher A. Shaw

"Why would I do that if I were a virus or a cancer cell, or the immune system? Before long, this internal dialogue became second nature to me: I found my mind worked this way all the time."

—Jonas Salk

6.1. Symptoms of COVID-19

In the early stages of a SARS-CoV-2 infection, it is the cells of the upper respiratory tract that are primarily affected. If the immune system is unable to clear the infection, then it can spread to the lower respiratory tract. If the lower respiratory tract is affected, this can cause inflammation of the alveoli in the lung, where gas exchange occurs, making breathing more difficult. The early symptoms of COVID-19 are very similar to other respiratory virus infections, largely because they reflect the body's protective responses to clear the infection. These include fever (37.8° Celsius or 100° Fahrenheit or higher), chills, headache, abdominal, muscle and other body aches, sore throat, cough, runny nose, shortness of breath or difficulty in breathing, diarrhea, fatigue, decreased or lack of appetite, rash, and pink eye (conjunctivitis). These symptoms may emerge two to fourteen days (with a median of three to four days) after initial viral exposure depending on the health and prior immune status of the person infected. Children tend to have milder symptoms than adults, with more than half of children being asymptomatic, but testing positive by PCR for the SARS-CoV-2 virus or possessing antibodies against the virus from a previous infection. A small number of younger children experience croup (laryngotracheobronchitis), which is characterized by sudden onset "barking cough," high pitched extra-thoracic breath sound (inspiratory stridor), and respiratory distress.

Unique symptoms of COVID-19 include a reduction or loss of taste (ageusia) or smell (anosmia); this occurred in about 12 percent of COVID-19 cases of those with European ancestry infected by the Omicron variant as compared to 1.9 percent of East Asians and 4.9 percent of Latino/Hispanic background.[1] This was linked with ethnic differences in the odorant-metabolizing glycosyltransferase enzyme encoded by the UGT2A1/A2 genes. However, compared with the Alpha and Delta variants, the Omicron variant tended to produce milder symptoms overall, and the altered sense of smell or taste loss was much less prevalent.

If the immune system is unable to keep the SARS-CoV-2 infection in check and the severity of the illness intensifies, systemic features such as shortness of breath (dyspnea) and altered levels of consciousness can result. Blood tests at this time may show a reduction in lymphocytes (lymphopenia) and albumin (hypoalbuminemia), with higher levels of alanine aminotransferase (a marker of liver damage), lactate dehydrogenase (marker of general organ damage with cell death), ferritin (marker of accumulation of too much iron), C-reactive protein (marker of inflammation), and D-dimer (a breakdown product of blood clots).

The severity of COVID-19 is linked with the production of a "cytokine storm," which includes elevated blood levels of several different immune cell activators such as interleukins (IL) IL-6 and IL-10, soluble IL2 receptor, and tumor necrosis factor-alpha (TNF-alpha).[2] Symptoms of a cytokine storm can include higher fever, chills, headaches, coughing, nausea and vomiting, diarrhea, fatigue, and low blood pressure. This overreaction of the immune system can ultimately result in multi-organ failure and death.

In infants and youth eighteen years old and under, multisystem inflammatory syndrome–children (MIS-C) has been identified as a rare complication of COVID-19 that occurs about two to six weeks after initial infection. Between March 11, 2020, and October 2, 2021, there were 269 cases of MIS-C reported to the Public Health Agency of Canada, with half seemingly linked to COVID-19.[3] About 58 percent of the MIS-C cases were in males compared to 42 percent in females. Although most of the cases required hospitalization, and a third required intensive care intervention, none of the cases were fatal.

A systemic review of all multisystem inflammatory syndrome–adults (MIS-A) cases in those over eighteen years old worldwide up to September 2021 identified 221 reports.[4] MIS-A had a median age of occurrence of twenty-one years and a 70 percent predominance in male adults. The most common symptoms were fever (96 percent), hypotension (60 percent), cardiac dysfunction (54 percent), shortness of breath (52 percent), and diarrhea (52 percent). Of the MIS-A patients that were hospitalized, 57 percent needed ICU care, 27 percent required respiratory support, and 4 percent died.

6.2. Blood Clotting Abnormalities and COVID-19

Soon after the first cases of COVID-19 infection were reported, it became apparent that this was not an airborne illness that exclusively caused death through respiratory failure and pneumonia. The infection appeared to initiate blood clotting (prothrombotic) and immune cell activation leading to complement activation, cytokine storms, endothelial destruction (the endothelium is comprised of cells of the inner layer of blood vessels), thrombosis of lung vessels, hypoxic respiratory failure, and death.[5] In addition, there were also many cases of blood clots occurring not only in the heart and brain but also unusual blockages of the large veins of the abdomen.[6] Consequently, COVID-19 caused by the spike protein has been described as inflammation of the endothelium (endothialitis). What follows are descriptions of how blood clotting in the body normally occurs, the way spike protein causes damage to blood vessels, typical clinical presentations of blood vessel damage, how these conditions are treated, and similarities and differences between SARS-CoV-2 infection and mRNA vaccine injuries, as well as unexplained findings.

6.2.1. Blood and Blood Vessels

Blood is the lifeline to the human body. Comprised of 70 percent saline, it also contains blood cells (red, white, and platelets), hormones, macromolecules such as albumin, antibodies, and thousands of different lower-abundance plasma proteins. In addition, blood transports oxygen, carbon dioxide, nutrients, and waste products to be eliminated. The volume of blood that each person has is around 7–8 percent of body weight. For the average person, this is approximately 5.25 liters. Red blood cells account for more than half of all of the cells (excluding bacterial) in the human body.

The heart and a network of blood vessels circulate blood throughout the body. With each contraction, arteries carry blood away from the heart and veins carry blood back to the heart. The veins also have a storage function; around 70 percent of the total blood volume is in the leg veins.

Each blood vessel consists of three layers. The innermost layer, or intima, is formed by the ultrathin endothelial layer that has multiple responsibilities for homeostasis (i.e., maintenance of temperature, pH, osmotic pressure, and protein levels, etc.) of blood; being a barrier to prevent fluid or cells moving into the extravascular space; regulating blood vessel contraction and relaxation and releasing substances to inhibit coagulation and or clot dissolution; and if punctured, acting as the site for platelets to attach and aggregate in order to seal the leak.

The middle layer, or media, is the smooth muscle cell layer that contracts and relaxes in response to chemical signals from the intima. Through these series of contractions and relaxations, pumped blood is moved along the vasculature.

The outermost layer, or adventitia, consists of loose connective tissue that sends and receives chemical signals to the surrounding soft tissue.

6.2.2. Blood Clots

Strictly speaking, the term "blood clots" refers to blood that has clotted outside of the blood vessel. For this to occur, the blood vessel must be punctured to allow blood to seep out. When contained in the surrounding tissue, this clotted blood is known as a hematoma, or bruise. Blood clots that occur within the blood vessel are known as thrombi, or a single thrombus.

The process of coagulation, or blood clotting, in a blood vessel is a complicated multi-step chemical process involving red blood cells, platelets, a cascade of plasma proteins responsible for coagulation, and the endothelium to produce an insoluble fibrin plug. Once the latter has been established, a reverse process of fibrinolysis, again involving multiple chemical pathways, starts to prevent the fibrin plug from becoming too large and blocking the vessel.[7] Thus, the endothelium is vital for normal homeostasis, as it secretes a number of chemicals that inhibit thrombus formation, much like the coating of a non-stick pan. Without this coating, there would be widespread thrombosis throughout the arteries and veins. The endothelium derives its nutrient supply from the circulating blood and, if blocked by a thrombus, will no longer function properly.

Once fibrin formation is initiated, if fibrinolysis cannot keep up, the formed thrombus will expand to either involve more of the blood vessel or completely occlude the vessel (complete thrombosis). Occasionally, a portion of the thrombus can break off (known as an embolus) and be carried by the blood to a downstream site and block another blood vessel. A common example of thromboembolism is thrombus that occurs in a large leg vein (deep vein thrombosis) and a portion of it breaks off to enter the lungs and occlude a lung blood vessel (pulmonary embolism).[8]

6.2.3. How Blood Clotting Occurs

The classic description of how thrombosis occurs is described by Wirchow's triad of three key factors: 1) stasis of blood flow, or blood flow that is slowed down which allows for prolonged interaction between blood and the endothelium; 2) hypercoagulability, or "thick blood" as a result of an abnormal increase in blood cells (such as red blood cells or platelets) or plasma proteins that are involved in blood clotting (either too many promoter proteins or too few inhibitory proteins); and 3) endothelial damage which may occur as a result of direct damage to the wall of the blood vessel.[9]

Normal coagulation is a dynamic process involving the endothelium, platelets, and blood. The process is initiated by damage to the endothelium with exposure of the subendothelial lining. Coagulation factors in the blood are activated and a cascade of chemical events ensues to produce thrombin, which converts soluble fibrinogen to insoluble fibrin.[10]

Platelets, the small bone-marrow-derived cells circulating in the blood, play a vital role in stopping bleeding or endothelial damage to the blood vessel. Much like debris that attaches to a non-stick pan once the coating has been damaged, platelets will adhere to a damaged intimal site and secrete chemical signals to attract more platelets to aggregate and combine with the fibrin plug, thereby extending the platelet plug until the tear is sealed. Once stabilized, platelets also secrete fibrinolytic proteins to melt away the platelet plug and allow remodeling to occur.[11] In diseases of platelets, too many may lead to early and repeated thrombosis, whereas too few can lead to excessive bleeding.

6.2.4. Inflammation

The body responds to trauma or any noxious agent with inflammation. Clinically, this is characterized by heat (fever), redness, swelling, and pain. The cells respond to inflammation by producing large amounts of white blood cells: neutrophils initially, followed by macrophages and monocytes to engulf toxins and dead cells, mast-cells that release histamine, and lymphocytes if the stimulus is unremitting. The process of cellular migration toward the inflamed area, proliferation of cells, and release of cytotoxic chemicals to produce inflammatory exudates is a complicated process. The goal of inflammation is to identify the foreign substance and isolate and destroy it by the innate immune system or, if persistent, with neutralizing antibodies that activate the complement system to facilitate its ingestion through the recruitment of scavenger cells, or macrophages. Although these cells need to recognize and not harm normal surrounding cells, collateral damage to surrounding tissue is usually seen whenever there is widespread inflammation.

Specialized white blood cells called antigen-presenting cells will identify the foreign protein and bring the key information to lymph nodes, which produces a proliferative response from B lymphocytes to produce specific antibodies to neutralize the foreign protein, as well as T cells that either release cytotoxic chemicals or develop into memory T cells to recognize the foreign protein should it return. The same processes are also evoked when the foreign proteins are parts of viruses and other infectious agents. More information about immune cells will be provided in chapter 7.

6.2.5. Infection with Spike Protein

Information gained from the last four years of COVID-19 has shown this disease to be highly complex. As an aerosolized pathogen, the SARS-CoV-2 virus gains entry into the body through the aerodigestive tract. Even early in the COVID-19 pandemic, for most people the viral infections were self-limited, and less than 5 percent required hospitalization, especially those that were elderly. About 3 percent of hospitalized patients with the Wuhan strain of SARS-CoV-2 that were symptomatic for COVID-19 had a fatal outcome.[12] In their review in the *International Journal of Immunopathology and Pharmacology*, Marik et al. (2021) showed that COVID-19 disease involves three pathological processes: lung macrophage activation with uncontrolled inflammation; complement-mediated endothelialitis, which is an immune response within the endothelium in blood vessels, in which these cells become inflamed; and a procoagulant state with thrombotic microangiopathy (i.e., the capillary walls become so thick and weak that they bleed, leak protein, and impede the flow of blood). The hyper-inflammatory state is exacerbated by the activation and degranulation of mast cells of the immune system.

In the upper airway, the SARS-CoV-2 virus infects body cells by binding to the ACE2 enzyme primarily found on the surface of the epithelial cells of the airway, macrophages, mast cells, and endothelial cells. Once fused, the RNA genome of the virus enters the cell and initiates viral replication. (See chapter 5.4.) Control of viral spread depends on the interaction between the epithelial (or endothelial) cells and the immune (white blood) cells. A battle between the host's innate immune system with recruitment of leukocytes, activation of interferon, and other cytotoxic proteins and the virus's chemicals that decrease interferon synthesis ensues. Patients with robust immune systems develop a brisk interferon response and eliminate the virus. Those with poor immune responses fail to prevent early viral replication, which leads to high viral loads and the potential for high viral transmissibility. Should this occur, white blood cells, primarily monocytes and macrophages, are attracted to the infected areas in the lung. Chemical messages (chemokines) released from macrophages promote further macrophage and platelet recruitment and activation. Appreciable levels of neutralizing antibodies are released about one week following initial infection with the virus.

Concurrently, as the virus gains entry into the bloodstream it will latch onto other cells rich in the ACE2 protein, which act as a receptor for the SARS-CoV-2 spike protein. These include endothelial cells, and an endothialitis and microvascular thrombosis occurs especially in the blood vessels of the lung, brain, skin, and fatty tissue. ACE2 is protective of the cardiovascular system by promoting oxygen species production and glycolysis (a metabolic pathway that converts sugars into pyruvate and the energy-storage compound ATP). The presence of spike protein, however, impairs endothelial function by down-regulating ACE2 and inhibiting mitochondria.[13] In addition, when examined in cell culture, spike protein also induces degradation of junctional proteins in the endothelium, which results in loss of the endothelial barrier function.[14] Thus, once fused to endothelial cells, the presence of the virus and surrounding dead and dying cells activates platelets, which clot the blood, destroying the endothelium and promoting thrombosis of the blood vessels.

6.2.6. Clinical Presentation

Paradoxically, both thrombosis (blood clotting) and excessive bleeding are complications of severe COVID-19 illness. Platelets have a central role in attaching to the damaged endothelium. A biomarker known as P-selectin that resides in platelets and red blood cells is monitored for evidence of increased adhesion of activated platelets to red blood cells (microclotting), which supports movement of white blood cells to the sites of inflammation. Initially, with abundant coagulation proteins such as fibrinogen and von Willebrand factor, there is thrombosis.[15] Blood clots that occur in medium-sized arteries have been noted to be platelet-rich.[16] Hospitalized patients often have thrombocytopenia (low platelet counts) and increased levels of D-dimer (a measurement of fibrinolysis as the body attempts to remove blood clots also known as thrombi). Further progression of this coagulopathy will consume clotting factors and platelets leading to a life-threatening condition known as disseminated intravascular coagulation (DIC), where there is a risk of serious bleeding. At the same time, because widespread thrombosis has occurred, there is a risk of venous thromboembolism. As most people with COVID-19 infections recover quickly, there may be no symptoms from these micro-clots. As the amount of thrombosis and inflammation increases, heart attack, stroke, or venous thrombosis presenting as deep vein thrombosis of the lower or upper extremities can result. Lodigani et al. (2020)[17] showed that symptomatic hospital patients admitted to the ICU for COVID-19 had a 28 percent prevalence of thromboembolic complications despite using heparin to prevent them. Venous thromboembolic complications were the most common, followed by heart attacks (2.5 percent) and stroke (1.1 percent). DIC occurred in 2.2 percent of patients.

Beyond thirty days and up to twelve months after acute COVID-19 infection, cardiovascular risks (stroke, heart attacks, dysrhythmias, and myocarditis) and thromboembolic disease (deep vein thrombosis and pulmonary embolism) continue. The risk is highest for those patients admitted to ICUs.[18]

6.2.7. Unusual Venous Presentations

At the outset of the COVID-19 pandemic, there were rare reports of clots occurring in unusual locations in the brain and abdomen. In the brain, delirium was the most common presentation.[19] Anticoagulation with "blood thinners" was the standard treatment, although fatality could be high as patients could also have excessive bleeding. The combination of stroke from blockage of a brain vessel combined with severe bleeding presents as a double jeopardy situation.[20]

Blockage of the blood vessels in the intestines is an acute event requiring surgery. The overall incidence is around one in one hundred thousand, although this increases with age. Of these cases, two-thirds are due to an arterial problem and the rest are due to blockage of veins (venous occlusion). In hospitalized patients with COVID-19, the persistent inflammation and thrombosis can lead to such blockage. Patients may present with agonizing abdominal pain, vomiting, diarrhea, and shock. Management requires prompt recognition of this condition (especially if the individual is already being treated for severe pneumonia), early surgery if required, and anticoagulation. The outcome will depend on the patient's general condition, the degree of blockage, and extent of surgery required.[21]

6.2.8. Diagnosis of Thrombosis

The diagnosis of arterial or venous thrombosis is based on standard diagnostic tools: accurate history, physical findings, laboratory tests, and imaging. Descriptions of history and physical findings can be found in many standard medical books. For laboratory testing, in addition to a hematology and chemistry panel, coagulation studies and D-dimer tests are frequently done.

The D-dimer test is a measurement of fibrinolysis, or how much breakdown of the clotting protein fibrin is occurring. The level is usually reflective of the amount of underlying thrombosis that is being removed by the fibrinolytic system. The test is very sensitive, meaning it can detect a very small amount. The problem with a slightly elevated level is that even a small bruise can raise the D-dimer level. D-dimer tests have been suggested to be used post-COVID-19 vaccination to determine if there is any underlying thrombosis as a result of the injection. However, this test is discouraged due to its lack of specificity for causality and its potential for revealing other injury, for example from COVID-19 vaccination.

Ultrasound is usually used for imaging studies of suspected venous blood clots unless they are located in an area that is not accessible with ultrasound, such as inside the skull. In that situation, and also for arterial imaging, computer tomographic (CT) scans with contrast agents are used.

6.2.9. Treatment of Thromboembolic Disease

Treatment of vascular complications from either the viral infection or vaccine is related to the severity of the complications. If patients are admitted to the hospital with evidence of poor perfusion and either severe COVID-19 or a COVID-19 vaccine complication, they should be evaluated for thromboembolic disease.[22] If thromboembolic disease is diagnosed, either unfractionated or low molecular weight heparin is initiated. Surgery may be required to repair the blood vessels. Afterwards, as the patient improves, conversion to an oral anticoagulant might be considered. Following discharge, unless the patient had a pre-existing condition that required long-term anticoagulation, there is no recommended duration of anticoagulation for COVID-19–related illness or vaccine injury. For patients who do not have proven thromboembolic disease, if their clinical condition is serious, preventative anticoagulation should be used unless there are contraindications.

6.3. Neurological Damage

Over 30 percent of elderly COVID-19 patients with Wuhan SARS-CoV-2 experience neurological symptoms,[23] ranging from mild symptoms such as headaches, dizziness, nausea, and loss of taste and smell, to severe conditions such as cognitive impairment, neuropsychiatric disorders, delirium, insomnia, cerebrovascular complications, stroke, seizures, and diseases of the brain (encephalopathy).[24,25] Many individuals infected with SARS-CoV-2 develop "long COVID," where clinical symptoms may persist for months after the virus has been cleared. Multisystem inflammation, neuropathic pain[26] as well as neurological,[27, 28, 29, 30, 31, 32, 33, 34, 35, 36] psychiatric,[37] and neurodegenerative conditions,[38, 39] are prevalent among long COVID patients. Hallmarks of neurological injury from SARS-CoV-2 such as central nervous system (CNS) inflammation, activation of microglia (resident macrophages of the CNS), and neuronal damage are also common features of neurodegenerative conditions such as Alzheimer's disease, Parkinson's disease, amyotrophic lateral sclerosis (ALS), multiple sclerosis, and HIV-associated dementia.[40, 41]

Mounting evidence indicates that the SARS-CoV-2 spike protein alone can lead to inflammatory and neurological conditions.[42] Spike protein can trigger systemic inflammatory responses,[43, 44, 45, 46] disrupt the blood-brain barrier,[47, 48] and impair endothelial function and integrity.[49] In addition, the spike protein is responsible for the virus's affinity for neural tissues, as its main receptor, ACE2, is found in glial cells and neurons of the CNS, and the vascular endothelium of the brain. [50] Other spike receptors such as the nicotinic acetylcholine receptor and neuropilin are also present in neural tissues.

Perhaps one of the most misleading claims regarding mRNA and DNA-based COVID-19 vaccines is that the production of spike protein in the body of vaccinees is a short-term process restricted to the injection site. Instead, a growing body of evidence indicates vaccine mRNA and spike protein can persist for weeks, even months, in the blood and lymph nodes of vaccinated individuals.[51, 52] Vaccine mRNA-encoding spike protein was found circulating in patients twenty-eight days after administration of Pfizer-BioNTech and Moderna vaccines.[53] Both vaccine mRNA and spike protein were detected in lymph nodes sixty days post vaccination,[54] and spike protein persisted in patients four months after vaccination. Biodistribution studies of mRNA and

DNA vaccines and their protein products are largely absent in humans. In mice, S1, the subunit of the spike protein, was found in virtually every organ, including the prefrontal cortex and in narrow niches of the brain where spike protein persisted for twenty-eight days, causing cell death and neuronal injury. Analysis of brain tissues from patients who died of COVID-19 showed the presence of spike protein in brain meningeal cells and in the vicinity of neurons in the cortex, but no viral RNA or nucleocapsid protein were found in these samples. In a post-mortem study of patients who died during the pandemic (from 2021–2022) of non-COVID-19 related causes, 29 percent had spike protein lingering in the brain.[55]

An autopsy performed on a seventy-six-year-old man who had received one dose of the AstraZeneca and two doses of Pfizer COVID-19 vaccines reported necrotizing encephalitis with signs of inflammation, lymphocyte infiltration, microglia activation, and vascular and neuronal damage. The S1 subunit of SARS-CoV-2 spike protein was detected in necrotic areas of the brain, within the endothelia and glial cells such as astrocytes and microglia, but nucleocapsid protein (a marker of natural infection) was absent, and the patient was negative for COVID-19 infection. This implies that the spike protein responsible for the injury was likely of vaccine origin.[56]

6.4. Long COVID

Long COVID refers to debilitating health symptoms that some people continue to experience following COVID-19 infection. The condition is also known as post-acute sequelae of COVID-19 (PASC).

The Canadian COVID-19 Antibody and Health Survey (CCAHS), covering the start of the COVID-19 pandemic through August 31, 2022, found that almost 17.2 percent of adults (approximately 1.4 million) who got COVID-19 said they continued to have symptoms three months or more after their original COVID-19 infection.[57] Nearly twice as many of these long COVID cases were female compared to males; 37.4 percent had four or more pre-existing co-morbidities prior to COVID-19, but 12.8 percent had no comorbidities. Of those with comorbitities, 27 percent were obese, 28.3 percent had disabilities, and 44.7 percent of hospitalized COVID-19 patients had longer-term symptoms. The survey also showed that long COVID was more common in those that were affected earlier in the pandemic (26 percent if infected before July 2021 and 15 percent from July 2021 to May 2022). The survey also indicated that 25 percent of adults that were not vaccinated prior to having COVID-19 reported long-term symptoms, compared to 13.2 percent of those with two vaccine doses and 12.2 percent with three vaccine doses. However, it should be recognized that most of the long COVID cases occurred before most people were eligible for double vaccination.

In the United States, long COVID occurs with a frequency ranging from 10–30 percent in non-hospitalized cases, 50–70 percent in hospitalized cases,[58]and about 9.5 percent of vaccinated cases with breakthrough infections compared to about 14.6 percent of unvaccinated cases with symptomatic COVID-19.[59] Most long COVID cases in the United States are in non-hospitalized patients with a mild acute illness, especially between thirty-six and fifty years of age. A higher prevalence of long COVID has been noted in people of Hispanic/Latino ancestry[60] and associated socio-economic risk factors including lower income and a need to return to work following inadequate recovery.[61, 62]

Over 20 percent of adults in Canada with long COVID reported that their symptoms impacted their ability to do daily activities. Almost half reported that they experienced symptoms for over a year and missed about twenty days of work or school.[63] Long COVID patients can experience a wide range of symptoms across multiple organ systems with numerous adverse effects. The most common outcomes reported by patients include cardiovascular, thrombotic, and cerebrovascular disease; type 2 diabetes; myalgic encephalomyelitis/chronic fatigue syndrome (ME/CFS); and dysautonomia (failure of autonomic nervous system function), particularly postural orthostatic tachycardia syndrome (POTS). Common symptoms include fatigue, muscle or body aches, shortness of breath or other difficulty in breathing, difficulty concentrating or focusing, and the inability to exercise (or be active).[64] While severity varies widely, long COVID can be a profoundly disabling condition as some sufferers cannot work and experience a very low quality of life. COVID-19 vaccination may exacerbate long COVID in some individuals.

Dawson's Creek writer Heidi Ferrer committed suicide after her Moderna vaccination dramatically worsened her long COVID symptoms.[65] Her husband stated in his eulogy for her:

> Then in March we were able to get the vaccine with the hope it would help you get all the way back. Within weeks it was clear something was very wrong. The tremors started in your hands. Small at first. You told me other people in your groups were getting them too . . . I'll never forget you literally collapsing in my arms as your whole body shook, but only lasting for a minute or two, they seemed manageable. But then the vibrations started in your chest every night, robbing you of your sleep almost immediately . . . I could see the shift in your outlook when this went on for more than a few days. A light was starting to dim. You were doubting a cure would come in time. I told you to hang on. That you, just existing, on our couch was enough for us. I didn't care if we ever left our neighborhood again. You were enough.

While this condition can be tragic in its severity, it is often poorly understood as most symptoms are not easily amenable to medical testing. Patients commonly report being mistreated by doctors who do not believe they are sick. Some medical professionals on Reddit have even openly mocked patients who insist that they have long COVID, claiming that many just believed they had COVID-19.[66]

Evidence-based practitioners offer a more realistic view on long COVID. Bisaccia and colleagues (2021) noted survey data where 19 percent of long COVID sufferers reported having POTS, a condition that can be objectively diagnosed with tilt table testing.[67] They described treatment strategies available for POTS such as the use of compression garments, the liberal intake of water and salt, etc. A few long COVID symptoms and co-morbidities can be found through medical testing so that appropriate treatment can be provided.

As most sufferers experience a long list of broad and poorly understood symptoms, the underlying mechanisms that lead to these effects have been elusive and are likely from multiple, overlapping causes. These include persistent SARS-CoV-2 infection; immune dysregulation that could include autoimmunity and reactivation of other pathogens such as, for example, Epstein-Barr virus and herpes viruses; disturbance of the microbiome in the gut; microvascular blood clotting; and defective signaling in the brain and/or vagus nerves. One of the other possibilities is that the COVID-19 vaccines actually exacerbate long COVID-19, since there is a lot of symptom overlap with the adverse effects of COVID-19 vaccines. Diexer et al. (2023) found that individuals infected with an Omicron variant of SARS-CoV-2 after three or more COVID-19 vaccinations were more likely to develop long COVID than unvaccinated individuals that had previously not been infected. [68] In their study undertaken in Germany, they tracked COVID-19 cases in 48,826 participants until June 15, 2022; about 70 percent of long COVID-19 cases following an Omicron infection occurred in those fully vaccinated for COVID-19 (about 50 percent with three doses). Those that had previously been infected with SARS-CoV-2 and fully recovered were the least likely to develop long COVID-19 after re-infection with the virus, whereas previous vaccination offered no meaningful protection against long COVID.

The relationship between long COVID and COVID-19 vaccination is filled with controversy. Some clinicians and researchers believe that vaccination can cause patients to develop long COVID-like symptoms. Two German clinicians argued that long COVID symptoms appeared following vaccination in 350 patients they had treated.[69] This contrasts to the recommendation on the US CDC website that staying up-to-date with COVID-19 vaccination is important to prevent long COVID.[70] However, there is no mention on the CDC website that COVID-19 vaccines could potentially cause long COVID or a long COVID-like syndrome.

Public Health Canada also recommends vaccination to prevent long COVID, claiming that evidence exists that "receiving two or more vaccine doses before infection helps to reduce the risk of developing post COVID-19 condition."

What does the scientific evidence indicate with respect to protection from long COVID from COVID-19 vaccination? Unfortunately, the overall risk-to-benefit ratio is unclear. The clinical trials for the COVID-19 vaccines did not anticipate the emergence of long COVID and did not collect data on endpoints related to it. Thus, it is necessary to rely on less reliable forms of evidence. The scientific literature contains reports of long COVID patients both worsening *and* improving following vaccination. Tsuchida et al. (2022) conducted a small prospective cohort study and found that long COVID (PASC) patients were slightly more likely to worsen following vaccination (nine of forty-two patients) than they were to improve (seven of forty-two patients).[71] More recently, Asadi-Pooya et al. (2024) from a survey of 1,236 long COVID victims interviewed in January and February 2022 noted that about 44 percent had experienced especially prolonged long COVID for over a year.[72] Of these, fifteen out of fifty-one people (29.4 percent) had not been vaccinated for COVID-19, and 528 out of 1185 participants (44.6 percent) had received at least one dose of a COVID-19 vaccine (eleven of twenty-four with only one dose; 181/392 with only two doses; and 336/769 with three doses) before acquiring prolonged long COVID-19. Prior COVID-19 vaccination and getting COVID-19 subsequently was significantly correlated with an increased risk of long COVID for over a year.

It is claimed that people with long COVID no longer have the virus and cannot spread it to others. However, it is interesting to note that some COVID-19 treatments such as ivermectin[73] and Paxlovid can provide relief in some cases of long COVID. One study showed that Paxlovid reduced the risk of long COVID-19 by 26 percent over a three-month period.[74] Effectiveness of an anti-SARS-CoV-2 replication drug on long COVID patients would support an underlying persistent, low-level infection with SARS-CoV-2 in some of these patients.

Another report noted that SARS-CoV-2 spike protein was detectable in twenty-four of thirty-seven patients with long COVID as compared to six of twenty-six patients just recovered from acute COVID-19, and their level rapidly declined to undetectable a month after recovery.[75] More than half of the long COVID cases appeared to have been vaccinated before or during their long COVID condition in this study. Elevated levels of spike protein in many of the long COVID serum samples were detectable even a year after the onset of the COVID-19 in the donors that provided the serum. However, the levels of interferons and various interleukins and tumor necrosis factor-alpha, which are markers of inflammation, were all in the normal range. This would indicate the development of immune tolerance to the spike protein, which could result in persistent SARS-CoV-2 infection.

A study of twenty-four long COVID patients found the activation of T cells; spike RNA and protein was detected 158 to 676 days after initial COVID-19 illness in all five patients who were tested.[76] It is noteworthy that the anti-nucleocapsid antibody marker for infection was not evident in about half of these patients, and all but one of the twenty-four patients had been vaccinated for COVID-19. When tested, there was also no evidence of the virus in rectal tissue biopsies that showed spike gene presence. Consequently, the presence of spike RNA and protein could as easily have been a consequence of COVID-19 vaccination as persistent infection with the SARS-CoV-2 virus.

Heidi Ferrer's eulogy notes that long COVID sufferers hoped that vaccination would heal them. But unfortunately for those like her, the development of safe and effective treatments for long COVID has not moved at warp speed. She was survived by her son and her husband.

6.5. Age Demographic of COVID-19 Cases, Hospital Admissions, ICU Admissions, and Deaths in Canada

Despite the risk of potentially serious symptoms and complications of COVID-19, including death, many Canadians remained completely asymptomatic following infection with SARS-CoV-2. According to Statistics Canada, by August 2022, 98 percent of Canadians had antibodies against SARS-CoV-2 and 54 percent had clear serological evidence of a natural infection with the virus.[77] Moreover, about 41 percent of adult Canadians and most children following infection developed immunity without any symptoms of COVID-19, i.e., they were asymptomatic. Clearly, those in the lower age groups are at much lower risk of hospitalization, ICU admissions, and deaths than the elderly.[78] Table 6.1 provides an assessment of the risks by Health Canada. The actual risks are at least an order of magnitude lower (i.e., one tenth) than these estimates because Health Canada numbers are based on the premise that less than 10 percent of Canadians have had COVID-19, whereas, serological testing indicates 50 to 90 percent of the population have antibodies that indicate prior infection with SARS-CoV-2. Furthermore, as much as half of recorded hospitalizations, ICU admissions, and deaths were from individuals that went to the hospital initially for reasons distinct from COVID-19.[79] Another issue is that there were 4.2-times more recorded deaths in those over eighty years old than ICU admissions (See Table 6.1.). On top of this, the current Omicron variants of SARS-CoV-2 induce less severe clinical disease and are accompanied by lower rates of hospitalizations, ICU admissions, and deaths from COVID-19 than seen with the earlier variants.[80] Overall, considering that close to 90 percent of around forty million Canadians have had COVID-19 at least once, and 35,079 deaths have been attributed to this disease, its average rate of lethality is close to one in a thousand, with it being closer to one in a hundred thousand for those from zero to twenty-five years of age, and one in two hundred for those over sixty-five years of age. This is a far cry from the 1 to 4 percent average lethality estimates of COVID-19 commonly cited.[81]

Table 6.1. Cumulative risks of COVID-19 cases, hospitalizations, ICU admissions, and deaths by age in Canada since the start of the COVID-19 pandemic to September 6, 2023.[82]

Age Group (Years)	Cases	Hospitalizations	Hospitalizations %	ICU Admissions	ICU Admissions %	Deaths	Deaths %
0–11	420,604	7,358	1.75	759	0.18	47	0.011
12–19	329,710	2,733	0.83	310	0.09	18	0.005
20–29	750,597	9,923	1.32	1,071	0.14	125	0.017
30–39	724,796	14,763	2.04	2,025	0.28	308	0.042
40–49	637,143	15,742	2.47	3,244	0.51	664	0.104
50–59	553,316	25,445	4.6	6,086	1.1	1,744	0.315
60–69	370,316	39,211	10.59	8,905	2.4	4,144	1.119
70–79	258,163	53,823	20.85	8,630	3.34	7,776	3.012
80+	347,257	80,501	23.18	4,860	1.4	20,253	5.832
All groups	4,391,902	249,499	5.68	35,890	0.82	35,079	0.799

CHAPTER 7

The Body's Defenses against Infectious Pathogens

Steven Pelech, Bonnie Mallard, & Niel Karrow

"Whenever the immune system deals successfully with an infection, it emerges from the experience stronger and better able to confront similar threats in the future. Our immune system develops in combat. If, at the first sign of infection, you always jump in with antibiotics, you do not give the immune system a chance to grow stronger."

—Andrew Weil

7.1. The Innate and Adaptive Immune Systems

With the constant threat of evolving and new infectious microbes, organisms have had to develop effective countermeasures. Every newborn baby is particularly vulnerable to pathogens, although mother's first milk, known as colostrum, is laden with protective antibodies and maternal immune cells that can confer significant immunity. As maternal protection wanes and the neonate is exposed to various environmental stimuli, hematopoietic (i.e., blood forming) stem cells in the body actively give rise to an extensive arsenal of diverse cells and molecules that form the immune system. The composition of the immune system and its functioning are complex, and involves hundreds of distinct immune-response proteins that affect over twenty different types of immune cells. What follows is a brief introduction to this amazing defense system against infectious pathogens and cancer.[1]

There are two main branches, known as the *innate* and the *adaptive* immune systems. The cells of the innate immune system are generally non-specific in their targeting. They develop very quickly, within minutes to days following exposure to a danger signal, and, therefore, are particularly useful for combating new pathogens. The innate immune system is especially strong in infants and children compared to adults. Over time, adaptive immune system cells called *lymphocytes* learn to recognize and remember foreign proteins and other structures called *antigens*. The specific portions that are targeted on an antigen are known as epitopes. The innate immune system, although still very active in adults, is less so due to increased activity by the adaptive immune system. Nonetheless, these two complementary systems work as a tightly coordinated defense force to protect the host against the diverse foreign agents that will be encountered over a lifetime.

7.2. The Production of Hematopoietic Cells of the Immune System

Hematopoietic stem cells reside primarily in the red bone marrow, which is the core of the bone, and generate many immune and other blood cells depending on how they are stimulated by intercellular mediators known as *cytokines*. These include a wide range of chemokines, interleukins, interferons, and colony-stimulating factors. Depending on which particular combination of cytokines interact with surface receptors on the stem cells, these cells undergo successive changes and differentiate into red blood cells (erythrocytes), platelets, or immune cells, which are collectively referred to as *white blood cells* or *leukocytes*. There is typically about one white blood cell for every seven hundred erythrocytes in the blood. Erythrocytes account for the majority of cells (excluding bacteria) in the body. The erythrocytes transport oxygen, carbon dioxide, and small molecules through the circulatory system. Platelets mediate the clotting of erythrocytes at sites of tissue damage to prevent loss of blood and initiate healing through the release of growth factors such as platelet-derived growth factor and transforming growth factor-alpha (TGF-alpha). Apart from acting as a growth factor to stimulate tissue regeneration, TGF-alpha can also promote the formation of new blood capillaries.

There are many distinct leukocyte populations, particularly in the innate immune system (Figure 7.1 in the insert). Whereas mammalian erythrocytes and platelets do not have nuclei (or DNA) or mitochondria, leukocytes are classified on the basis of their progenitor cell (myeloid or lymphoid) or on the morphology of their nucleus (mononuclear cells have rounded nuclei and polymorphonuclear cells have multilobed nuclei) and the presence or absence of granules in their cytoplasm. This results in two general groupings: 1) blood mononuclear cells (BMCs, also known as agranulocytes), which includes monocytes and lymphocytes; and 2) polymorphonuclear leukocytes (PMNs, also known as granulocytes). Granulocytes feature granules in their cytoplasm that are loaded with inflammatory and cell toxic factors, which are released from these cells when they are activated. For example, eosinophils contribute to attacking multicellular parasites, such as worms, through the release of cytokines, positively-charged peptides, and hydrolytic enzymes. Basophils release the anticoagulant heparin to reduce the rate of blood clotting and the vasodilator histamine to increase blood flow to tissues. Neutrophils are among the first recruits to a site of inflammation, where they attack and engulf viruses and other microbes.

At the early stages of differentiation into leukocyte subpopulations, the stem cells are prompted by specific cytokines to transform into a variety of different lymphoid or myeloid cell types. From myeloid progenitor cells, erythrocytes and platelets are generated to comprise most blood cells, but granulocytes are also produced to form monocytes such as dendritic cells and macrophages or other cells that produce substances that aid in the killing of foreign cells as well as recruiting other leukocytes. The lymphoid precursor cells mature to form lymphocytes, of which B cells (antibody-producing) and T cells comprise the adaptive immune response. Other cells that are closely related to T cells, such as natural killer cells, are effective in attacking cancer cells and certain microbe-infected cells. These cell types have some characteristics of both the innate and adaptive immune responses, thereby helping to bridge coverage between these two systems to ensure no chinks exist in host defense armor.

The existence of cells associated with innate host defense was first reported in starfish larvae that were irritated with small citrus thorns in 1886 by Russian scientist Elie Metchnikoff.[1] The thorns were attacked and digested by macrophages, which are highly mobile, phagocytic cells. Since starfish have been on the Earth for over a billion years, this demonstrates just how ancient and critical immune systems are.

The development of B and T cells starts before birth *in utero*. In newborns, these lymphocytes are naïve to the extra-uterine environment and undergo major transitions. The populations of B and T cells, for example, learn to differentiate between *self* and *foreign*, or *non-self*. If the immune system is unable to recognize normal cells of the body as "self," then autoimmune disease could arise as immune cells would target the components of the body that are misjudged as "foreign." The lymphocyte population also learns to ignore harmless molecules in food and the non-dangerous substances that are commonly and continuously encountered in the environment to avoid being constantly and unnecessarily activated; for example, this would include the non-dangerous substances encountered in the gut and airways. The development of tolerance occurs via several unique mechanisms before and after birth. The ability of the immune system to distinguish between an enormous range of harmless (self) and harmful (non-self) molecules is a unique feature that is critical for survival.

Activation of the immune system is a double-edged sword; a careful balance must be found in order to remove the foreign agent without harming the host in the process. For example, too much acute or prolonged activation of the immune system may cause severe inflammation and overt tissue damage to the host. Therefore, the immune system has a large number of regulatory mechanisms to detect when a pathogen has cleared and it is appropriate to turn down immune activation. This is also the reason why any B and T cells that inappropriately recognize the body's normal cells, resident flora of bacteria and microbes, or common substances in the environment are committed to self-destruction early in development or are carefully regulated throughout life.

The B and T cells remaining after this careful "education" process form a diverse pool of naïve lymphocytes that are sensitive to foreign pathogens. Selective stimulation of these naïve cells with antigens on the novel pathogen triggers their activation and successive divisions into a clonal army of identical cells that have high specificity for an antigenic epitope. As the amount of foreign antigen in the environment declines, such as the successful eradication of a pathogenic virus, the stimulated lymphocyte clones undergo programmed cell death or contract to an inactive resting state. During this process, memory lymphocytes also develop, which survive for various prolonged periods of times—in some cases even a lifetime—following exposure to a foreign entity. These memory cells can rapidly awaken from their slumber to engage with the pathogen once again when presented with the same or very similar antigens on the pathogen. This allows much faster and more effective immune responses than in their first encounter. This unique feature of long-term immunological memory is why recovery from a pathogenic infection often provides sustained protection against future encounters with that specific pathogen. This is referred to as naturally acquired immunity.

7.3. The Nature of Antibodies

The specific parts of the foreign antigens that T and B cells recognize are called epitopes. They can be very small, down to just a few amino acids in unique combinations. Such epitopes should be distinct in structure from those found in the normal proteins of the body. Any T and B cells that would target *self-antigens* are weeded out early in the development of the immune system. Antigens can be proteins, sugars, fats, or nucleic acids.

As part of the *humoral* immune response, B cells produce *immunoglobulins*, which are relatively large proteins that bind to specific epitopes on antigens. These *antibodies* are among the most common classes of globulin proteins found in the plasma of blood after albumin. Each B cell initially produces a specific antibody that has affinity for a distinct epitope. Since the body has a broad repertoire of billions of different B cells to recognize the various foreign antigens that it will encounter in a lifetime, at the start there can only be one of each unique antibody producing B cell. However, in a process known as clonal expansion, engagement of a B cell with an antigen can induce its rapid proliferation into an army of identical B cell clones that target exactly the same epitopes on the antigen. Different B cells may produce antibodies that bind to different epitopes on the same antigen; this is referred to as a *polyclonal antibody response*. In short, the body does not have the capacity to hold large numbers of each clone, so it expands and contracts the number of clones as required.

The pathogen itself might have many different proteins and other structures to which antibodies can bind. The binding of antibodies to a virus, bacteria, or even the toxins produced by them can block their functional interactions, such as attachment to host receptors. Bound antibodies also attract other immune mediators such as *complement proteins* to support the attack against antibody-coated infectious pathogens and cells that are infected with these pathogens.

The specificity of a single B cell to produce an epitope-selective antibody is exploited in the production of monoclonal antibodies. When a B cell is chemically fused with a special type of cancer cell, the resulting hybridoma cell can be immortalized to constantly grow, divide, and keep producing identical antibodies in future generations of that cell. This has been extremely useful for production of therapeutic antibodies that can specifically attack cancer cells or pathogens, and even for blocking the ability of a pathogen like the SARS-CoV-2 virus to bind to host receptors, thus preventing its entry into cells. However, minor changes in the structure of the SARS-CoV-2 spike protein due to evolutionary pressure can reduce the efficacy of such highly specific antibodies. By contrast, mutations would be less problematic for the polyclonal antibodies that would be found in the blood of a person who has been infected with the virus. This is because the polyclonal antibodies work together to recognize a wide range of structures on the pathogen. For example, with regard to SARS-CoV-2, a set of antibodies will recognize its spike protein, another set the membrane protein, another set the envelope protein, and so on. Therefore, changes in the spike protein will not impact broad-based, naturally acquired immunity to the same degree as a focused vaccine-induced immunity to a single spike structure. This is one of the reasons that mirroring naturally acquired immunity is often considered the gold standard in vaccine design. T cells also play a role and will be discussed in the next section.

Antibodies are amazingly durable proteins. There are different classes of antibodies that vary in their primary locations of action, ability to dock multiple antigens, and stability (Figure 8.2). In the blood, IgG antibodies predominate, and these can survive for three weeks or more at 37° Celsius (98.6° Fahrenheit), cruising at high speed through the sixty thousand-plus miles of the arteries, veins, and capillaries in the circulatory system as well as the lymphatic system. Kept at 4°Celsius (39.2° Fahrenheit) with antibiotics to prevent bacterial growth (bacteria like to eat proteins), these antibodies can retain their structure and binding properties for over a decade. In the nasopharynx, airway passages, lungs, and lower digestive tract, secreted IgA and IgM antibodies can last for about five to six days. These latter antibodies are the most useful for fighting a respiratory virus infection. There are also IgD and IgE class antibodies that tend to work primarily in the gut.

All human antibodies are composed of two identical large (heavy) chains and two identical small (light) chains linked together with disulfide atoms. These interwoven protein chains take on a "Y" shape where the branching portion (called the Fab portion) features two separate, identical binding regions at its tips for recognition of an epitope. This region is unique, with differences in amino acid sequences that define the specificity of an antibody. Due to the presence of two copies of epitope-binding domains in each antibody, antibodies are *bivalent* and can bridge two separate viruses simultaneously to cluster them into larger inactive complexes. The other end of the antibody, which is almost identical for antibodies of the same class, is known as the "Fc" portion and acts as a tail-piece. Many different cells of the innate immune system have specific Fc receptors, and so are directed to antibody-coated pathogens to facilitate their destruction. Antibodies of the IgD, IgE, and IgG types are bivalent as they occur only as monomers, or single units. However, IgA type antibodies can occur in units of two (dimers), three (tetramers), or five (pentamers) as well, and IgM antibodies exist in complexes as pentamers or hexamers (Figure 7.2 in the insert). This and other unique features of IgA- and IgM-class antibodies strengthen the mucosal antibody response to pathogenic microbes. These classes are better able than IgG-class antibodies to sequester viruses and bacteria for destruction by roving macrophages. However, vaccines that are injected intramuscularly predominately generate IgG-class antibodies.

7.4. The Nature of T cells

In circulating blood, about 80 to 90 percent of the lymphocytic cells are T cells. Whereas monocytes account for only about 5 to 10 percent of the peripheral blood mononuclear cells (PBMCs), B cell numbers vary from 5 to 10 percent, and dendritic cells represent only about 1 to 2 percent. The dendritic cells are important for processing and presenting antigens to T cells. T cells feature unique receptors (T cell receptors) for antigens, which, like antibodies, have specific recognition of epitopes. However, these antigens generally must be presented by cell surface membrane receptors called *major histocompatibility* (MHC) *proteins* on *antigen-presenting cells*, including dendritic cells, macrophages, Langerhans cells, and B cells, in the central nervous system by astrocytes and microglia (macrophages in the CNS), and by perivascular macrophages.

There are at least three major classes of T cells that are distinguished by marker proteins on their surfaces:

1. Helper T cells that coordinate adaptive immunity through the activation and regulation of other immune cells, including B cells;

2. T cells that can destroy damaged, pathogen-infected and cancerous cells; and
3. A small subset of *gamma-delta* (γδ) T cells that are less common in humans but have their highest abundance in the gut mucosa where their unique features allow them to quickly recognize and respond to foreign antigens.

To activate the destruction of pathogen-infected cells, the antigenic epitopes must be "presented" (on MHC class I molecules) and recognized by a specific T cell receptor. For this reason, T cells primarily attack cells that are actively infected with a pathogen, but rarely a pathogen directly, which is the main job of the antibodies.

There are many other T cell subsets, as well as related cells, such as natural killer (NK) cells, with the ability to destroy cells. The NK cells have a large array of unique activating and inhibitory surface receptors, but not classic MHC molecules that allow them to detect and kill specific viruses and cancer cells. There are also various regulatory T cells and NK-cells that ensure these highly potent killing mechanisms are tightly controlled so as not to harm the host.

In short, the immune system is an amazing set of cells and molecules educated to distinguish "self" from "non-self" so it can detect, remember, and protect the host from cancers and every kind of foreign invader. In chapter 14.3 on immunoceuticals, various ways to empower the immune system so it can function optimally to provide protection from infections and cancer will be discussed.

7.5. The Consequences of a Too Active Immune System

The immune system is highly active under conditions of infection, and many of the symptoms of disease are a consequence of its activation. For example, at higher temperatures, the immune system is more efficient, and many viruses can only survive within a defined temperature range, so a metabolically costly fever is induced to help protect the host. Redness and swelling at a site of infection reflects the protective inflammatory response. Overproduction of mucus and coughing is a strategy to restrict the spread of pathogens (within the body) and clear it. Likewise, postnasal drip is a means of cleansing the nasal cavities of microbes by flushing them out. Unfortunately, these actions can also help the spread of pathogens to others, which is one of their strategies for survival. All of this can induce discomfort and takes a toll on the body but helps remove the foreign invaders. This is especially undesirable when a benign *allergen* that is a common element in the environment, such as pollens or peanuts, inappropriately activates immune mechanisms to cause hay fever or anaphylactic shock, respectively.

Most of the time, the host defense mechanisms work harmoniously to protect the host, but there are times when the immune system overreacts or fails to distinguish self from non-self. For instance, there can be too much or inappropriate immune activation where the production of antibodies, T cells, or other immune meditators can trigger autoimmunity, allergy, immunopathology, or other diseases. For example, while antibodies are highly specific, at very high concentrations they can cross-react with off-target proteins that are normally present in the body, and this can induce inflammation and tissue damage. Also, if all B cells produced antibodies at the same time, the viscosity of blood would be so great that it would flow poorly. Therefore, when individuals are infected and mount an effective immune response that successfully eliminates the pathogen, it is imperative that antibody levels naturally wane, but a degree of residual immune protection remain. Antibodies typically decline in blood once a pathogen is eradicated by the immune system over a period of weeks or months. Importantly, despite low antibody levels, the B cells that produced these antibodies remain alive in a dormant state as memory B cells that reside in tissues and circulate in blood ready to respond should the same invader return. Upon re-infection with the pathogen, these "hibernating" B cells are individually stimulated to grow and divide to generate identical daughter cells that produce the same antibody with an improved specificity for attacking the invading pathogen. Plasma and memory B cells can survive for decades and still produce antibodies upon reinfection with the same pathogen.[2] Symptomatic disease occurs when the infectious pathogen can propagate faster than the immune system can mount an effective response. However, upon re-infection, the immune system usually overcomes the pathogen in a few days with fewer symptoms, and full recovery is usually achieved, once again demonstrating the power of naturally acquired immunity.

7.6. Evading the Immune System

The immune system is the only body system with the ability to match pathogen diversity and deal with the plethora of strategies employed by foreign invaders. The mammalian immune system employs thousands of immune response genes as needed depending on the pathogenic encounter. Conversely, each type of pathogen has many fewer genes and therefore is more restricted in its own arsenal. Nonetheless, each type of pathogen has developed strategies to subvert or even destroy the immune system. For example, the human immunodeficiency virus (HIV) that causes AIDS selectively infects and destroys T helper cells until their numbers decline below functional levels. Since these cells are critical in coordinating the adaptive immune response, their loss eventually leads to a collapse of the immune system and allows this virus and other viruses to spread largely unimpeded.

Antibody-dependent enhancement (ADE) should also be mentioned here as another instance when the immune response may actually inadvertently aid the pathogenic invader. This is a mechanism, sometimes referred to as immune enhancement or disease enhancement, by which the coating of the pathogen, such as a virus, with suboptimal antibodies actually helps the pathogen invade the host by binding to Fc or other receptors on the host cells. ADE can happen following vaccination or natural infection, particularly when non-neutralizing or sub-neutralizing concentrations of antibodies are elicited. ADE has often been observed with positive-strand RNA viruses such as those causing dengue fever, yellow fever, and Zika, as well as betacoronaviruses. Prior to the COVID-19 pandemic, ADE was noted in rodents vaccinated against the SARS-CoV-1 coronavirus. The more targeted the antibody response, the greater the risk of ADE. When few antibodies are bound to a virus and it is still functional, the antibodies can act as a bridge between the virus and the Fc receptor of immune cells. Once attached to the surface of these immune cells, the virus can enter their cytoplasm where it can replicate. Normally, the phagocytic cell would engulf the virus in a process called *phagocytosis* and demolish the virus in digestive vesicles called lysosomes. This potential to induce non-appropriate immune responses illustrates the critical importance of monitoring for ADE and related phenomena when developing vaccines. As will be evident in chapter 13, the phenomena of ADE is a serious concern with COVID-19 vaccines that have focused solely on the spike protein as an antigen.

CHAPTER 8

Tracking SARS-CoV-2 and the Immune Response

Steven Pelech & Christopher A. Shaw

"We see what we want to see. Tunnel vision limits your perception and common sense. You see just what's in front of you, not what you need to see."

—Gustavo Razzetti

8.1. Contact Tracing

Contact tracing is described by the World Health Organization (WHO) as a public health tool for "identifying, assessing, and managing people who have been exposed to someone who has been infected" with any virus of concern.[1] The recent WHO posts on contact tracing regard the COVID-19 virus and the later variants of the same as requiring contact tracing. In brief, the idea behind contact tracing is that health professionals might be able to prevent some portion of the spread of an infectious disease in a local population, in this case COVID-19, by first identifying a person infected with the disease early enough to prevent them from spreading it to others not yet infected. The means to prevent onward spread involves several interrelated parts: verify that the person has the disease, stop onward transmission by isolating or quarantining that person, and finally by tracing the immediate contacts of that person in the days leading up to either the onset of symptoms or a positive test for the causal disease agent.

The effectiveness of this strategy is dependent upon two things: timeliness of the diagnosis and the accuracy of the testing. It is also critical that the contact tracing be used in the earliest stages of a pandemic. Once the disease is rampant in the community, as during a wave of infections, this strategy is ineffective. In the right circumstances, such as preventing the spread of Ebola virus, contact tracing can be very effective. However, Ebola is not spread through casual contact, air, food, or water, but only through someone who is symptomatic.

The Mayo Clinic posts instructions for contact tracing on their website.[2] They advise the following steps: 1) Identify those who have been diagnosed with a disease, e.g., COVID-19 diagnosed in a clinic, hospital, or laboratory; 2) Send the name of the person infected with SARS-CoV-2 based on signs and symptoms of disease, along with either PCR or the so-called "rapid antigen" tests to the health department for that area; and 3) The health authority will follow up with those named to trace "close contacts," that is, someone who has been within two meters of the infected person for fifteen or more minutes within two days of the infected person's diagnosis and may include family members, friends, coworkers, or others.

The follow-up by the health department asks the contacts questions about symptoms and may request that the contacts also be tested for COVID-19 by the described methods. The further follow-up of the contacts is divided into those who test negative and/or cannot be tested for the disease versus those who test positive. For those that have been in contact with a confirmed case of COVID-19, but are not symptomatic, the health department is advised to make four requests:

> Ask them to self-quarantine at home for [fourteen] days after they were exposed; request that they keep social distance from others or even isolate themselves from family and pets, and use a separate bedroom and bathroom; request that they monitor their health and watch for any COVID-19 symptoms; ask them to check their temperature twice a day; ask them to let their doctor and health department know right away if they develop any symptoms; request that they send doctors and the health department daily health updates.[3]

For those in the second category, e.g., "those who have symptoms," they are to request the following:

> Ask them to self-isolate and recover at home if illness is mild. People with symptoms will likely be asked to isolate themselves from family and pets and use a separate bedroom and bathroom; ask them to seek medical care if they have any emergency warning signs, such as trouble breathing or persistent chest pain; give them specific instructions to monitor their symptoms and avoid spreading the COVID-19 virus to others.[4]

The reader may have noticed the two follow-up actions are practically identical. How well does contact tracing work in theory versus practice?

While in principle contact tracing could be useful to break the infection cycle with newer victims, its success depends on how rapidly the initial tracing is done to correctly identify whether a person suspected of harboring the disease actually has it. If this is not done rapidly, the potential case will have acquired many more potential contacts, individually or through family and friends, who can, in turn, infect others.[5] As discussed in chapter 6.1, the symptoms of COVID-19 are very much the same as other common respiratory illnesses. Any symptoms, mild to severe, will show considerable overlap with many infectious viral respiratory diseases, including other members of the coronavirus family, influenza, RSV, and a host of others. So, if symptoms alone will not suffice, what analytic tests can be performed to complement the symptoms and give an accurate diagnosis of disease?

Only two types of COVID-19 tests have been widely adopted. The first is PCR tests (further discussed in detail in chapter 9.2). The second is rapid antigen tests (also further detailed in chapter 9.3). Blood tests for antibodies (further presented in chapter 9.4) are far more accurate but cannot discern *when* an infection occurred, and for this reason will not be addressed further in this section. Viral spread can be exponential after "patient 0" is first identified if not prevented from adding further potential victims.

The first problem is the accuracy, or inaccuracy as the case may be, of the diagnostic tests. Both PCR and rapid antigen tests may be highly inaccurate (see in chapter 8.3 for PCR and 8.4 for rapid antigen tests). For example, PCR performed at thirty-eight thermal cycles (Ct) and above will give over 90 percent false-positive results. Active virus can be detected at Ct's of twenty-five or less, but if higher Ct numbers are needed for detection, then it is more likely dead virus or RNA fragments are being picked up. Using thermal cycles above twenty-five generate false positives for active virus, and the higher the Ct amplification number, the greater the error. Ct of thirty-five or higher are essentially useless for quantitative estimates of disease status for individuals and populations. What this means in practice is that the contact tracers will be wasting time tracking people who do not actually have COVID-19 or had it and have since recovered. These people are unlikely to have the disease when tested and thus those they contacted immediately before the PCR are also not likely to have the active disease either, unless they acquire it from another source. In other words, PCR used improperly may subject healthy individuals to restrictions that cause more harm than good.

The accuracy of the rapid antigen tests is problematic for the opposite reason, since they can be insensitive and miss the early stages of a SARS-CoV-2 infection. Both PCR and rapid antigen tests should only be used to confirm diagnosis in someone who has or recently had COVID-19-like symptoms. It remains unclear whether those without symptoms are infectious or have been infected. A prior infection with SARS-CoV-2 could be revealed by a blood test for antibodies, but those who test positive will probably not be actively infectious any longer.

For these reasons, unless both timeliness and accuracy are ensured, contact tracing is mainly an exercise in "virtue signaling," unable to prevent disease spread, especially during an active wave of SARS-CoV-2 infections.

The assumption that contact tracing would prevent the spread of COVID-19 was based on a hypothetical situation of very limited disease vectors with clear symptoms and accurate testing. Neither of these has been true for COVID-19. Effectiveness claims made by the Mayo Clinic and others also ignore the reality that any diminution of disease spread may more likely be due to acquired herd immunity.

The Government of Canada website for the Public Health Agency of Canada, last updated on November 3, 2021, stated the following with respect to the "infectious period": "The time period in which an individual with COVID-19 is infectious remains uncertain. A person may be infectious for up to 3 days before showing symptoms (pre-symptomatic infectiousness)."[6]

With respect to the "incubation period": "The incubation period ranges from 1 to 14 days. The median is 5 to 6 days between exposure and symptom onset. Most people (97.5%) develop symptoms within 11.5 days of exposure."[7]

With respect to "reinfection": "There is emerging evidence of human reinfection with SARS-CoV-2. This has been documented by individuals confirmed to have been infected by different strains of the virus. Further research is required to fully comprehend the relationship between positive antibody tests and any protection against reinfection."[8]

And, "Currently, we do not know: whether the presence of antibodies indicates immunity to re-infection, and if it does, how long that potential immunity lasts; or the potential severity of subsequent infections [reformatted for clarity]."[9]

None of this should give the public much assurance as written and could be roughly translation from Government of Canada-ese as, "We don't really know if you have or had COVID-19 because the time frames are incredibly broad and our tests, which we are not discussing, don't work as advertised."

Similar concerns are echoed in the Canada Communicable Disease Report (CCDR) issued on November 5, 2020, and also produced by the Public Health Agency of Canada (PHAC):

> **Background:** COVID-19 cases need to be isolated long enough to prevent further transmission but no longer than needed. Determining the infectious period of COVID-19 is complicated by four factors: 1) people can be diagnosed when they are symptomatic, pre-symptomatic or asymptomatic, 2) the

> common diagnostic test, RT-PCR, is accurate for diagnosis as it is able to detect viral genetic material, but it cannot document when someone is no longer infectious because it cannot distinguish whether viral particles are still infectious or not, 3) cell culture is the best way to confirm whether infectious virus is present, but it takes time and requires specialized laboratory facilities, and 4) although transmission is primarily respiratory, virus has been found in feces and eye secretions.[10]

In other words, the authors of the CCDR knew all the difficulties in 2020, but they were clearly not communicated in any effective way to PHAC, with the consequence that government health authorities continued to do things that simply could not work to diagnose or control COVID-19. Even non-government organizations like the Mayo Clinic did not have a sound approach to the problem.[11] Alas, they proposed the same PCR methods (without specifying Ct to be used) and antibody tests, again, without any clear specificity for those tests that are most effective or used long after the symptoms of the disease have subsided and the person is no longer infectious.

For the covered reasons, in both Canada and the United States, the tactics used by health authorities during the pandemic essentially meant they had no realistic ability to determine who was infected with COVID-19 or whether their control measures were effective. With this conclusion, should the public be surprised that COVID-19 policies in both countries were largely *ad hoc*, inconsistent, and highly ineffective?

8.2. PCR Tests for SARS-CoV-2

To establish whether a person has an active ongoing infection with SARS-CoV-2 and not another pathogen that produces similar symptoms to COVID-19, specific tests are necessary. Likewise, other tests are required to determine whether an individual has immunity from future infections with SARS-CoV-2 and is protected from getting COVID-19 again. Such specific tests have been feasible since the release of the genome sequence of the original Wuhan strain of SARS-CoV-2 in January 2020.

There are two major types of testing used to determine whether a person is actively infected with SARS-CoV-2. A nucleic acid test (NAT), most commonly the Reverse Transcription-Polymerase Chain Reaction (RT-PCR)-based test, has been used for detection of the RNA component of the virus. It relies on amplification of the viral nucleic acid material through repeated heating and cooling cycles of separation and annealing of the nucleic acid strands, with a doubling of the genetic material with each thermal cycle. The other type of test is the rapid antigen test, which detects the presence of a viral protein.

As mentioned earlier, the main issue with the RT-PCR test is that it often employs a high number of thermal cycles, which can generate a large percentage of false positive results. Individuals can still test positive with the RT-PCR test two weeks after they have fully recovered from COVID-19 and are non-infectious. It is not possible to amplify the viral protein material in a rapid antigen test, so it suffers from a lack of sensitivity and can often generate false negatives. Depending on the specificity of the antibody detection reagent used, it may also cross-react with related proteins found in other (common cold) coronaviruses and produce false positives.

The polymerase chain reaction (PCR) test is a commonly used molecular diagnostic tool used to detect the presence of DNA or RNA in a sample. For the clinical detection of SARS-CoV-2, all clinical virology laboratories use reverse-transcriptase real-time PCR (RT-rtPCR) for the detection of SARS-CoV-2 viral RNA in nasopharyngeal swabs (NPS), mid-turbinate swabs (MTS), or saliva.[12] In this method, a reverse transcription step is first performed, which copies the genetic code of the viral RNA into DNA, which is much more stable than RNA. The PCR can then be performed, which involves using what are called *primers*, short pieces of DNA that are designed to bind to unique complementary sequences present in a viral genome. The primers are designed to bind at either end of a segment of the viral genome.

If the primers bind, an enzyme known as a *polymerase* will use the viral genome as a template to extend the primers until the target gene segment has been completely copied. This works by varying the temperature of the sample. A high temperature is used to get double-stranded DNA to separate into single strands. Next, an *annealing* temperature is used to allow the primers to bind to the single strands of DNA. Finally, a third temperature is used to promote extension of the primers until the targeted gene sequence has been copied. This constitutes a single thermal cycle of the test. Multiple cycles are employed to increase the copies of the targeted gene segment exponentially, essentially doubling the amount of DNA with each thermal cycle.

A fluorescent dye is usually added to the sample that incorporates into the targeted gene segment. If enough gene segments get amplified, a special machine can detect the amount of the fluorescent dye. The amount of dye usually correlates with the number of viral genomes in the clinical specimen. An important piece of information generated with the RT-PCR test is the *cycle threshold* (Ct) value. The Ct value is the number of thermal cycles that had to be performed for the fluorescent signal to exceed background levels.

While RT-PCR tests are based on a remarkable technology, they never should have been used as a standalone "gold standard" test for defining cases of COVID-19. In fact, it is wholly inappropriate to diagnose COVID-19, which is an illness with clear symptoms, based only on the presence of SARS-CoV-2

RNA as detected by the PCR test. A positive result with a PCR test does not mean a person has COVID-19 and is able to transmit the disease. First of all, every laboratory conducting RT-PCR tests for the detection of SARS-CoV-2 should have determined an appropriate Ct cut-off through parallel testing of samples using the gold standard functional virology assay in which evidence of replication-competent, potentially infectious virus particles is obtained by looking for evidence of cytopathic effect (killing) in what are known as *permissive cells* (cells stripped of their antiviral properties so that viruses can readily infect them). This was done by Canada's National Microbiology Laboratory, with the Ct cut-off determined to be only twenty-four, meaning that tests showing positive results at Ct values greater than twenty-four failed to demonstrate the presence of potentially infectious viral particles.

Secondly, the presence of replication-competent viral particles in a sample does not necessarily equate to a case of COVID-19, which is a disease with symptoms. The latter can only be diagnosed if an active infection is present in conjunction with signs and/or symptoms of illness, which would require assessment by a physician. Remarkably, however, entities like Public Health Ontario categorized samples with Ct cut-offs of up to thirty-eight cycles and, in some cases, in the absence of clinical data, as representing positive cases of COVID-19 with greater than 90 percent inaccuracy. This is highly ill advised, especially in the absence of publicly available data proving that the Ct cut-off was established using the functional virology assay. Consequently, overall cases of COVID-19 have likely been dramatically overestimated, and to an unknown degree. This inflation of the problem of COVID-19 resulted in unnecessary pressure to force COVID-19 vaccines in both public and private venues. It also led to diagnosis of COVID-19 cases that may have been due to other respiratory viruses.

Studies have shown that if more than thirty cycles of PCR amplification are required to detect the presence of SARS-CoV-2 RNA, the viral content is insufficient to propagate in optimal cell culture conditions in a laboratory.[13] Unfortunately, many results reported in the scientific literature are based on the use of thirty-five thermal cycles or greater. This is true for the clinical Phase 3 trials used to test the efficacy of the COVID-19 vaccines. This undermines public health data on the number of people infected with SARS-CoV-2, as well as many clinical studies intended to determine the effectiveness of a vaccine to prevent COVID-19. For example, a Substack essay by Dr. Byram Bridle listed forty-eight of the most influential publications cited by public health officials to mislabel asymptomatic people as sources of SARS-CoV-2 infection.[14]

It is also worth mentioning that PCR testing of sewage water for the presence of nucleocapsid RNA became a common strategy to monitor community levels of SARS-CoV-2 infection. It should be appreciated that such an application of the PCR method is highly non-quantitative. Apart from the accuracy of the test at high Ct performance numbers, sewage water levels vary significantly depending on the weather and season, which would result in variable dilution of the RNA. RNA is also very unstable. At best, such measurements might be useful for identifying the presence of new variants of SARS-CoV-2 relative to other variants.

8.3. Rapid Antigen Tests for SARS-CoV-2

Unlike PCR tests that monitor for the presence of SARS-CoV-2 viral mRNA, antigen tests detect the presence of target proteins within the virus particle. This relies on the availability of premade antibodies that bind specifically to one or more of the virus's proteins, most commonly the spike or nucleocapsid protein. Such antibodies may be generated in animals inoculated with target viral proteins artificially manufactured in cells, described as *recombinant* versions of the proteins. These recombinant proteins are believed to be essentially identical to the original viral proteins, although they may be subjected to minor modifications. A major difference between the antigen tests and the genetic tests is that the number of viral protein molecules cannot be amplified as it is using the PCR method.

Many Canadian provinces recommended widespread use of rapid antigen tests, especially for those who did not receive at least two injections of a COVID-19 vaccine. One of the most used test kits is manufactured by Abbott Panbio.[15] The Ontario government recommended this test only for asymptomatic (apparently healthy) individuals. Remarkably, however, as indicated in the printed material provided by the government of Ontario, the kits were only tested on and approved for use in symptomatic individuals. No evidence was provided that screening with the kit was effective for use in asymptomatic individuals. Finally, the printed materials stated that a negative test result (expected when testing asymptomatic people) does not exclude that a person has been infected with SARS-CoV-2. However, by definition, an asymptomatic person cannot have COVID-19, because COVID-19 is a disease characterized by symptoms and signs of illness.

Interestingly, the booklet accompanying the rapid antigen test kit that was approved by the government of Ontario contradicts the government's general messaging regarding PCR testing for SARS-CoV-2. Whereas the government claimed that people who test positive with the PCR test at cycle thresholds of up to thirty-eight can transmit SARS-CoV-2, the rapid antigen test kit stated that people who test positive at cycle thresholds above thirty-three are not contagious.

The inability of the Abbott rapid antigen test to detect SARS-CoV-2 in asymptomatic people was confirmed in a study conducted by the Canadian

Public Health Laboratory. The test kit was unable to detect SARS-CoV-2 in samples that tested positive with RT-PCR cycle thresholds greater than twenty-two. People testing positive at cycle thresholds of twenty-two or less would clearly be sick (i.e., symptomatic).[16]

Many Canadians, especially those who did not receive a COVID-19 vaccine, were forced to use these kits between two to five times per week to maintain their jobs, volunteer positions, etc., often at their own expense. Each kit cost about CDN$16 from the manufacturer. Pharmacies charged CDN$40 (and up to CDN$99) per test. This resulted in substantial extra costs for working people and substantial profits for those in the testing business. To reiterate, these rapid antigen tests would usually be positive only when someone had such a high viral load that they would be clearly symptomatic.

The requirement that asymptomatic working people have rapid antigen tests (which were rarely positive) as a condition of employment made it appear that due diligence was being practiced with respect to public health. In reality, a lot of money and time was wasted on products that could not reliably detect early infection. Meanwhile, the manufacturers made massive profits from something with little public health value. People who did not receive a COVID-19 vaccine should not have been forced to take these tests in order to work. This was especially true in 2022 and 2023 in Canada, when most reported COVID-19 cases were in double- and triple-vaccinated individuals and many people already had natural immunity.

8.4. Serological Tests for Antibodies against SARS-CoV-2

Once the SARS-CoV-2 virus is cleared by the immune system of recovered COVID-19 survivors, evidence of immunity is established by the presence of antibodies in their blood and other body fluids such as saliva, or less commonly, by the presence of specific T lymphocytes in their blood.

The blood tests for antibody detection have the advantage that they are highly sensitive and can provide a measure of the immunity present in a previously infected individual, even years after the initial exposure to the virus. However, it is also possible to pick up immunoreactivities with antibodies produced against related viral proteins found in other coronaviruses. Historically, the PCR test was most used due to its accuracy and sensitivity, but antigen testing is more convenient and can even be performed in the home or workplace for rapid analysis of SARS-CoV-2 infection status. Relatively little serological antibody testing has been performed in Canada; it was primarily offered commercially by just a few companies.

Serological tests work by immobilizing a purified protein from a pathogen on a surface such a cellulose membrane, or glass or plastic slide. If an antibody present in a blood or saliva sample recognizes the protein or peptide as an antigen, then it may tightly bind to it. The binding of that antibody is then detected with a secondary antibody that recognizes the Fc portion of the primary antibody being tracked. For example, this could be an anti-human IgG antibody made in sheep. The secondary antibody is tagged with a dye, or an enzyme that generates a dye, which will be visible on the surface of the antigen-coated membrane or slide.

While rapid antigen testing for SARS-CoV-2 infection is strongly encouraged by public health authorities in Canada, testing for SARS-CoV-2 antibodies in blood or saliva samples has been discouraged by many of the same agencies, including the BC Centre for Disease Control.[17] Whereas over forty million dollars was allocated by the Canadian federal government for genome sequencing of SARS-CoV-2 isolates (e.g., the CanCOGeN Project),[18] little funding was provided in Canada for the development and application of antibody tests to determine the extent of natural immunity or immunity provided by the COVID-19 vaccines. A small number of serological testing projects in Canada were funded by the COVID-19 Immunity Task Force (CITF).[19]

One early project to evaluate antibody-based immunity was funded through the Angus Reid Group and conducted by the University of Toronto and was called Action to Beat Corona Virus (Ab-C).[20] Using over twenty-two thousand dried blood spot samples provided by over eleven thousand Canadians, the detectable spike and nucleocapsid antibodies in these samples were used to ascertain vaccine-induced and naturally induced levels of immunity, respectively, against the virus. The Ab-C study reported that by August 2021 only about 6 percent of tested Canadians had natural immunity.[21] These findings revealed that the study's methodology markedly underestimated the degree of natural immunity in the Canadian population. For example, about 3.9 percent of Canadians who had COVID-19-like symptoms had tested positive for SARS-CoV-2 infection using PCR-based tests by this time.[22] Due to underreporting of COVID-19 cases, recorded PCR results were already believed to underestimate actual SARS-CoV-2 infection rates by at least another four-fold.[23] Moreover, at least 40 percent of SARS-CoV-2 infections are asymptomatic.[24] Consequently, the actual percentage of SARS-CoV-2-infected Canadians was substantially higher than the Ab-C study estimates.

In the Ab-C study, recombinant versions of only the spike and nucleocapsid proteins were used for testing the dried blood samples. Dried blood already has a problem with low sensitivity; since antibody levels normally begin to decline in the months following the elimination of a viral infection, they may decline to below the threshold of detection with these tests. Also, as will be discussed in the following, antibodies against the nucleocapsid protein are often not detectable in the blood of recovered COVID-19 patients.

Fresh blood or serum samples can provide much better yields of active antibody than dried blood specimens. Serological tests, like those provided by LifeLabs with fresh blood samples,[25] tracked antibodies against the nucleocapsid and spike proteins. These tests utilized recombinant proteins that are expensive to manufacture and used at dilute concentrations to minimize costs, but at the sacrifice of sensitivity. LifeLabs has since discontinued its COVID-19 antibody testing service.

8.5. Antibody Neutralization Assays for Spike Binding

Testing for SARS-CoV-2 spike and nucleocapsid protein antibodies were viewed by health authorities as of limited value in assessing the public's immunity against COVID-19, it was still considered to be considered highly relevant in evaluating the efficacy of vaccines to prevent COVID-19. In particular, vaccine manufacturers and health agencies were particularly fixated on the measurement of "neutralizing" antibodies against the spike protein as a surrogate for overall immunity to SARS-CoV-2. Due to the location of the spike protein on the surface of the viral particle and the importance of its receptor binding domain (RBD) for attachment to the ACE2 protein on the surface of host cells, the ability of antibodies to block this binding was considered a measure of the degree of immune protection afforded.

A few different strategies were developed to test the degree of "neutralization" of the spike protein. The first was simply to evaluate whether antibodies in recovered patients were able to block the ability of SARS-CoV-2 to infect and kill monkey or human cells in culture. However, this kind of testing was expensive, since Biosafety Level (BSL) 3 or 4 laboratories are required for handling the SARS-CoV-2 virus in Canada and the US. Consequently, alternative approaches were developed that relied on a surrogate virus that could express the SARS-CoV-2 spike protein on its surface, allowing it to enter and kill animal or human cells transfected with human ACE2.

Lentiviruses were especially popular for this application because, as safe, non-pathogenic viruses, they are commonly used in biomedical research.[26] When genes necessary for replication are deleted, these viruses can be used safely in BSL-2 laboratories to create surrogate viruses useful for neutralization testing. Such neutralization assays were instrumental in the original identification of cells that produce therapeutic monoclonal antibodies that could block SARS-CoV-2 infection in COVID-19 patients. The only difficulty was that minor changes in the amino acid structure of the target virus, as occurred with subsequent variants of SARS-CoV-2, rendered many of the early therapeutic monoclonal antibodies ineffective.

Another strategy was to use enzyme-linked immunosorbent assay (ELISA) plates to test the ability of antibody-containing serum samples to block a dye-labeled recombinant spike protein from binding to the ACE2. The presence of such neutralizing antibodies results in a reduction in detected spike protein due to the antibodies' binding to the spike protein.

While such neutralizing antibodies would be a desirable outcome from immunization with a vaccine or natural infection with the SARS-CoV-2 virus, it is important to appreciate that over 95 percent of the antibodies produced against the spike protein do *not* target its RBD, but still provide immune protection, in part by guiding different classes of innate immune cells directly to the virus particles and to virus-infected cells that express spike protein on their surface. Furthermore, T cells also recognize epitopes throughout the spike protein, which facilitates their killing of SARS-CoV-2-infected cells.

8.6. Results of the Kinexus Serological Tests for Natural Immunity to SARS-CoV-2

The clinical studies conducted by the Vancouver-based company Kinexus Bioinformatics Corporation have provided important insights into the adaptive antibody response to SARS-CoV-2 infection and COVID-19 vaccination. In the interests of full disclosure, one of the authors and editors of this book, Dr. Steven Pelech, is a majority shareholder, the president, and the chief scientific officer of Kinexus.

In February 2020, Kinexus began its research to identify the parts of the various proteins encoded by the genome of SARS-CoV-2 that elicited strong immunoreactivities with antibodies in people who had recovered from COVID-19. With the availability on January 10, 2020, of the full sequence of the SARS-CoV-2 genome, it was possible to predict the amino acid sequences of all twenty-nine of the viral proteins encoded by its genes.

Using its automated peptide-synthesis capability, Kinexus created cellulose membranes upon which overlapping fifteen-amino-acid-long pieces of these viral proteins were tiled out as arrays of distinct peptide spots of defined composition. This permitted the detection of antibody epitopes as small as two amino acids long. Over six thousand distinct, but overlapping, parts of all twenty-nine viral proteins were robotically synthesized. The concentrations of these peptides were at least fifty-times higher than could be achieved with recombinant versions of the same SARS-CoV-2 viral proteins. This permitted detection of antibodies that might specifically bind to these peptides at much lower concentrations than other serological tests. Kinexus identified over four hundred viral peptides that generated strong antibody production following infection by SARS-CoV-2, then reduced the number of best common markers to 120 peptides. The company then further tested samples from another 450 recovered COVID-19 patients, as well as healthy adults with no history of COVID-19 illness, to identify forty-one peptides that served as the most commonly targeted parts of ten of the SARS-CoV-2 proteins. This allowed the creation of a forty-one-marker test that was the size of a postage stamp. With these forty-one-marker peptide spot arrays, Kinexus then screened more serum or dried blood spot samples from over four thousand additional individuals. This permitted exploration of the degree of natural and COVID-19-vaccine induced immunity in people primarily located in British Columbia and Ontario.

Figure 8.1, found in the insert, provides an example of one of the earlier serological antibody tests for SARS-CoV-2 proteins, in this instance the spike, membrane, and nucleocapsid proteins. A dark spot in this test indicated that this region of the targeted protein was immunogenic and elicited antibodies against this part of the virus protein. Interestingly, the RBD region of the spike protein, specifically targeted by COVID vaccines, was not particularly immunogenic in people who successfully recovered from COVID-19. Peptides that are expected to feature Omicron BA.1 mutations are highlighted in shading. Apart from the D796Y and N969K mutations in the Omicron spike protein, none of the other thirty-two mutations were in parts of this viral protein that elicited strong antibody responses and the establishment of lasting immune memory from natural infection.

The Kinexus SARS-CoV-2 antibody clinical study with the various SARS-CoV-2 peptide spot arrays revealed that almost everyone tested had a unique antibody response evident from very diverse spot patterns of immunoreactivities with selected SARS-CoV-2-based peptides between people. Also, when about a hundred of the study participants were retested nearly a year later, from when they were initially screened following an earlier SARS-CoV-2 infection, the spot patterns were very similar and reproducible for the same person. Furthermore, the study found the presence of multiple antibodies against the SARS-CoV-2 protein that were clearly evident in people even thirty months after their initial infection with SARS-CoV-2, which was consistent with establishment of immune memory or ongoing exposures to the virus.

Another important insight from the Kinexus clinical study was that following infection with the SARS-CoV-2 virus, each person's antibodies could collectively recognize hundreds of very different parts of the virus proteins. This polyclonal antibody response underlies the immune system's ability to combat mutated versions of the virus. Scores of different antibodies against different parts of the spike protein alone may be detected in the serum from a single recovered COVID-19 patient. Another striking finding is that when the locations of the amino acid mutations in the Alpha, Beta, Delta, and Omicron variants of SARS-CoV-2 are mapped, it turns out that these mutations rarely occur in the parts of the SARS-CoV-2 proteins that people usually make antibodies against. Therefore, most of the antibodies made against the original Wuhan strain of the virus should, and do, work effectively against any of the variants, and *vice versa*. This is why the COVID-19 vaccines that were produced with the original Wuhan strain of the spike protein could still produce protection from even the Omicron BA.4 and BA.5 strains of SARS-CoV-2 for at least a few months. In fact, the bivalent vaccines with the Wuhan/Omicron BA.4/5 Spike RNA combination proved to be no better for eliciting antibody responses than the original Wuhan spike RNA vaccines.

The Kinexus clinical study also revealed that the RBD region of the spike protein was poorly immunogenic. Since all the subjects who had COVID-19 had fully recovered, this demonstrated that antibodies against the RBD, which would likely be considered "neutralizing" antibodies in tests with lentiviruses, were not really reliable markers of effective immunity against SARS-CoV-2.

Another significant finding from the Kinexus clinical study was that over 90 percent of the more than 2,900 people who were asymptomatic for COVID-19 clearly possessed antibodies that could recognize SARS-CoV-2, with numbers and intensities of visible immunoreactive spots similar to those seen with PCR-test-confirmed recovered COVID-19 patients. This was already evident in a preliminary study Kinexus conducted with the BC Children's and Women's Hospital that was published in the flagship journal of the American Society for Clinical Investigation, *JCI Insight*.[27] In this *JCI Insight* report, which included serum samples collected in Spring 2020 from 276 healthy adult participants, half of whom were health-care workers, about 90 percent of those tested had detectable antibodies that immunoreacted with many of the targets on the Kinexus forty-one-marker SARS-CoV-2 peptide spot array and also reacted with recombinant preparations of the spike and nucleocapsid proteins. The Kinexus SARS-CoV-2 antibody test results were cross-validated with another SARS-CoV-2 antibody test developed and marketed by the US company MesoScale Diagnostics.[28] The Kinexus SARS-CoV-2 antibody tests are likely among the most sensitive and accurate serological antibody tests available. No other reported tests have detected antibodies against so many different SARS-CoV-2 proteins.

In the Majdoubi et al. (2021) *JCI* study, it was suggested that the high rate of detection of antibodies in the serum of healthy adults in late Spring 2020 was due to the presence of pre-existing antibodies.[29] This was subsequently tested by Kinexus with serum samples obtained from thirty people who had confirmed COVID-19 and strong antibody responses. The corresponding spike protein amino acid sequences that were the most immunoreactive were tested against equivalent, but slightly different amino acids sequences in SARS-CoV-1, MERS, and four cold coronaviruses. While some of the antibody responses were clearly stronger with SARS-CoV-2 spike peptides, responses were often as strong or stronger with sequences derived from other coronaviruses. This indicated that many of the antibodies that reacted with SARS-CoV-2 may have arisen from

B cells that were previously stimulated by other coronaviruses. Exposure of these individuals to SARS-CoV-2 likely re-activated memory and plasma B cell that recognized spike protein from past infections with one or more of the other coronaviruses. Since most of the participants in the Kinexus study were apparently asymptomatic for COVID-19, it would appear that their antibodies were sufficiently robust to provide effective protection against SARS-CoV-2. These results likely account for why so many people remained asymptomatic for COVID-19 despite becoming infected with SARS-CoV-2.

Despite clear detection of antibodies against the spike and other proteins from this virus in those with PCR test-confirmed symptomatic COVID-19, Kinexus observed that nearly half of the participants had little or no detectable antibodies against the nucleocapsid protein of the SARS-CoV-2 virus. There have also been cases of people who were hospitalized for COVID-19 who failed to exhibit anti-nucleocapsid antibodies in their blood when tested a couple of months later using LifeLabs' serological test, which relied on whole recombinant nucleocapsid protein as an antigen. Consequently, the absence of anti-nucleocapsid antibodies is not a reliable indicator that someone has not already been infected with SARS-CoV-2. The most robust and consistent antibodies that Kinexus identified were generated against the membrane protein of SARS-CoV-2. Since the membrane protein is present in greater abundance on the surface of the SARS-CoV-2 particle than the spike protein, this would have been a better marker of seroprevalence of SARS-CoV-2 infections than the nucleocapsid protein, and possibly a more suitable target than the spike protein for COVID-19 vaccine development, since the spike protein can induce blood clotting on its own. While anti-spike protein antibody detection could also be used early on to establish the seroprevalence of SARS-CoV-2 infections, once mass vaccination was underway, this antigen could no longer be used to distinguish between vaccine- and natural infection-induced immunity.

8.7. Seroprevalence to SARS-CoV-2 during the COVID-19 Pandemic in Canada

According to seroprevalence studies funded by the Canada COVID Immunity Task Force (CITF), in March 2020, only 0.3 percent of tested Canadians had antibodies against the SARS-CoV-2 virus.[30] As mentioned in the previous section, the Ab-C study determined that a year later, in March 2021, only around 6.5 percent of tested Canadians had natural immunity.[31]

With CITF funding, the Canadian Blood Services, using highly sensitive Roche Elecsys anti-SARS-CoV-2 spike protein antibody and anti-nucleocapsid antibody tests, determined that 99.65 percent of 13,189 unique donors had anti-spike antibodies, and 22.65 percent had anti-nucleocapsid antibodies by mid-February 2022.[32] Anti-spike antibodies could have been produced as a consequence of natural infection and/or COVID-19 vaccination. Anti-nucleocapsid antibodies, which could only arise from natural infection, were evident in 36.59 percent of blood donors between seventeen and twenty-four years of age across Canada. Despite nearly all donors having vaccine-related antibodies as of December 2021, with the emergence of the Omicron variants, by mid-February 2022, the infection-related antibody rate was more than four times the monthly seroprevalence rate for the anti-nucleocapsid antibodies observed for the year of 2021. Evidently, vaccination was not protective against infection by SARS-CoV-2. By June 2023, more than 90 percent of blood donors in the seventeen to twenty-four years of age group had anti-nucleocapsid antibodies.[33] About 80 percent of the general Canadian population was found to have anti-nucleocapsid protein antibodies by this date.

In a meta-analysis of Canadian seroprevalance studies from the Ab-C study group, Canadian Blood Services and others that was published in the *Canadian Medical Association Journal*, in November 2021, there was over 95 percent seropositive prevalence of anti-spike protein antibodies, but only 9 percent seropositive prevalence of anti-nucleocapsid protein antibodies.[34] By March 15, 2023, 74 percent of Canadians were determined to have anti-nucleocapsid antibodies, due to the dramatic increase in the rate of infection during the Omicron wave of the COVID-19 pandemic. It is also noteworthy that the rate of natural infection was higher among younger than older people during the course of the pandemic. This is not surprising, in part because younger people are more socially outgoing and have more robust immune systems.

The Ab-C findings of low anti-nucleocapsid protein antibody seropositivity during the first two years of the COVID-19 pandemic accounts for the lack of appreciation of the actual extent of natural immunity in the Canadian population by health authorities. Natural immunity was not factored into projected models of the COVID-19 pandemic, and policies such as implementation of vaccine passports also discounted natural immunity. By contrast, natural immunity was recognized in the issuing of vaccine passports in many European countries.

Were Canadian researchers and health authorities misled by these studies, which relied on a single marker for past SARS-CoV-2 infections, i.e., anti-nucleocapsid antibodies, and were most often performed with dried blood samples? Several other studies certainly challenge the notion that SARS-CoV-2 infections were low in Canada prior to the emergence of the Omicron variants.

Early studies performed by Ichor Blood Services in Alberta found that about 51 percent of the serum samples from unvaccinated people tested by August 2021 had detectable spike and nucleocapsid antibodies comparable to levels in samples from those who had PCR-confirmed COVID-19.[35] Subsequently, by December 23, 2021, Ichor Blood Services found spike protein antibodies in 89 percent of unvaccinated people, even in distant rural areas around La Crete in northern Alberta with much lower population densities than cities.[36] With such high rates of natural immunity in remote rural settings, it is reasonable to expect comparable or even higher rates sooner in urban, higher population-density settings.

In the Kinexus clinical study of SARS-CoV-2 antibody prevalence in primarily the Vancouver area, over 1,600 of the participants who clearly tested positive for a previous SARS-CoV-2 infection and had COVID-19-like symptoms first experienced these symptoms between November 1, 2019 and March 31, 2020.[37] Since Kinexus first started testing people in March 2020, about 90 percent of those tested have consistently had antibodies that were immunoreactive with peptides patterned after hundreds of regions in the SARS-CoV-2 protein as partly documented in Figure 8.1 (in the insert). The number and intensity of immunoreactive antibodies against the smaller forty-one marker tests that Kinexus conducted remained consistent with over four thousand people who tested positive with multiple markers throughout the course of the three-year study, very unlike the results from the CITF-funded studies mentioned earlier. The lack of nucleocapsid immunoreactivity detected in the pre-Omicron period with these studies is likely due to the poor sensitivity of those tests that relied on low concentration of recombinant nucleocapsid protein and less robust immune responses early in the pandemic for most people who were infected. With secondary Omicron infections, the antibody titers against this target were finally boosted to levels that became detectable in most people with the nucleocapsid antibody-based tests funded by the CITF.

By early 2022, the majority of people in Canada and the United States had been infected by SARS-CoV-2, and about a quarter of those had experienced COVID-19 twice. In British Columbia, using a serological test for antibodies against the spike and nucleocapsid proteins of SARS-CoV-2, the BC Centre for Disease Control (BCCDC) reported that by August 2022, at least 70–80 percent of children younger than nineteen years old, 60–70 percent of adults from twenty to fifty-nine years, and only approximately 40 percent of adults older than 60 years had been infected.[38] In the United States, seroprevalence studies found that about 75 percent of US children that were tested had infection-induced antibodies following Omicron infection, meaning that there was clearly widespread naturally acquired immunity in this population by early 2022.[39, 40] Likewise, in England, SARS-CoV-2 antibody testing of unvaccinated school pupils from January to February 2022 showed that 62.4 percent of primary and 97 percent of secondary students were serologically positive for previous infection with the virus.[41]

8.8. T Cell Tests against SARS-CoV-2

In the adaptive immune response, humoral immunity with B cells producing antibodies directed against the SARS-CoV-2 proteins is only part of the protection against the virus. T cells are also important in thwarting the propagation of the virus by attacking and destroying the host cells that have been hijacked into becoming virus-producing factories. Measuring the T cell response is more time-consuming and expensive than serological testing studies. Firstly, fresh blood needs to be used, and techniques must be applied to separate the peripheral blood mononucleocyte fraction of blood cells from the other over 99 percent of blood cells, which are erythrocytes. Commercial testing for these in Canada was difficult to obtain, but at least one company called Immunity Diagnostic Inc. (Immunity Dx) based in Vancouver, BC conducted a clinical study to evaluate the extent of natural T cell immunity against the SARS-CoV-2 virus.[42]

Immunity Dx developed two methods to monitor the presence of T cells that are immunoreactive with SARS-CoV-2 proteins. With both methods, synthetic peptides based on SARS-CoV-2 proteins or recombinant virus proteins were spotted onto membranes, and these were used to capture T cells with antigen receptors that specifically recognized SARS-CoV-2 antigens. Following engagement of their T cell antigen receptors, these T cells grew and propagated and were subsequently detected and quantified. The more T cells that were detected, the higher the levels of T cell immunity in the person from which the blood sample was obtained.

Dr. Ismael Samudio, the president of Immunity Dx, spearheaded a collaboration with Kinexus to evaluate whether clinical blood samples in some of the Kinexus clinical trial participants that were being tested for SARS-CoV-2 antibody levels also had T cells that recognized the virus. In the blood samples from over thirty participants, there was a very strong correlation between the level of antibody response and the degree of T cell recognition of the same viral proteins. These findings indicated that monitoring SARS-CoV-2 antibody responses served as a good surrogate for overall immunity, including T cell immunity, although it must be acknowledged that this study was likely underpowered. It took about a week to perform the T cell profiling of a participant's blood sample, and with the high costs of the reagents to perform each test, it was an expensive assay to perform. Ultimately, Immunity Dx had to close in 2022. At present, T cell antigen testing is available through Ichor Blood Services, through a contract with the US Seattle-based company Adaptive Biotechnologies.[43]

8.9. The Natural Immune Response to SARS-CoV-2

As has been discussed in chapter 7, the immune system has an effective combination of innate and adaptive immune responses to fight an infection by a virus like SARS-CoV-2. For a respiratory infection, the ability of the immune system to mount its defenses at the initial site of infection is critical. The innate immune response with phagocytic cells that consume foreign pathogens is instrumental in producing a robust follow-up adaptive immune response. Memory B cells present in the tissues in the upper airways may become activated to produce antibodies if these cells have previously encountered the same or similar pathogens. With the whole pathogen, there are many different parts that provide for a broad spectrum of epitopes that can be targeted for antibody production. The more antibodies bound to the pathogen, the greater the opportunity to take it down by interfering with the pathogen's ability to bind to cells and by improving innate immune cell and T cell recognition of the pathogen. In the nose, mouth, throat, and upper lungs, these antibodies are primarily of the IgM and IgA classes. Because these antibodies are multivalent, they are very effective for clumping the pathogen so that it can be more effectively eliminated in mucus-enriched nasal secretions, and by sneezing, coughing, and ingestion. These antibodies will also facilitate better recognition of the pathogen by innate immune cells and T cells. Ultimately, the presentation of portions of the digested pathogen on innate immune cells along with major histocompatibility antigens in these cells triggers the activation of highly specific B cells and T cells with even greater affinity and at higher levels than prior to the infection. In a coordinated effort, this will effectively eliminate the pathogen and set up the immune system for an even faster and more robust immune response in the future, usually without any disease symptoms.

As will become evident in the later chapters, COVID-19 vaccines were rapidly developed in an attempt to educate the adaptive immune system to prevent COVID-19 following exposure to SARS-CoV-2. In North America and Europe, the strategy was to employ totally new types of unproven genetic vaccines that were developed in a hurried fashion and inadequately tested for efficacy and safety. The immune responses that were produced from these vaccines relied on production of antibodies of the IgG class, which are present at much lower concentrations in the upper airway passages and upper lungs than IgM and IgA antibodies. These vaccines required regular boosting due to their directed response to spike protein only, mutation of the spike protein in the evolving SARS-CoV-2 variants, and the poor establishment of immune memory.

The original Wuhan SARS-CoV-2 strain appears to have been much more virulent in causing death than the variants of concern that arose later. The early limited COVID-19 mortality data guided later public health responses and prompted the vast majority of unvaccinated recipients in Phase 3 clinical studies to quickly get vaccinated within a few months of the onset of these trials when they were unblinded. A private organization in the United Kingdom established the Control Group Cooperative with tens of thousands of unvaccinated individuals to ascertain the effectiveness of natural immunity.[44] In a survey of 18,497 unvaccinated members that reported their health status between September 2021 and February 2022 (during the Delta and Omicron BA.1 and BA.2 predominant periods of the COVID-19 pandemic), 25.1 percent had SARS-CoV-2-like symptoms (14.4 percent mild; 8.7 percent moderately severe; 2 percent severe; 1.4 percent hospitalized) and another 3 percent had confirmed SARS-CoV-2 infections, but were asymptomatic.[45] Because the survey findings were self-reported, there were not data for those that would have died from COVID-19. However, these findings do indicate that the likelihood of hospitalization as a consequence of SARS-CoV-2 infection was only 0.4 percent during the six-month study period, which encompassed one of the largest waves of COVID-19 cases during the pandemic. Consequently, the Omicron variants were not particularly virulent, and/or there was already a high degree of natural immunity already in the unvaccinated population prior to their predominance.

The protection against COVID-19 conferred by natural immunity following recovery from a SARS-CoV-2 infection, especially with the less virulent Omicron subvariants, is now very evident. In a large Israeli retrospective study that tracked 124,500 individuals from June 1 to August 14, 2021, the SARS-CoV-2-naïve vaccinees were six- to thirteen-fold more likely to experience a breakthrough SARS-CoV-2 Delta infection compared to previously infected unvaccinated persons.[46] In another United Kingdom study with 25,661 participants, conducted from June 18 to December 31, 2020, the risk of a new SARS-CoV-2 infection and COVID-19 was reduced by 81 percent if the participant had previously been infected and recovered.[47] For those that became re-infected, the median interval between the primary and reinfection was about 7.9 months, and about half of these participants were asymptomatic for COVID-19. The robustness and durability of natural immunity for protection against illness from new SARS-CoV-2 infections, including subsequent variants, is well documented in other studies.[48, 49]

CHAPTER 9

The Effectiveness and Risks of Masks

Steven Pelech & John Hardie

"No one can wear a mask for very long."

—Seneca the Younger

"If you can get a cotton material like a T-shirt, you cut it up, you fold it and put elastic bands around it—this is a non-medical facial covering."

—Dr. Theresa Tam

Before the development of COVID-19 vaccines, the primary strategies employed by public health officials to slow the spread of SARS-CoV-2 were quarantining, restrictions of congregations of peoples, and masking. The mandatory wearing of masks to prevent the spread of SARS-CoV-2 infection was one of the most controversial public health measures instigated in response to the COVID-19 pandemic. Despite the widespread adoption of masking, the purpose of this chapter is to critically analyze the scientific literature to assess the merits and caveats that have been identified for this practice. At this juncture, there appears to be little justification from randomized controlled trials and other measures of a significant benefit from mask wearing with respect to reducing the spread of the SARS-CoV-2 virus. By contrast, growing data indicate many physiological and psychological outcomes from extended mask wearing in hospital and community settings.

9.1. History of Masking for Protection against Environmental Assaults

The use of masks to prevent disease goes back to at least ancient Roman times when the naturalist and philosopher Pliny the Elder suggested fashioning masks out of animal bladders to protect minors from poisonous lead oxide.[1] During the seventeenth and eighteenth centuries, plague doctors in Europe used masks with beaks stuffed with aromatic spices and herbs to protect against contagions in the air that were described as bad odors.[2] This later evolved in the nineteenth and twentieth centuries into tight-fitting gas masks with protective eye glass sockets, and with charcoal and other filters to block passage of gases and microbes into the mouth and nose. During World War I, it became critical to wear gas masks made of gauze, cloth, and other materials to fend off attacks with poisoned gases. Early on, Canadian soldiers used urine-soaked rags as makeshift gas masks against German advances employing chlorine gas. During the Spanish Flu pandemic of 1918–1920, cloth mask wearing was mandatory in some American jurisdictions, including San Francisco.[3]

9.2. Masks to Prevent Viral Transmission

The utility of masks to prevent the spread of diseases caused by viruses has been questionable ever since it was observed that viruses could penetrate fine-mesh filters that stopped bacteria. Bacterial cells are typically more than ten times smaller than human blood cells, and viruses are easily an order of magnitude (one tenth) smaller than gut bacteria such as *Escherichia coli*. Influenza and SARS-CoV-2 virus particles are very similar in size, with diameters that are around 0.08 to 0.12 microns and 0.06 to 0.14 microns, respectively.[4, 5] Both are tiny respiratory-disease viruses that are spread in aerosols. (By comparison, even the finest human hair is seventeen microns in width.) Decades of research into the use of masks during influenza pandemics have consistently called into question their effectiveness for prevention of transmission outside of a hospital setting.

Here is what the Canadian Pandemic Influenza Plan for the Health Sector (2006) describes about masks:

> Although there is a lack of evidence that the use of masks prevented transmission of influenza during previous pandemics; in the early phase of an influenza pandemic, it may be prudent for HCWs (healthcare workers) to wear masks when interacting in close face-to-face contact with coughing individuals to minimize influenza transmission. This use of masks is advised when immunization and antivirals are not yet available but is not practical or helpful when pandemic influenza has entered the community. There is no evidence that the use of masks in general public settings will be protective when the virus is circulating widely in the community.[6]

This was followed up in the Government of Canada publication *Surveillance Annex: Canadian Pandemic Influenza Preparedness: Planning Guidance for the Health Sector*, which was updated in December 2015. The word "mask" was only used once in the entire document, and it was in the context that the use of masks still required evaluation as a protective measure.[7]

With the arrival of COVID-19 in Spring 2020, many public health officials initially advised against the implementation of masks as a necessary protective strategy for the public. For example, Dr. Theresa Tam, the chief public health officer for Canada, advocated against asymptomatic people wearing masks and expressed concern over the findings that wearing a mask, and touching it or removing it, increased the risk of contracting the virus.[8] But by September 2, 2020, she argued that Canadians should "stop kissing, avoid face-to-face closeness, wear a mask that covers your mouth and nose, and monitor yourself and your partner for symptoms ahead of any sexual activity. . . . The lowest-risk sexual activity during COVID-19 involves yourself alone."[9]

Dr. Bonnie Henry, the chief public health doctor (titled the Public Health Officer) of the Canadian province of British Columbia also initially argued against mandatory public masking for COVID-19, although on March 16, 2020, she advocated health professionals should use surgical masks.[10] Then on March 19, 2020, Dr. Henry claimed that if a person is not sick, wearing a mask is not effective. She also said wearing a mask in public does not protect a person in any way. On June 22, 2020, Dr. Henry said that people cannot rely on wearing a mask, because "wearing a mask is not what keeps us safe." She reiterated this view on September 11, 2020.[11] Right up to November 18, 2020, she stated that "Ordering universal mask use in all situations creates unnecessary challenges with enforcement and stigmatization." A day later, in a Public Health Order, Dr. Henry proclaimed sweeping mandatory measures that included mandatory masking.[12] This Public Health Order was rescinded on March 11, 2022.[13] On November 17, 2022, Dr. Henry rejected calls for mask mandates for COVID-19 for the public.[14] The Public Health Order for mandatory masking in health-care settings such as hospitals, long-term care, and assisted living facilities in British Columbia was finally lifted on April 6, 2023.[15] However, despite relatively few COVID-19 cases in British Columbia, she re-imposed mandatory masking once again in health-care facilities on October 3, 2023.[16] However, this was only mandatory for health-care workers and not for their patients and visitors.

This mixed messaging was not unique to Canadian health officials. For example, Dr. Anthony Fauci, then director of the US National Institute of Allergy and Infectious Diseases (NIAID), advised in early 2020 that people do not need to wear masks.[17] He later explained that he was worried about the supply of masks for health-care workers, and that the NIAID was unaware at the time that 40 to 45 percent of people were asymptomatic with SARS-CoV-2 infections and that they could still transmit the virus to others (the validity of this conclusion remains highly debatable, as discussed in chapter 3.6). He argued that the data later became very clear about the effectiveness and importance of mask wearing.[18]

The World Health Organization (WHO) also delayed recommending the adoption of masks for reducing COVID-19 transmission until June 2020 due to a lack of clear evidence from community-based, randomized-controlled trials.[19, 20] The WHO had concerns that mask-wearing might create a false sense of security against SARS-CoV-2 infection. In April 2020, the WHO recommended masking only for health-care workers and those that were symptomatic for COVID-19 or otherwise medically compromised. The WHO did not recommend the widespread use of masks. In a follow-up meta-analysis study that was commissioned by the WHO, there was no scientifically justified evidence to support mask wearing.[21] The Chu et al. (2020) analysis contained no randomized controlled trials for COVID-19, but rather used a mixture of data about associations of ill-defined factors. Their appraisal of "certainty" regarding their conclusions about masks was "LOW," and they stated that "our confidence in the effect estimate is limited; the true effect could be substantially different from the estimate of the effect" (from their Table 2). Another subsequent meta-analysis that year further confirmed that there was weak evidence for any benefits of masking for protection against COVID-19.[22]

Since then, the argument put forth by the public health officials has been that the "science" has changed and that the mounting data related to COVID-19 spread showed the effectiveness of even simple cloth masks. Proponents of masking have suggested with little evidence that even asymptomatic individuals with a SARS-CoV-2 infection can shed high viral loads, and 40 to 45 percent of those infected with the virus are asymptomatic.[23, 24] However, none of these studies appear to have specifically evaluated "live" virus. Moreover, it was claimed that masks can filter out 65 to 85 percent of aerosolized SARS-CoV-2 particles depending on the mask type.[25] However, the evidence for the effectiveness of masks to prevent the spread of COVID-19 was not so black and white.[26]

Much of the published evidence has relied on small studies that focused on physical properties of masks, often with robotic mask wearers, and examined the spread of solid particles rather than the spread of infection. Furthermore, much of the evidence for the efficacy of masks to prevent COVID-19 transmission is supported by PCR testing, which at the thermal cycle numbers typically used, can generate 90 percent or more false-positives.[27] The viral RNA detected might correspond to fragments of inactive virus rather than the intact virus. It is important to appreciate that only the intact virus can replicate in the new host to propagate an infection. In hospitals or in households with symptomatic members there can be high concentrations of these non-infectious RNA fragments floating in the air, which could very easily pass through masks and generate false-positive PCR testing results in people that are not actually infected with intact virus.

Even if masking could be shown to have a significant effect on blocking COVID-19 transmission, many of the mandated masking policies simply did not make sense. Some examples of the illogical rules included: wearing masks to enter a restaurant but not when eating; wearing masks while outside, even at beaches and alone, and masking children in day care except during sleep time. Rancourt (2020) challenged many of the assertions about mask wearing to prevent the transmission of COVID-19.[28] In consideration of the effectiveness of masks as barriers to viral entry and exit via the mouth and nose, it is important to consider the physical properties of masks and the SARS-CoV-2 virus.

9.3. The Physics of Mask Wearing and Aerosolized Viruses

Previous experiences with influenza pandemics likely caused skepticism as to how effective standard medical masks truly were at preventing SARS-CoV-2 infections. As mentioned above, influenza and the SARS-CoV-2 virus are similar in size and are primarily transmitted in suspended droplets in the air. A person symptomatic with COVID-19 might, through coughing and sneezing, expel infectious virus particles in droplets that have the velocity and viral load to be effective in transmission. Most larger droplets from sneezing or coughing range from sixty to a hundred microns in size and can travel up to two meters (at ten meters per second) before they either fall to the ground or disappear completely due to evaporation.[29] Extremely large droplets can be up to a thousand microns in size and will drop even faster. With normal breathing (at one meter per second) and viral particles in a suspended aerosol form, which is less than sixty microns, the range for a possible transmission to occur is a meter or less.[30] Moreover, such tiny droplets evaporate within seconds at room temperature, and the survival of the SARS-CoV-2 virus in a dried out, desiccated form is unclear, although depending on temperature and humidity, the virus has been proposed to last with infectious potential for two to three days.[31] Inhaled particulates that are larger than a hundred microns do not usually pass beyond the nose and larynx, whereas those that are ten microns or less can travel into the upper lungs.[32]

It is indeed reasonable to conclude that someone who is physically sick with COVID-19 may reduce transmission of the virus by wearing a face covering that can capture large droplets generated by sneezing or coughing. Presumably, such an individual would be unlikely to be out and about and interacting with the public. The argument has been advanced that, since surgical masks are routinely used in operations to prevent transmission of infectious diseases, they must work. However, it should be appreciated that surgical masks are really used to prevent large droplets from the surgeons and support staff from falling into sterile surgical sites and as personal protection for the surgical staff from splashes of body fluids from their patients. They are aware that these are not intended for protection against viruses.

The real question is how likely is it that cloth face masks, surgical masks, and even N95 masks will be able to block the exit of aerosolized SARS-CoV-2 virus from an infected person and prevent the entry of these suspended viral droplets through these masks? This depends on the pore sizes of these masks, which are effectively holes that will still allow the wearer to breathe. The pore sizes in each of these masks vary over a ten-fold range, and it is important to determine the sizes of the majority of pores. Evaluation of the filtration performance of masks is determined by their microstructures (such as fiber diameter, thickness, and porosity), surface charge density, and environmental conditions (such as air velocity, aerosol particle diameter, temperature, and humidity).

In a study by Du et al. (2021), the pore-size distributions of cloth face masks, surgical masks, and N95 masks were carefully examined with solid particulates to evaluate pore sizes.[33] The investigators used X-ray tomographic imaging, which is a non-destructive approach to characterize the pore distribution in the mask materials. In all tested masks, most of the pores were thirty microns or greater in size (Table 9.1). In view of the size of the SARS-CoV-2 virus particle relative to the sizes of most of the pores in these masks, the analogy has been made that the masks are just as likely to block virus entry and exit as a chain-wire fence is to stop mosquitos.

Table 9.1. Aerosol permeability of commercial face masks.[34]

Face Mask Type	Peak Pore Size (microns)	Porosity (%)	Breathability	Permeability (per micron^2)
N95	30	65	Low	0.26
Surgical	35	77	Medium	0.34
Reusable	45	82	Medium	0.37

The flow resistance of masks also plays a role in the aerosol permeability of commercial face masks. The flow streamlines during exhalation through three types of face masks have been modeled.[35] This provides information on the highest relative velocity of the aerosol particles. It was evident that higher air permeability occurs in the reusable masks, which demonstrates lower blocking efficiency. The N95 masks have the most heterogeneous flow in the outlet plane, and droplets have the slowest diffusion rates through this type of mask. Ultimately, air flow resistance provided especially by N95 masks will necessitate some rebreathing of expired air and reduce the passage of fresh air. Other experiments have shown an increase in airway resistance by a remarkable 126 percent on inhalation and 122 percent on exhalation with an N95 mask.[36] Moisturization of the N95 masks can increase the breathing resistance by a further 3 percent,[37] which can ultimately increase the airway resistance up to

2.3 times the normal value. The greater the airway resistance, the more likely it is that a person will be re-breathing their exhaled air.

Another significant consideration is the breathability of commercial masks, which can be monitored by real-time infrared thermal imaging. Both the reusable cloth mask and the surgical mask exhibit better breathing comfort than the N95 mask as higher temperatures are observed with the N95 masks by this method.[38]

Many videos demonstrate that reusable cloth masks and surgical masks permit particulates to escape at the upper and side-ends of these masks. While coughing, jets of aerosols are generated toward the backend of tightly fitting masks. Air venting past the ears, which is the other common location of leakage with low-cost masks, means that aerosols are generally directed behind a person. Public health policies usually recommend that people turn away from others in close proximity when they cough. This increases the chance of someone being exposed to pulmonary aerosols with a higher flow rate than if they did not wear a mask. The principles of distributing pulmonary aerosols over the eyes and behind the mask wearer also holds true for face shields. Even if low-cost masks could be properly sealed around the neck and face, SARS-CoV-2-laden aerosols can still readily pass through the relatively large pore sizes of the filtering material.

For over fifty years prior to World War I, the wearing of mustaches was mandatory in British soldiers and common in European soldiers by the early 1800s.[39] With the use of lethal gases in World War I, the gas mask became critical for survival in the battlefield. However, fulsome mustaches interfered with the proper fitting of gas masks. Adolf Hitler, who served in the German army in World War I, was apparently ordered to shave his full mustache, which was transformed into a "toothbrush" moustache, although near the end of that war he still experienced ill effects from being gassed.[40] Then and now, beards have been fashionable. This is why the use of looser fitting cloth, surgical, and N95 respirator masks on persons sporting a beard today were rather pointless even if it was able to prevent entry or exit of the SARS-CoV-2 through these facial barriers. It is also noteworthy that respiratory viruses are also able to gain entry through the eyes and ears, which these masks are not designed to prevent.

Some caution must be exercised in assessing video evidence of the passage of water droplets through masks, although there are videos that demonstrate solid particulate matter passing through masks, including dust from sanding dried gypsum mud. Some videos have shown that aerosols can pass through five surgical masks that are layered over each other. However, the interpretation of these videos is complicated by the fact that most of the water in exhaled breath is in a vapor form that easily penetrates through masks. Once the water vapor passes through the mask into cooler air from the 37° Celsius (98.6° Fahrenheit) temperature in the lungs, it condenses into tiny liquid droplets that become visible on a cold day in the air or on a cool surface.

Some materials used in face masks such as polypropylene may enhance filtering effectiveness by generating a triboelectric charge (a form of static electricity), which enhances the capture of charged particles.[41] Other materials such as silk might help repel moist droplets and reduce fabric wetting and thus maintain breathability and comfort.[42]

Another issue worthy of mention is related to the frequent reuse of masks by the public. Some aerosolized viral particles exhaled by an infected person will accumulate on the mask. While the mask was worn, the humidity generated from breathing might permit the virus particles to remain hydrated. However, when the mask is off, these aerosol droplets will shrink in size from evaporation, and the reuse of the mask permits a sufficient concentration of viral particles to re-infect the person at a higher viral load, especially if such viruses are insensitive to desiccation.

In consideration of the effectiveness of masking to prevent infection and the spread of SARS-CoV-2, it is worthwhile to appreciate that the virus is considered by the Public Health Agency of Canada as a biosafety level (BSL) 3 pathogen. There are about a dozen research facilities that handle SL3 pathogens in Canada and only one in Winnipeg that can work with BSL4 pathogens such as the Marburg and Ebola viruses. In a BSL3 laboratory, the requirements that scientists must use to ensure safe handling of SARS-CoV-2 typically include the following:

1. Handling of SARS-CoV-2 can only be done inside a certified BSL3 or BSL4 facility.
2. Anything containing SARS-CoV-2 can only be opened inside a biological safety cabinet, which is designed to provide a barrier between the virus and the scientist by sucking air into the cabinet and passing the air through HEPA filters before it is exhausted out of the cabinet.
3. The scientist must wear a full body suit, including shoe covers and gloves. A head covering attached to a clear face shield that seals around the neck and face must be worn. The head covering is connected by a tube to a pump that delivers filtered air into it, thereby maintaining positive pressure (i.e., ambient air cannot flow into the head covering).

Figure 9.1 (located in the insert) shows a photograph of the personal protective equipment required to prevent the wearer from becoming infected with a BSL3 pathogen, such as SARS-CoV-2. A person wearing a low-cost mask would simply not be allowed to enter a BSL3 laboratory due to a profound lack of protection. Clearly there is a large disconnect between what is truly considered to protect an individual from SARS-CoV-2 and the public health messaging surrounding cloth and surgical masks, which falsely implies a substantial amount of protection.

9.4. Key Studies that Support Mask Wearing to Prevent COVID-19 Spread

A few published studies have been cited by public health officials to support the contention that masks are a useful means to reduce infection and transmission with SARS-CoV-2 and the spread of COVID-19. The conductance of clinical and field studies is more generally discussed in chapter 10 in the context of drug and vaccine studies. A key issue with studies of the effectiveness of masks, as with other epidemiology studies, is the influence of confounding variables. It is often hard to disentangle whether any of the moderate reduction in COVID-19 spread with masking is not instead due to unmeasured confounding factors such as the practices of increased physical distancing and hand hygiene. At the end of June 2023, eighteen such studies had been profiled on the US Food and Drug Administration (FDA)'s website.[43] Several of the more notable studies are considered next.

Leffler et al. (2020) based on analysis of data from 169 countries and modelling reported that in countries with cultural norms or government policies supporting public mask-wearing, the per-capita coronavirus mortality increased on average by just 16.2 percent each week, as compared with 61.9 percent each week in remaining countries.[44] In countries with high morbidity from COVID-19, the duration of peak COVID-19 cases without masks had a mean of 6.69 weeks compared to countries with low morbidity without masks, which had a mean of 4.74 weeks duration. However, there were many other confounding factors that complicated the interpretation of these findings. Firstly, by May 9, 2020, low-mortality countries had performed one test for every 575 members of the population, whereas high-mortality countries had performed one test for every eighty-three members of the population. Therefore, more deaths might have been attributed to COVID-19 in those countries with higher morbidity rates. Those countries that had lower morbidity rates also had younger populations with 60 percent more of their population under fourteen years of age. The death rates were also affected by other differences, including more urbanization of the population in countries that experienced higher mortality. Increased urbanization results in greater population density and increased opportunity for viral spread. Most countries that adopted masking early with lower mortality were Asian. Interestingly, in the same study, time since the start of international travel restrictions tended to be statistically inversely associated with mortality.

Chernozhukov et al. (2021) reported that employee mask mandates reduced mortality by 34 percent based on mathematical modelling. The authors stressed that their study was "observational and should be interpreted with great caution."[45] They further noted that their "approach explicitly recognizes that policies not only directly affect the spread of COVID-19 (e.g., mask requirement) but also indirectly affect its spread by changing people's behavior (e.g., stay-at-home order). It also recognized that people react to new information on COVID-19 cases and deaths and voluntarily adjust their behavior (e.g., voluntary social distancing and hand washing) even without any policy in place." Thus, in this and most other studies, it is difficult to ascribe reductions in COVID-19 morbidity and mortality as being solely due to the use of masks.

Li et al. (2021) conducted a systematic review and meta-analysis that was ultimately based on six case-control studies that were conducted in China, the United States, Thailand, and Bangladesh. They concluded: "in general, wearing a mask was associated with a significantly reduced risk of COVID-19 infection (Odd Ratio (OR) = 0.38, 95% Confidence Interval (CI): 0.21–0.69)."[46] An OR of 0.38 could be interpreted as a 62 percent reduction of COVID-19 incidence. The relatively low number of case studies used in this analysis is somewhat problematic but does reflect the strict criteria that the authors tried to employ in selecting suitable data sources. Nevertheless, two of these studies were extremely underpowered, as shown in Table 1 of the review, with only forty participants in the masked group and thirty-two in the unmasked group in one Chinese study, and in the only US investigation, three and thirty-four participants, respectively. It was only known for two of these studies which kind of masks (i.e., N95) were used. When only healthcare workers were considered, the effect of masking was more statistically significant (OR = 0.29, 95 percent CI: 0.18–0.44). When the data in aggregate are considered, the relative risk reduction by masking was 43 percent and the absolute risk reduction was 8.6 percent for getting COVID-19 during the study periods. Absolute risk reduction better reflects the true impact of the intervention on the population.

In another systematic review and meta-analysis from the same group,[47] the authors did not apply PRISMA-P (Preferred reporting items for systematic review and meta-analysis protocols),[48] nor did they perform GRADE (Grading of Recommendations, Assessment, Development, and Evaluations) reliability analysis,[49] which is the established standard when such medical research is intended to be used for policy guidance. If Liang et al. (2020) applied GRADE to their investigation it would be invalid, because the studies that were included were not random controlled trials (RCTs), and because its confidence intervals encompass outcomes that would fail to support the recommendation of masks.[50] RCTs are the gold standard on which to base reliable clinical data.

In the Li et al. (2021) meta-analysis, one of the larger studies was performed in Bangladesh by Khalil et al. (2020) from May to June 2020.[51] The data were collected from hospital physicians that recalled events and filled out a survey form. Of the COVID-19 positive physicians, 59.8 percent had worn face-shields and/or goggles, compared to 77.3 percent of the COVID-19-negative physicians. The use of medical surgical masks was essentially the same in the COVID-19 positive and negative groups (96.7 percent and 95.5 percent, respectively) during the routine care of COVID-19 patients. During aerosol-generating procedures, despite a wide range of possible measures, including face shields, only the use of N95 masks was determined to statistically significantly reduce COVID-19 incidence, and this was by 27.8 percent.[52]

Another major study in Bangladesh by Abaluck et al. (2020) has been cited by public health agencies to justify COVID-19 mask mandates.[53] Between November 2020 and April 2021, 342,183 adults were examined across 572 villages where various mask promotion strategies were tested. However, there was only a 9 percent reduction in symptomatic seroprevalence of SARS-CoV-2 evident in villages that received mask interventions when compared to other villages without implementation of such measures. The proportion of individuals with COVID-19–like symptoms was 7.63 percent (N = 12,784) in the intervention arm and 8.60 percent (N = 13,287) in the control arm, which indicates an over-all absolute risk reduction of around 1 percent. In this study, the campaign to promote mask wearing increased usage to 42.3 percent in villages with in-person interventions compared to 13.3 percent when intervention measures were not introduced. It has been argued that if there were a greater adoption of masking, the reduction in symptomatic COVID-19 could have been higher. Social and physical distancing were also encouraged in the villages exposed to the masking campaigns, so it was difficult to evaluate how much of the modest reduction on COVID-19 cases was solely due to the masks. The authors noted that while they believed that surgical masks were effective in reducing symptomatic seroprevalence of SARS-CoV-2, this reduction did not appear to achieve statistical significance for cloth masks.

Leung et al. (2020) studied surgical mask-wearing in 246 symptomatic individuals with influenza, rhinovirus, and seasonal coronaviruses infections.[54] Using PCR tests, they recorded a significant reduction in detectable virus in exhaled breath droplets and aerosols in the 124 individuals that were randomized to wearing masks (four of ten versus zero of eleven, $p = 0.04$). However, this study did not confirm that the observed viral RNA was from intact and infectious virus. It is likely that fragmented, inactive SARS-CoV-2 was primarily detected.

Interestingly, Spiegel and Tookes (2021) reported mask recommendations increased deaths by 3.1 percent, whereas mask mandates reduced deaths by only 5.9 percent over a two-week testing period.[55] In this comprehensive study, a time-series database was constructed of business closures and related restrictions including masking for every county in the United States from March 1 through December 31, 2020. Fatalities were examined rather than COVID-19 cases to avoid bias introduced by substantial variation in testing capacity over time and region.

9.5. Studies that Do Not Support Mask Wearing to Prevent COVID-19 Spread

While masking has been widely adopted and even mandated as a major measure to control the spread of COVID-19, over a hundred studies challenge the validity of this approach compared to the few investigations that support it.[56,57] The following publications document a few of the many studies that question the benefits of masking for the prevention and control of COVID-19.

The DANMASK-19 study in Denmark was one of the first RCTs to investigate the effectiveness of masks to mitigate SARS-CoV-2 infections.[58] In follow-up studies after one month, 1.8 percent (forty-two of 2392) of participants in the mask group and 2.1 percent (fifty-three of 2470) in the control group developed infection. This small 14 percent decline was not statistically significant ($p = 0.38$).

Hunter et al. (2021) reported no effect of mandating or recommending masks on reducing COVID-19 mortality in thirty European countries during 2020.[59] Surprisingly, the mask mandates correlated with a slight increase in the incidence of COVID-19 cases, although the authors cautioned against drawing strong conclusions due to differences between the countries when mask recommendation advisories were introduced and mask mandates were imposed.

Lyu et al. (2020) examined mandated face mask use in sixteen US states and compared these to states without mask mandates from April 8 to May 15, 2020. They reported that "daily COVID-19 growth rates significantly declined, but only by 0.9%, 1.1%, 1.4%, 1.7%, and 2.0% at 1–5, 6–10, 11–15, 16–20, and 21 or more days following the state mandate, respectively." However, a significant impact of employee-only mask mandates (no public community requirement) was not evident.[60]

Liu et al. (2021) concluded that "fourteen of sixteen identified randomized controlled trials comparing face masks to no mask controls failed to find statistically significant benefit in the intent-to-treat populations."[61]

Studies looking at the effect of face masks on the spread of influenza have shown little if any benefit. Barasheed et al. (2014) carried out a study randomizing tents at the Hajj (an annual Islamic pilgrimage event to Mecca, the holiest city for Islam) to "supervised mask use" (mask use 76 percent) or "no supervised mask use" (mask use 12 percent) for individuals with influenza-like illness (ILI) and also their contacts who slept within two meters.[62] It should be noted that "flu-like illness" or "influenza-like illness" means non-laboratory-confirmed infection, based on reported symptoms or clinical observations. Such determinations are not "verified outcomes" and are thus more susceptible to bias. The authors observed less ILI among contacts in the mask group (31 percent versus 53 percent, $p = 0.04$), but there were no differences in laboratory-confirmed respiratory virus detections.

Aiello et al. (2012) performed a cluster RCT in university residents and found no effect in the primary analysis of influenza-like illness or laboratory-confirmed respiratory infections with masking alone.[63]

Cowling et al. (2009) conducted a cluster RCT of 259 households with confirmed influenza patients to evaluate the effectiveness of surgical masks with and without hand hygiene.[64] There were no statistically significant differences in either laboratory-confirmed or clinical influenza infection with the masks or the combination of mask with hand hygiene. However, if the intervention was applied within thirty-six hours of symptom-onset in the index case, mask and hand hygiene together reduced laboratory-confirmed influenza infections but not clinically defined influenza.

MacIntyre et al. (2009) performed a cluster RCT of adult household members masking after a child in the household was diagnosed with a respiratory illness. They compared surgical and N95 masks to no-mask controls. There were no significant differences between either type of mask versus the unmasked controls.[65]

Dugre et al. (2020) conducted a systematic meta-analysis of the effectiveness of masks in health-care workers and the public.[66] They used eleven systematic reviews, with eighteen RCTs, of which twelve were in the community. In their meta-analysis, mask-wearing by the public did not reduce clinical respiratory infection or confirmed influenza or any other viral respiratory infection.

Another meta-analysis by Aggarwal et al. (2020) using pooled controlled trials failed to identify a significant effect for either mask use alone or in combination with hand hygiene versus control in reducing influenza-like illness in household and university settings.[67]

The research group of Dr. MacIntyre has published several studies that have evaluated the effectiveness of masks in different settings to control respiratory infections. Dr. MacIntyre had received substantial grant funding from 3M, which is a major manufacturer of surgical and N95 masks. In an earlier study with 1,441 doctors and nurses in fifteen Beijing hospitals, the same researchers reported that the rates of respiratory tract infection were approximately double in the medical mask group compared to the N95 group in health workers who continuously wore masks throughout their shift.[68] However, there were no statistically significant differences with other interventions such as use of medical masks, vaccination, and handwashing.

MacIntyre et al. (2013) determined in RCT studies that ordinary cloth masks are thirteen times less efficient than medical-type surgical masks for prevention of influenza-like illness.[69, 70] Penetration of cloth masks by influenza and other respiratory viruses, including common cold coronaviruses, was almost 97 percent and with medical masks was reduced to 44 percent. They also described less than 0.01 percent penetration of N95 masks, which seems to be at odds with many other studies. The authors stressed in 2020 that cloth masks would not be desirable for protection against SARS-CoV-2 compared to surgical masks.[71] Remarkably, in these clinical studies, the cloth masked group had 3.5-fold more respiratory infections than the control group with a 58.5 percent reduction in mask use.

MacIntyre et al. (2016) performed a cluster, randomized, controlled trial of surgical masks for patients with ILI (n = 123) compared to controls (n = 122) and evaluated the risk of secondary cases in household contacts.[72] There were no statistically significant differences in clinical respiratory illness, ILI, or laboratory-confirmed viral infections in the study groups. Since a third of the controls wore masks, the authors carried out a post-hoc per protocol analysis and noted that masks had a statistically significant protective effect in reducing clinical respiratory infections, but not laboratory-confirmed respiratory infections.

In a more recent review, MacIntyre and Chughtai (2020) examined nineteen RCTs and concluded that respirators (N95 masks) were effective in healthcare workers (but not in community settings). They stated that respirators "if worn continually during a shift, were effective but not if worn intermittently. Medical masks were not effective, and cloth masks even less effective." The results were claimed to have been reported according to the Preferred Reporting Items for Systematic Reviews and Meta-Analyses (PRISMA) criteria.[73] However, Rancourt (2020) pointed out at least eight PRISMA directives that were failed to be adopted in this meta-analysis.[74]

In non-health care settings, masking to protect the wearer is unlikely to be effective. Existing evidence indicates that wearing a mask within households after an illness has begun is largely ineffectual at preventing secondary respiratory infections. Ultimately, decades of research have confirmed that masks do not work for an influenza pandemic, and more recently this has been shown to be so for SARS-CoV-2.[75, 76] This is not surprising, since the influenza and SARS-CoV-2 virus are similarly sized and transmitted. In a recent Cochrane Collaboration meta-analysis done by Jefferson et al. (2023),[77] the authors concluded that masks probably make little or no difference in the transmission of influenza-like or COVID-19–like illness (risk ratio, 0.95 [95 percent CI, 0.84 to 1.09]) and were uncertain if there was any difference between N95 respirators and medical or surgical masks in preventing the spread of viral respiratory illness. On its publication, this Cochrane study received much adverse criticism as the conclusions ran counter to the strong masking narrative offered by public health officials at the time of publication. Note that previous publications from the group offering similar conclusions did not receive the same degree of criticism. The Cochrane editorial board could not arrive at a firm conclusion on the benefits of masks, apparently because there were not enough high-quality randomized trials with high rates of mask adherence.[78, 79] Of the seventy-eight studies assessed, only ten focused on what happens when people wear masks versus when they did not, and another five compared various masks for blocking viral transmission. Many of the studies examined mask use in parallel with other protective measures like hand hygiene and disinfection.

Bowing to political pressure, Karla Soares-Weber, editor in chief of the Cochrane Collaboration, published a communiqué reinterpreting the results of the review. She did this without consulting the twelve authors of the review, the peer reviewers, or the editors who approved its publication, all of whom continue to support the review's original conclusions. Understandably annoyed by the editor's unprofessional behavior, Dr. Jefferson was adamant in a subsequent interview concerning masks that "There is just no evidence that they make any difference. Full stop."[80]

9.6. Studies of Masking in Children to Prevent COVID-19 Spread

The studies that have evaluated the benefits of masking in children are fewer in number and have demonstrated variable, but generally limited results with respect to their effectiveness for source control. Again, many of these studies are performed to evaluate the effectiveness of masks for influenza, but these findings can be extrapolated for SARS-CoV-2. There have also been consistently lower rates of adherence, especially in younger children. The masks currently used for children are adult masks that are manufactured in smaller geometric dimensions and not specially tested nor approved for use with children.

RCTs have been undertaken for evaluating mask use for influenza prevention in the community that included children as the index cases. Two studies, where implementation was within thirty-six hours of symptom-onset in the index case, found a possible protective effect for a combination of masking and hand hygiene together.[81, 82] However, two other studies failed to demonstrate any protective effect from mask wearing.[83, 84]

Suess et al. (2012) conducted a cluster of RCTs comparing masking, masking with hand hygiene, or unmasked controls in eighty-four households, including starting (index) cases, with influenza infection in the 2009/10 and 2010/11 seasons. There were no significant effects from masking with or without hand hygiene in the primary analysis. Almost all index cases were children under fourteen years of age (eighty-one of eighty-four [96 percent]). However, the average daily adherence to masking by index patients ranged from 40–60 percent and decreased over time.

Canini et al. (2010) conducted a cluster RCT of the effect of masking five days after patients (33 percent under age fifteen years old) tested positive for influenza with a rapid test. ILI was found in 16.2 percent of contacts where the index case was masked and 15.8 percent when the index case was not masked. There were no significant differences between surgical mask wearers and control groups. The children in this study were significantly more likely to report mask discomfort (such as feeling pain), compared to adults (three of twelve [25 percent] versus one of thirty-nine [2.6 percent], $p = 0.036$).

Simmerman et al. (2011) conducted a cluster RCT of 442 households in Thailand during the influenza H1N1 pandemic comparing hand hygiene only, hand hygiene with masking with surgical masks, or unmasked controls to prevent influenza transmission in households with an influenza-positive child.[85] Half of the index patients were under six years of age. There were no differences in clinical or laboratory confirmed influenza in either intervention arm compared to the controls.

Uchida et al. (2017) completed an observational questionnaire-based study with 10,524 school-aged children in Japan, of whom 5,474 (52.0 percent) reported wearing masks.[86] Using a multivariable logistic regression model, it appeared that wearing a mask was associated with very moderate reduced risks of influenza infection; 21.3 percent of non-mask-wearing children in grades 1–3 were diagnosed with influenza, compared to 20.2 percent of mask-wearing children (relative effectiveness 5.3 percent, absolute risk reduction 1.1 percent); 21.5 percent of non-mask-wearing children in grades 4–6 were diagnosed with influenza compared to 18.9 percent of mask-wearing children (relative effectiveness 12.0 percent, absolute risk reduction 2.6 percent).

Sandlund et al. (2023) performed a systematic review of the scientific literature up to February 2023 and identified twenty-two published studies that assessed the effectiveness of masking to reduce transmission and severity of COVID-19 in people under eighteen years of age.[87] The authors reported that:

> six observational studies reporting an association between child masking and lower infection rate or antibody seropositivity had critical (n = 5) or serious (n = 1) risk of bias; all six were potentially confounded by important differences between masked and unmasked groups and two were shown to have non-significant results when reanalysed. Sixteen other observational studies found no association between mask wearing and infection or transmission.[88]

No randomized control trials have yet been performed to assess whether mask wearing offers any protection from COVID-19 for children.

9.7. Physiological Risks of Mask Wearing

The decision to support the wearing of masks to protect against the infection and transmission of respiratory diseases such as COVID-19 and influenza must consider the benefits and harms—potential and realized—from this course of action. The previous sections examined whether masking has a substantial impact in reducing the spread of these diseases. At this juncture, it is very questionable whether mask recommendations or mandates provide any significant benefit. Whatever benefit they might provide has to be considered in the face of what harms might also be produced by this practice.

The US CDC has acknowledged, but underplays, that there are adverse effects associated with the wearing of masks to prevent SARS-CoV-2 transmission.[89] These include: "Some studies have found that during intense exercise, especially when approaching the aerobic threshold, wearing a mask can increase dyspnea (difficulty breathing), perceived exertion, and claustrophobia, and produce modest negative effects on measured cardiopulmonary parameters."[90]

It is important to bear in mind that most physiological and subjective physical effects of masks have been observed with healthy people at rest and under exertion.[91, 92] Similar effects of masks are likely to be more pronounced on sick and elderly people even without exertion.

> In some people, face masks worn for longer durations might be associated with skin reactions such as acne, itching, dry skin and worsening of existing dermatoses. Wearing a surgical mask and N95 respirator may have a higher risk of skin reactions compared with a cloth mask.[93]
>
> In children aged 10–17 years who wore masks for 6–7 hours during the school day, some children self-reported general (4–7%) or situation-specific (2–4%) side-effects such as skin irritation, headache, or difficulty breathing during physical education.[94]

Over time, the external surface of a mask might become contaminated with SARS-CoV-2 as well as other viruses, bacteria, and fungi. Self-contamination by face touching is a common practice, especially in children. Continuous mask use has been associated with irritant dermatitis, facial skin lesions, worsening acne, and impaired vision in those wearing glasses.[95, 96, 97] Lan et al. (2019) reported skin irritation and itching when using N95 masks among 542 test participants and a correlation between the skin damage that occurred with the time of exposure (68.9 percent at six hours/day and 81.7 percent at more than six hours/day).[98]

The skin problems associated with masks could be caused by the chemicals used in their manufacture. There are different types of surgical masks. Most are made of polypropylene, but some are made from other polymers such as polycarbonate or polystyrene. As phthalates are common additives to polymers, the face mask could be a potential source of phthalate exposure. Exposure to phthalates has been linked with asthma, attention-deficit hyperactivity disorder, breast cancer, obesity, damage to the liver, kidney, lungs, and reproductive systems, prenatal mortality, and low birth weight. Phthalates are used as plasticizers to reduce shear in the polymer production process and to improve flexibility and versatility of the polymers. A commonly used phthalate is polyvinyl acetate phthalate (PVAP). In a study by Xie et al. (2022),[99] twelve possible phthalates were measured in fifty-six mask samples collected from different countries. The phthalates were detected in all the samples, with total levels that ranged from 0.115 μg/g to 37.7 μg/g. Estimated daily intakes (EDIs) of the phthalates from the masks ranged from 0.0037 to 0.639 μg/kg body weight/day, and the EDIs of the phthalates from masks for toddlers were approximately four to five times higher than those for adults. Although non-carcinogenic risks in relation to the phthalates in masks were found to be within safe levels, 89.3 percent of the mask samples exhibited potential carcinogenic effects to humans.

Contact eczema and urticaria can arise from hypersensitivities to other ingredients of the industrially manufactured masks (surgical mask and N95) such as formaldehyde (an ingredient of the textile fabric of the mask) and thiram (an ingredient of the ear bands).[100, 101] Formaldehyde is a biocide and a known carcinogen. The hazardous substance thiram, originally a pesticide and corrosive, is used in the rubber industry.

A study of intensive care-unit nurses observed physiologic respiratory changes from the prolonged use of N95 masks, but these findings were subtle and not considered clinically relevant.[102] In a study of New York health-care workers that described various subjective complaints (e.g., headache, impaired cognition), only skin effects (e.g., irritation, acne) were commonly reported.[103] Wearing surgical or N95 masks caused headaches in 71.4 percent, drowsiness in 23.6 percent, detectable skin damage in 51 percent, and acne in 53 percent of the mask users. In a Singapore investigation of 322 participants using N95 masks, acne was detected in up to 59.6 percent of them, with itching in 51.4 percent and redness in 35.8 percent reported as side effects.[104]

Studies performed with children have identified low adherence to proper use in school settings,[105, 106, 107] but the impact of mask use on the quality of children's education is less clear.

Long-term prevention of exposure to the microbial world and natural environment in children has been associated with an increased incidence of allergies, asthma, and autoimmune diseases based on an immunological principle known as the "hygiene hypothesis."[108, 109] On the one hand, the wearing of the masks during the COVID-19 pandemic, even if masks are ineffective against respiratory viruses that are the size of coronaviruses, should reduce exposure to bacteria, fungi, and other larger immunogens such as pollens. While the concept of the "hygiene hypothesis" is less favored today because it conveys a sense that hygiene is not as desirable for a developing immune system, moderate and targeted exposure to pathogens is still desirable for preventing infectious diseases. However, government COVID-19 policies that restricted children from sports and other outdoor activities, as well as closure of schools and encouragement to stay home, wear masks, and use hand sanitizers frequently, have likely undermined the development of children's adaptive immune systems with possible long-term adverse consequences. This could result in a generation of "pandemic youth" that will grow up to experience even higher than average rates of allergies, asthma, and autoimmune diseases due to being raised in isolated and highly sanitized environments during a critical period of their immunological development.

On the other hand, the warm and humid microclimate environment created in and underneath masks might offer ideal growth and breeding grounds for pathogenic bacteria and fungi, and for the accumulation of viruses on and in masks.[110] At these mask sites, immune and other protective body defenses, such as the complement system, innate and adaptive immune cells, antibodies, and pathogen-inhibiting peptides on mucous membranes, are unable to be effective.[111, 112] The longer a mask is worn or reused, the germ density increases, by as much as ten-fold after only two hours of use.[113]

Another undesirable consequence of masking is "mask mouth," which is associated with increased inflammation of the gums (gingivitis), bad breath (halitosis, fungal infection with *Candida albicans* (candidiasis), lip inflammation especially in the corners of the mouth (cheilitis), dental plaque accumulation, and dental caries.[114, 115] This is attributed in part to reduced saliva flow and increased breathing through an open mouth under the mask to improve oxygen uptake. The presence of accumulating germs in and under the mask is also likely to contribute to these phenomena.

Ironically, since masks can muffle speech and make it harder for listeners to hear, there is also a tendency for mask wearers to speak louder,[116] and the increased volume of speech contributes to increased aerosol production by mask wearers.[117] This might counteract any benefits masks provide in preventing the spread of infectious virus.

Moreover, there is evidence that people wearing fabric, surgical, and N95 masks release significantly and proportionately smaller particles into the air than maskless people, when breathing, speaking, and coughing.[118] Apparently, masks can act as nebulizers and produce very fine aerosol droplets of three microns or less that can spread faster and further than those that are produced by unmasked people. In this 2020 study by Asadi et al.,[119] test subjects that wore single-layer fabric masks released 384 percent more particles when breathing than unmasked participants.

9.8. Impact of Masking on Blood Oxygen and Carbon Dioxide Levels

An important consideration with respect to potential issues of mask wearing relates to the inspiration of oxygen (O_2) and expiration of carbon dioxide (CO_2). The concentration of O_2 in the atmosphere is around 20.95 percent, whereas the concentration of CO_2 is a mere 0.04 percent. Human exhalation contains about 14–16 percent O_2 and 4–5.3 percent CO_2 under resting conditions. The more physically active a person is, the higher the O_2 requirement with a corresponding increase in CO_2 production. Consequently, with tighter-fitting masks, which are necessary, in principle, to block entry of aerosolized viruses, the rebreathing of exhaled air will reduce O_2 availability and increase CO_2 production. The availability of O_2 in the blood and body tissues is critical to fuel the metabolic reactions in the body, and especially in the brain. If these levels are too low, the breathing and heart rates will increase to compensate for the hypoxia (decrease in O_2). Over time, red blood cell production may also increase to provide further compensation, which occurs in people that live at high altitudes where O_2 levels are lower in the atmosphere.

Over the past century, surgical masks have been used routinely by healthcare workers, sometimes for eight hours or more per day. One might expect that if they caused problems, this would certainly be evident by now. As it turns out, they can cause problems for some individuals. In view of the importance of maintenance of O_2 levels for healthy breathing and clearance of CO_2, this is not surprising. During surgical operations where surgeons and their support staff wear surgical masks for very long periods, it is important to note that the operating rooms are well ventilated and have extra O_2 that can be as high as 23.5 percent. This usually results from leakage of the oxygen delivered to anesthetized patients. Higher concentrations of O_2 than 23.5 percent increase the risk of a fire in a surgical area.

The oxygenation of blood from aeration of the lungs and the removal of CO_2, which is produced by mitochondrial respiration, is critical to maintain healthy cells in the body. The consumption of O_2 is necessary for most of the production of adenosine-triphosphate, which is the major compound used to drive most biochemical reactions in the body and is essential for making the cellular nucleic acids DNA and RNA. The build-up of excess CO_2 in the blood, known as hypercapnia, is also harmful, particularly in people with chronic obstructive pulmonary disease. Hypercapnia causes shortness of breath, and can produce tiredness, fatigue, irritability, headaches, fever, and sweating during wake time. In more extreme cases, it can also result in disorientation, confusion, paranoia, depression, and seizures.[120]

Several studies have tried to evaluate just how much masking for various times and levels of physical activity affects respiration. In one study performed with twenty-two infants (under two years of age) and twenty-five children (two to twelve years of age), the effect of wearing masks for up to sixty minutes was compared to sixty minutes of not wearing masks.[121] Young children have much higher metabolic rates and O_2 demand than adults, which results in higher respiratory rates. In this study, which included a walking test with the children, the O_2 saturation in the blood was maintained, but after completion of the walking test with masking, there were statistically significant increases of 9.4 percent in the heart rate (beats per minute) and 18.2 percent in the number of breaths per minute to compensate for the effects of the masks.

In another study by Shaw et al. (2021), twenty-one male and five female hockey players with an average age of 11.7 years were examined for the effects of a three-layer surgical face mask on the arterial O_2 levels over the course of seven simulated hockey shifts.[122] The authors claimed that there were no significant differences in blood oxygenation, but there was evidence of lower oxygenation of tissues, especially in the seventh shift for the females. In the males, there was a lower tissue oxygenation index with masking in the first six shifts, but not the seventh shift. Heart rates were higher with masking. Two of the participants vomited after they wore masks. When reviewing the arterial O_2 saturation data for each shift, it is evident that there were huge differences among the players with respect to their individual measurements, which accounts for why statistical differences in blood oxygenation were unlikely to be evident with such a low number of participants.

In a study that was conducted prior to the COVID-19 pandemic, Roberge et al. (2012) tested twenty adult subjects exercising on a treadmill for an hour with and without surgical masks and measured a variety of physiologic parameters.[123] With regard to blood oxygenation, they found that the mean O_2 concentration of hemoglobin during mask wearing was 97.6 percent whereas without masking it was 97.5 percent. However, the surgical mask use resulted in statistically significant increases in heart rate (by 9.5 beats/minute), respiratory rate (by 1.6 breaths per minute), and transcutaneous carbon dioxide (PtcCO2) (by 2.17 mm of mercury (Hg)), and decreased temperature of uncovered facial skin (by 0.40° Celsius). A 1.76° Celsius (increase in temperature of the skin covered by the mask was associated with a mask dead space apparent heat index of 52.9° Celsius (127.2° Fahrenheit).

In a meta-analysis performed by Kisielinski et al. (2021), the authors reviewed sixty-five publications, of which forty-four had experimental data, to evaluate the known side-effects of mask wearing in what has been described as mask-induced exhaustion syndrome.[124] They observed a wide range of respiratory changes in mask wearers with significant correlation of O_2 drop and fatigue ($p < 0.05$), a clustered co-occurrence of respiratory impairment and O_2 drop (67 percent, in six of nine studies), N95 mask and CO_2 rise (82 percent, in nine of eleven studies), N95 mask and O_2 drop (72 percent, in eight of eleven studies), N95 mask and headache (60 percent, in six of ten studies), respiratory impairment and temperature rise (88 percent, in seven of eight studies), and also temperature rise and moisture (100 percent) under the masks. They concluded that "extended mask-wearing by the general population could lead to relevant effects and consequences in many medical fields."

These effects are not surprising in view of the extra airway resistance introduced with the wearing of a mask, especially after a prolonged period of use. The disturbance of breathing by masks easily explains the observed compensatory reactions with an increase in breathing frequency and simultaneous feeling of breathlessness from increased work of the respiratory muscles. This extra burden due to the amplified work of breathing against larger resistance caused by the masks also leads to intensified exhaustion with a rise in heart rate and increased CO_2 production. Along with significant respiratory impairment, a significant drop in O_2 saturation especially in tissues was commonly found in studies.

Of some concern is the potential effect of masking on a pregnant mother and her unborn child, since there is a requirement to maintain a fetal-maternal CO_2 gradient. The mother's CO_2 blood levels must be lower than that of her baby to ensure diffusion of CO_2 from fetal blood into the maternal circulation. Roberge et al. (2014) reported in a study with twenty-two pregnant women wearing N95 masks during twenty minutes of exercise that there were significantly ($p = 0.04$) higher percutaneous CO_2 values, with average Ptc CO_2 values of 33.3 mm Hg compared to 31.3 mm Hg than in twenty-two pregnant women without masks.[125] The sensation of heat experienced by masked expectant mothers was also significantly increased ($p < 0.001$) in this study.

9.9. Psychological Side Effects of Masking

While masking can produce hypoxia and hypercapnia, which can have effects on the cognitive abilities and reduced responsiveness of individuals, masking can induce many other psychological harms. Impairment of the field of vision (especially the lower field) and of habitual actions such as eating, drinking, touching, scratching, and cleaning, which is perceived consciously and subconsciously as obstruction and restriction, induces discomfort. Resentment and anger are fostered especially when the wearing of masks is imposed by others through mandates. While the wearing of masks for several hours can induce many physical symptoms such as headaches, skin irritation, acne, itching, sensations of heat and dampness, etc., the face area is especially sensitive due to the large representation that the face and head occupy in the cerebral cortex of the brain.[126]

Masks are very effective visual tools to signal danger in the environment during an infectious disease pandemic, thereby alerting the populace that there is danger in their midst, and to act accordingly. However, this can incite an appreciable level of fear and paranoia in many people. In one study by Prousa (2020), masks were found to frequently cause anxiety and psycho-vegetative stress reactions in children and adults along with an increase in psycho-somatic and stress-related illnesses and depressive self-experience, reduced participation, social withdrawal, and lowered health-related self-care.[127] In this study, at least 50 percent of the participants expressed having at least mild depressive feelings.

The loss of facial expression induced by a mask disrupts non-verbal communication due to feelings of insecurity, discouragement, and numbness, as well as isolation. This can be extremely stressful for the mentally and hearing impaired.[128] The wearing of masks is problematic for those who are deaf or hard of hearing and rely on lip-reading to understand a speaker. The covering of faces can interfere with the normal development of facial recognition in infants. As well, in Canada with a large immigrant population, mask wearing by teachers and students can diminish language acquisition.

Adult mask wearing has profound psychological effects on children. In one study, masks and face shields caused fear in 46 percent of children (thirty-seven out of eighty).[129] When the children were given the choice of whether the doctor examining them should wear a mask, they rejected this 49 percent of the time. Both the children and their parents preferred the practitioner to wear a face visor.

In an observational study of 25,930 mask-wearing children in Germany, 53 percent complained of headaches, 50 percent of difficulty concentrating, 49 percent of joylessness, 38 percent of learning difficulties, 37 percent of fatigue, and 25 percent had new onset anxiety or nightmares.[130] The potential of psychosomatic and stress-related illness was evident in a stress survey that found on a scale of one to ten, 65 percent of mask wearers reported the highest score of ten, and less than 10 percent had stress scores less than eight.[131]

While masks might have been promoted originally for their hygienic potential, they have become transformed into visual symbols of conformity and solidarity, signifying a shared responsibility to protect the community for some people. This reduces possible stigmatization of mask wearers who are extra fearful of severe disease and potential death following infection or who are concerned about adversely affecting others with whom they have contact.

For those that are healthy and have a very low risk of severe disease, the wearing of masks does not appear to be sensible. The donning of masks by such individuals has been portrayed as "virtue signaling" whether such labeling is valid or not, since their compliance may have really been an effort to protect the most vulnerable or out of fear for themselves. In any event, when people are walking around wearing masks in isolated places, outdoors, or driving alone in cars, especially when COVID-19 cases numbers are very low, such behavior approaches being a psychosis.

Although the masks were originally intended to protect people from infectious pathogens, they have also come with a heavy economic and environmental toll. The WHO has estimated that during the early phase of the COVID-19 pandemic in 2020 the need for masks was around eighty-nine million per month.[132] However, around fifty-two billion disposable masks were produced in 2020, and about 1.6 billion masks entered the oceans that year.[133] These masks degrade into microfiber plastics in about two years, which will take about another 450 years to ultimately breakdown.[134] Mask pollution from 2020 was calculated to be equal to 7 percent of the Great Pacific Garbage Patch, which floats in the Pacific Ocean. Klemeš et al. (2020a,b) estimated that the production of a single mask consumes about ten to thirty watt-hours of energy and releases fifty-nine grams of CO_2-eq greenhouse gas to the environment.[135, 136] Clearly, the continued use of masks in this manner is unsustainable and will not only cause harm to the human population, but also to much of the other life on the planet Earth.

CHAPTER 10

Evaluating the Efficacy and Safety of Vaccines

Steven Pelech

"Americans broadly consent to funding clinical research because they believe in the promise of medical research. But people support scientific work only if they trust that it serves societal interests, respects patient dignity and operates with guardrails."

—Scott Gottlieb

"Absence of evidence is not evidence of absence."

—Martin Rees

10.1. Pre-Clinical and Clinical Studies

Some studies report on only one patient (case study) or a small sample of patients (clinical or case series). These studies offer some knowledge about novel medical conditions, but are not considered high quality as there is no control group for comparison. For clinical studies that have control groups, the designs are case control studies (sometimes known as retrospective studies), cohort studies (usually prospective studies that compare two groups of patients but not randomized), and the gold standard randomized controlled trials (RCTs). The latter provides the best information as the two groups treated and untreated (control) are balanced by randomization, and usually blinded to the trial participants and often administering physicians (double-blinded) to eliminate bias.

For the testing of a drug, vaccine, or medical device, the underlying principles of the scientific method are rigorously applied. Because the stakes are much higher with human subjects, patient safety as well as the efficacy of the intervention are critical in the evaluation process. There is no point in introducing an intervention that causes more problems than the condition that needs to be treated. These tests are typically divided into pre-clinical studies in animals, and Phase 1, 2, 3, and 4 clinical studies in humans. Most government regulatory agencies require compelling results from Phase 3 human trials before permitting a drug, vaccine, or other medical treatment to be offered to the public. In the context of a pandemic crisis like COVID-19, balancing the need for speed against safety presented major challenges.

Typically, promising potential treatments are performed on at least two species of animals during pre-clinical studies. This is long before any human trials are normally considered and implemented. Rats and mice are usually the favored animals for experimentation, so a huge body of prior studies with these particular rodents is available for comparative purposes. These are also relatively inexpensive for conducting studies that require many individual animals for statistical purposes. Should the studies with rodents be promising, then further work may be conducted on larger animals such as dogs, pigs, or monkeys. Particular animals may be selected, because they possess characteristics or propensities that are more similar to humans with respect to the particular disease under investigation.

Based on promising efficacy and safety in pre-clinical animal studies, a product manufacturer would normally register a proposed set of clinical trials with a government regulatory agency such as Health Canada or the US FDA and then commence with Phase 1 human trials upon approval. In these small-scale, short-duration studies, the main objective is to establish safety of the intervention in healthy individuals. These usually involve small numbers, on the order of twenty to a hundred people, tested over several months, to establish any gross toxicity issues.

In Phase 2 studies, the drug or other intervention is tested on diseased patients with different dosages to maximize the therapeutic effects and minimize any undesirable side effects. Ideally for drugs, toxic dose concentrations are much higher than those that produce the desired therapeutic effects. Such drugs are described as having a high therapeutic index and may be considered as effective and safe, at least in the short term. Several hundred people may be enrolled in a Phase 2 study.

Phase 3 studies are usually long and involve the enrollment of several thousands of people in multiple treatment centers, often in more than one country. These randomized controlled trials provide the best information, since they reduce bias by having two groups (treated and control), are balanced by randomization, and blinded to the participants and the testing doctors. These trials typically extend over one to four years. They ideally involve comparable numbers of carefully matched participants and the placebo controls, who have the disease condition but are not treated with the intervention under evaluation. Clear evidence of significant clinical benefit from Phase 3 studies with no evidence of major side effects may compel government regulatory agencies to permit the marketing of the product to the general public. However, further long-term safety testing data in Phase 4 clinical studies may be required to be ongoing for a few more years to allow continued approval. This may require the manufacturer to provide the results from extended monitoring of the product for side effects within the general population. This is described as "Post-Approval Research and Monitoring."

It should be appreciated that around 90 percent of promising therapeutics that enter into Phase 1 clinical studies fail to receive regulatory approval at the end of Phase 3 studies.[1] For most drugs that do succeed, the pre-clinical and clinical trials typically take between ten to fifteen years to complete, with clinical trials alone taking on average six to ten years.[2] The typical cost for development of a successful drug, including the cost of the failures to get to a successful drug, is on the order of US $2 billion.[3] This, along with high advertising costs, is why new drugs are exceedingly expensive when they are first released on the market. However, the typical patent life of a new drug is only a few years, since three-quarters of the twenty-year patent protection has usually elapsed by the time the new drug first reaches the market. Thereafter, any generic drug company can produce exactly the same compound much more cheaply without infringing on any patents related to the drug. However, drug manufacturers can reap several billions of dollars per year for the remaining duration of their patent without competition after regulatory approval.

The market for a drug is limited by the number of people who have the illness that it is designed to ameliorate. By contrast, vaccines are a prophylactic measure, where the market includes both healthy as well as diseased individuals. Thus, the potential markets for vaccines are an order of magnitude larger than traditional therapeutic drugs. For example, one of the most successful of all drugs in history, Lipitor, generated for Pfizer around US $10 billion annually in sales over fourteen years.[4] By contrast, in its first year of sales, Pfizer received over US $37.8 billion in 2021 and once again the same amount in 2022 in revenues from their COVID-19 vaccine.[5, 6] This made the Pfizer COVID-19 vaccine the top-selling pharmaceutical product in 2021, grossing 78 percent more than its closest competitor, Abbvie's Humira, which is a monoclonal antibody drug used to treat rheumatoid arthritis and other autoimmune diseases.[7] In close third as the best-selling pharmaceutical product in 2021 was the Moderna COVID-19 vaccine, with about 48 percent of Pfizer's COVID-19 vaccine total profit.

In 2019, the revenue from the worldwide pharmaceutical market was about US $1.278 trillion.[8] In 2022, it climbed to US $1.482 trillion. Most of this increase came from COVID-19 vaccine sales.

Prior to the COVID-19 pandemic, the timeline for development of vaccines was typically ten to fifteen years, and in some instances, even longer.[9] Historically, the durations of Phase 1, 2, and 3 trials and the number of participants tested for each phase for vaccines are similar to those of drug trials. As shall be discussed later in chapter 12, several of the COVID-19 vaccines were developed, tested, and approved for distribution to the general public in less than a year.

10.2. Post-approval Drug and Vaccine Safety Monitoring

Several governments have established databases whereby doctors, their patients, and others may report adverse effects from the medications after their approval and release to the public. These databases were intended to provide warnings about products with safety issues that may not have been apparent from clinical studies, which may have been underpowered with respect to the numbers of participants tested to detect rarer side effects. These databases can also facilitate detection of bad batches of a particular drug or vaccine.

One of the largest regulatory agency databases is the Vaccine Adverse Event Reporting System (VAERS) established by the US Congress in 1990 and operated by the US Centers for Disease Control and Prevention (CDC) and the FDA.[10] It is a voluntary reporting system that typically received reports of about thirty thousand vaccine adverse events per year prior to the COVID-19 pandemic. While most reports of injury are less serious, 10 to 15 percent of them describe hospitalization, life-threatening illness, disability, or death. Although most filed reports are provided by doctors and health-care professionals, anyone can report an association between a vaccination and an adverse event. However, these reports are monitored, and the CDC often follows up to investigate whether the vaccination may have actually caused the adverse event, since these associations may be coincidental in many cases. A forensic analysis of a large sample of VAERS death reports by McLachlan et al. (2021) showed that most reports were submitted by health service employees and in only 14 percent of the COVID-19 cases could a vaccine reaction be ruled out as a contributing factor in their death.[11] One study, conducted by Harvard Pilgrim Health Care, Inc. for the Agency for Health Care and Quality of the US Department of Health and Human Services, indicated that less than 1 percent of likely adverse reactions are reported in VAERS.[12]

One of the other major adverse reporting databases for medical products is VigiAccess, which was set up by the WHO in 2015.[13] It records adverse drug reactions (ADRs) and adverse events following immunization (AEFIs) that are reported to national pharmacovigilance centers or national drug regulatory authorities. The latter are members of the WHO Programme for International Drug Monitoring (PIDM), which was created in 1968. Like VAERS, VigiAccess warns users that a high association of side effects with particular drugs or vaccines does not necessarily indicate a causal relationship. Unlike VAERS, individual cases reports cannot be viewed in VigiAccess due to strict data protection laws and agreements between PIDM members and the WHO.

The European Medicines Agency (EMA) created the EudraVigilance system in 2001 for the European Union medicine regulatory network to manage and analyze information on suspected adverse reactions to medicines and vaccines that have been authorized in the European Economic Area (EEA).[14] The data in EudraVigilance are provided by EMA authorization holders and sponsors of clinical trials, who must report and evaluate adverse medicinal product reactions during their development and following their marketing authorization in the EEA.

In the United Kingdom, the Yellow Card scheme provides for the reporting of suspected side effects to drugs, vaccines, and medical devices to the UK Medicines and Healthcare products Regulatory Agency (MHRA).[15] This scheme collects and monitors information on suspected safety concerns involving health-care products, which are filed by the public and health-care professionals. It serves to provide an early warning that the safety of a product may require further investigation by the MHRA. A forensic analysis of a random sampling of fifty-seven death reports in the Yellow Card system in the 1980s showed that at least forty were true positives (77 percent) while none of the remaining could be proved to be false positives.[16]

The Canadian Adverse Events Following Immunization Surveillance System (CAEFISS) specifically tracks reports of possible vaccine injury, and it is managed by Health Canada and the Public Health Agency of Canada (PHAC).[17] CAEFISS collects information from provincial and territorial health authorities that is passively reported to local public health units primarily by nurses, physicians, and pharmacists, as well as from federal authorities that provide immunization within their jurisdiction. Data into CAEFISS is also provided by the Canada Vigilance Program (CVP) within the Health Products and Food Branch (HPFB) of Health Canada, which tracks reports filed by market authorization holders for vaccines to the Marketed Health Products Directorate (MHPD) CVP whenever there are serious adverse events following immunization. The Advisory Committee on Causality Assessment (ACCA) reviews the reports of adverse events following immunization received through these national surveillance systems and assesses whether an event was likely to be causally linked to a vaccine using strict criteria developed by the Brighton Collaboration.

The Brighton Collaboration was originally conceived in 1999 at a vaccine conference in Brighton, England, and was initially funded by the WHO. Later funding was provided by many other organizations, including the European Center of Disease Prevention and Control, the Bill & Melinda Gates Foundation, the CDC, and, most recently, the Coalition for Epidemic

Preparedness Innovations (CEPI). CEPI was founded in Davos by the governments of Norway and India, the Bill & Melinda Gates Foundation, the Wellcome Trust, and the World Economic Forum, but has since received funding from over thirty national governments and the European Union, as well as several private sector organizations. The Brighton Collaboration criteria for vaccine injury has become stricter over the years and is heavily influenced by input from CEPI's Scientific Advisory Board and its Vaccines Research & Development & Manufacturing Committee, which receives input from various vaccine manufacturers.

One of the reasons why the VAERS was set up and is so important in the United States is the very limited liability that vaccine manufacturers have for their products as compared with pharmaceutical drugs. This stems back to increased litigation against vaccine manufacturers in the United States in the mid-1980s and a reluctance of the pharmaceutical industry to continue producing new as well as off-patent vaccines, which threatened a vaccine shortage at that time. The US Congress responded by passing the National Childhood Vaccine Injury Act (NCVIA) in 1986. This included the establishment of the National Vaccine Injury Compensation Program (VICP) to compensate those injured by vaccines on a "no fault" basis.[18, 19] In 2005, the US Public Readiness and Emergency Preparedness Act was passed, which empowered the Health and Human Services secretary to provide legal protection to companies that manufacture or distribute critical medical supplies in an emergency, including drugs and vaccines, unless there is "willful misconduct" by the company. This was first invoked for countermeasures against COVID-19 on March 17, 2020, and was to be in effect until the COVID-19 pandemic was no longer a declared emergency or by October 1, 2024, at the latest.[20] On May 11, 2023, the US Federal COVID-19 Public Health Emergency declaration was terminated.[21]

Ultimately, a great deal of expense and effort has been expended in establishing and maintaining these vaccine adverse event reporting systems. It has been suggested that less than one percent of all vaccine adverse reactions are reported to systems like VAERS.[22] Nevertheless, as shall be shown later in chapter 13, they have documented to date unprecedented levels of signals for COVID-19 vaccine injuries and deaths that are magnitudes higher than any prior approved vaccine to date. Despite this, most of these vaccine adverse event reporting systems still state that the risks of vaccine injury are outweighed by the risks of severe disease from COVID-19. As shall be evident in the next three chapters, there have been serious breaches in the production and testing of the COVID-19 genetic vaccines.

CHAPTER 11

Production of COVID-19 Vaccines

L. Maria Gutschi, David J. Speicher, Susan Natsheh, Philip Oldfield, Philip Britz-McKibbon, Neil Karrow, Bernard Massie, Bonnie Mallard, Glenn Chan, & Steven Pelech

"Sometimes when you innovate you make mistakes. It is best to admit them quickly and get on with improving your other innovations."

—Steve Jobs

"Nothing but the natural ignorance of the public, countenanced by the inoculated erroneousness of the ordinary general medical practitioners, makes such a barbarism as vaccination possible . . . . Recent developments have shown that an inoculation made in the usual general practitioner's light-hearted way, without previous highly skilled examination of the state of the patient's blood, is just as likely to be a simple manslaughter as a cure or preventive. But vaccination is nothing short of attempted murder. A skilled bacteriologist would just as soon think of cutting his child's arm and rubbing the contents of the dustpan into the wound, as vaccinating it in the same."

—George Bernard Shaw with respect to smallpox vaccination

11.1. Historical Vaccine Development

As explained in chapter 7, the body has evolved a highly sophisticated and effective immune system that learns to recognize and specifically counteract novel infectious pathogens. In particular, the adaptive immune system relies on the combined actions of B cells that produce specific antibodies and T cells that attack pathogen-infected cells. Such recognition depends on the ability of these lymphocytes to target tiny portions of a pathogen called epitopes. As shown in chapter 7.6, some parts of a pathogen are very immunogenic, i.e., elicit a strong immune response, whereas other portions are ignored by the immune system. Infectious pathogens such as viruses, bacteria, and fungi are constantly evolving, and previous exposure to an earlier version of the pathogen can provide immune protection against future infections, including other highly related pathogens.

For example, the science of vaccinology made a major leap in 1796 with the observation by the English physician and scientist Edward Jenner that milkmaids who had mild cowpox rarely got the more severe smallpox disease.[1] One of his patients, Sarah Nelmes, had developed a slight rash following milking a cow that was recently afflicted with cowpox. On May 14, 1796, using a sample made from the pocks on Sarah's hand, Jenner scratched the skin of an eight-year-old boy, James Phipps, who had not yet suffered from smallpox. (Dr. Jenner could have used the pocks from the udder of the infected cow instead for his experiment.) The young boy became mildly sick with cowpox a few days later and then fully recovered within a week. On July 1, 1796, Jenner then exposed the boy to the smallpox virus by a method known as variolation, and the child did not get sick and develop smallpox. He appeared to be protected against the more virulent smallpox.

Variolation against smallpox goes back to at least the mid-1500s, when it was used as a prophylactic to reduce the severity of future smallpox infections in China. With this variation of variolation, smallpox scabs were dried, ground down, and blown with a pipe into a nostril of the recipient. In Britain and New England in the eighteenth century, variolation was practiced to protect people likely to be at risk of smallpox infection, even though the procedure had extremely high rates of adverse effects, including getting smallpox. Dr. Jenner himself was subjected to variolation as a youth. About 1 to 2 percent of those who were variolated died from smallpox compared to around 30 percent of those who contracted the virus naturally. Safer vaccination with cowpox completely replaced variolation in England by 1840, when variolation for smallpox became prohibited.[2] Hypodermic syringes were also developed about sixteen years later.

Afterward, the introduction of a related or less virulent form of an infectious pathogen became a standard way of conferring resistance to future infections with deadly pathogens. Before there were methods to artificially produce the proteins of these pathogens for direct injection into vaccine recipients, the use of weakened, attenuated strains elicited an immune response with much lower risks of severe disease.

Heat or chemical inactivation of a pathogen may be used for such vaccines but has the disadvantage that the level of pathogen is restricted to what is injected. With a live pathogen that has retained its ability to multiply, ideally very slowly to give the immune system time to develop counter-defenses before the pathogen can do too much damage, stronger immunity can be achieved. This is why traditional vaccines have typically contained a few dozen copies to thousands of copies of a particular pathogen.

The immune response in vaccines is also commonly accentuated with the use of adjuvants, which are substances that attract immune cells to produce a better inflammatory response and may help keep the injected pathogen localized. Some of the more commonly used adjuvants in vaccines include aluminum salts, such as aluminum hydroxide and aluminum potassium sulfate, along with more complex compounds such as MF59 and AS03. These latter adjuvants are known as emulsion adjuvants and are based on squalene found in shark liver oil. MF59 and AS03 have been used in some influenza vaccines and recently, in some of the COVID-19 non-genetic vaccines.[3]

11.2. How COVID-19 Vaccines Work

With the advent of recombinant DNA technology in the 1970s, it became feasible to isolate the genes that encoded the proteins of pathogens and start to produce them in larger quantities in bacteria like *Escherichia coli* (E. coli). Purified preparations of these recombinantly produced pathogen proteins or short artificial pieces of these proteins created by chemical synthesis in the laboratory provided large quantities of antigens that could be injected into animals to induce antibody production against the foreign proteins. However, the immune response would be focused on the specific proteins that were inoculated into the animals and not the whole pathogen, which results in a narrower immune protection. Nevertheless, a polyclonal antibody response would be induced, because a population of different B cells would be stimulated to produce different antibodies against different parts (i.e., epitopes) of an injected protein or peptide fragment (see chapter 7 for more details). Incidentally, preparations of monoclonal antibodies can be developed by creation of hybridoma cells where an antibody producing B cell is fused with a cancer cell, isolated, and then repeatedly propagated to give rise to a pure population of identical cells that generate exactly the same antibody specific for a single epitope. Such monoclonal antibodies can be effective therapeutics when they target specific oncoproteins on cancer cells or proteins on the surface of pathogens.

Over two hundred COVID-19 vaccines were developed, with over seventy-one reaching Phase 3 trials, and at least thirty-eight were approved.[4] The Chinese Sinovac (CoronaVac) and Sinopharm vaccines, which use chemically inactivated whole SARS-CoV-2 virus with an aluminum adjuvant for injection, are essentially traditional vaccines. However, most of the COVID-19 vaccines used in North America and Europe exclusively target the spike protein of the SARS-CoV-2 virus as the sole antigen to evoke an immune response to achieve immunity. In these latter vaccines, either the inoculation features the spike protein or it contains messenger-RNA (mRNA) or DNA to instruct the recipient's own cells to manufacture the viral protein. Novavax's Nuvaxovid (also known as Covovax) and Medicago's Corifenz vaccines are protein subunit vaccines that use recombinant purified spike protein as the antigen. Such preparations of spike protein may be about 95 percent pure, as achieved with the histidine-tagged spike protein in the Novavax product (the other 5 percent are insect proteins from the Sf9 caterpillar cells used to produce the recombinant spike protein). It is possible that the contaminating proteins can also elicit an immune response. All of the aforementioned COVID-19 vaccines have tended to offer poorer initial efficacy for production of anti-spike protein antibodies than is achieved with COVID-19 genetic vaccines.[5] This is likely due to the inability of these vaccines to provide as high levels of the spike antigens as can be generated with the lipid nanoparticle (LNP)/mRNA or adenovirus/DNA-based vaccines.

The Russian Sputnik V, AstraZeneca's Vaxzevria, and Janssen's Jcovden (Johnson & Johnson) COVID-19 vaccines contain spike DNA that triggers synthesis of the spike protein in host cells. They use modified adenoviruses to deliver the DNA to the cells. Adenoviruses can cause colds and even cancer, but the versions used as delivery vehicles are genetically engineered so as not to replicate and not to cause cancer by removal of viral genes that are necessary for these outcomes.[6] A significant advantage of these adenovirus-based vaccines is that the DNA is fairly stable, and multiple copies of RNA can be produced from each spike DNA molecule. Multiple copies of each spike protein can then be generated from a single mRNA molecule. However, the mRNA that is produced is very labile, and production of spike protein from that mRNA is presumed to be transient. But integration of the DNA into the host cell genome is a possibility that could potentially turn cells cancerous if the integration is near cancer-related genes (known as proto-oncogenes or tumor suppressor protein genes) in the genome. The risk for this may be low, and as discussed later, such cells are likely destroyed by the immune system. Another disadvantage of this type of vaccine is that the immune system also learns to recognize the adenovirus vector with its own viral proteins. Consequently, a different strain of the delivery adenovirus may be required for booster shots, since the immune system can produce antibodies that may inactivate the ability of the adenovirus to enter into cells or facilitate the adenovirus's removal by innate immune cells. This might be alleviated by inoculation of the delivery adenovirus through the mucosal route, either in the airway or by intrarectal administration.

Pfizer-BioNTech's BNT162b2 (later named Comirnaty and tozinameran) and Moderna's mRNA-1273 (later named Spikevax and elasomeran) are mRNA-containing vaccines that deliver a genetically modified mRNA (modRNA) gene for production of the spike protein. These modifications permit high stability of the mRNA through the incorporation of non-natural nucleotides (i.e.; N1-methyl pseudouridine for uridine) and an altered nucleic acid sequence, particularly to increase the nucleotide base content in the RNA for more cytidine and guanidine nucleotides. Cytidine and guanidine nucleotides pair with greater affinity for each other than does adenine and uracil (or N1-methyl pseudouridine) pair in double-stranded nucleic acids. Higher content of cytidine and guanidine nucleotides can improve the stability of the RNA. Despite the different RNA sequence from the original spike gene, the resultant spike protein should be identical in conformity to the genetic code of life (see chapter 3.3).

The replacement of N1-methyl pseudouridine for uridine also reduces the ability of the foreign mRNA to induce the activation of Toll receptors inside of cells that mediate production of proinflammatory cytokines such as tumor necrosis factor-alpha and interleukins 8 and 12, which would otherwise elicit too strong an immune response against the cells taking up the vaccine mRNA.[7]

The genetic COVID-19 vaccines work to produce an immune response through very different mechanisms of action from traditional vaccines, and while there is overlap in many of the intervening steps, the differences have profound implications for the efficacy and safety of these products. In the case of the traditional COVID-19 vaccines, innate immune cells directly consume and digest the spike protein and then present pieces to T cells and antibody-producing B cells. By contrast, the COVID-19 genetic vaccines have a pharmacological phase in which they penetrate normal body cells, the mRNA are released from the LNPs into the cytoplasm, and they are then translated into spike protein by the ribosomes. Some of the LNPs are not processed and are secreted out of the cell in extracellular vesicles or exosomes. The pharmacological phase is then followed by an immunological phase where the spike protein that is expressed on cell surfaces elicits immune cell attack and damage to the spike protein-producing cells. The debris produced from the damaged or destroyed cells are then engulfed by immune cells and degraded into pieces of the spike protein, which are complexed on their surfaces with major histocompatibility antigens for presentation to T cells and B cells. Exosomes with spike protein have been detected in the circulation even four months after the second dose of a COVID-19 mRNA vaccine.[8] The immune cells that take up the exosomes ultimately travel to lymph nodes and the spleen. Memory B cells are also widely distributed in the bone marrow, Peyer's patches, gingiva (gums), mucosal epithelium of tonsils, the lamina propria of the gastro-intestinal tract, and in the circulation.

In the typical descriptions of how the COVID-19 genetic vaccines work, it has been suggested that the lipid nanoparticles or adenovirus in these vaccines are directly taken up by host innate immune cells such as dendritic cells and macrophages. Although the LNPs used in the Pfizer/BioNTech and Moderna RNA vaccines have no specific targeting proteins on their surface, a biocorona is formed upon exposure to bodily fluids, rich in lipoproteins, which tend to fuse preferentially with liver cells but allow fusion with most cell membranes that they encounter. Likewise, the adenovirus-based COVID-19 vaccines can bind to a wide variety of different cell surface receptors to gain entry into diverse cell types. Only a very tiny portion of the LNPs or adenoviruses in the COVID-19 vaccines would end up in immune cells directly. The more likely scenario is presented in Figure 11.1 (in the insert), where almost any cell could be penetrated by an LNP or adenovirus. It should be appreciated that pre-existing antibodies to the spike proteins of other coronaviruses or anti-spike antibodies generated from the first inoculation with a COVID-19 vaccine will elicit a more powerful inflammatory and destructive response with booster injections, unless the mechanisms of immune tolerance are induced.

11.3. COVID-19 Genetic Vaccine Production

Large-scale production of vaccines comes with major challenges to ensure consistency in the final product to maintain batch stability, efficacy, and safety. Since the Pfizer/BioNTech COVID-19 vaccine is the most commonly used vaccine in Canada and the United States, the next few subsections provide a summary of the main findings of a more detailed technical assessment concerning the development and manufacturing of BNT162b.[9] A number of deficiencies in the product's development were identified by regulatory agencies and appear to have either been ignored or glossed over. Substantial differences in Pfizer's manufacturing (Process 1 versus Process 2) led to worrisome quality differences between the clinical trial product (manufactured with Process 1) and what most people received in the commercial rollout of the Pfizer vaccine (manufactured with Process 2). Vaccine approval for the declared COVID-19 pandemic was given "fast-track" conditional approval to address "a seriously debilitating, rare or life-threatening disease devoid of a viable treatment," and approval was granted on the condition that additional information would be forthcoming after the vaccine was rolled out. Much of these data have not been fully provided to date.

Data for the following portion of this chapter was primarily obtained from the European Medicines Agency European Public Assessment Report (EPAR) for the BioNTech/Pfizer vaccine.[10] Additional information was obtained through email leaks from December 2020 that were released to journalists and to the *British Medical Journal*.[11, 12] It should be appreciated that the information provided to the EMA by Pfizer was very similar to what was provided to other health regulatory agencies, including Health Canada and the FDA.

As mentioned earlier, traditional vaccines contain a known amount of the target antigens found in attenuated or dead versions of pathogens or proteins derived from them to evoke an immune response. They do not require a person's cells to manufacture and present them on their membrane surface at an uncontrolled rate and level. It is this very difference that has been overlooked when assessing the safety, dosage, and pharmacokinetics of BNT162b2 (Pfizer-BioNTech mRNA vaccine) and its by-products, including the mRNA-encoded spike protein. Therefore, BNT162b2 and the other COVID-19 genetic vaccines are not like any other vaccine that has ever been used successfully in the past, as the innate immune response is initially targeted directly against one's own cells rather than against the invading pathogen. The mRNA directs the body's cells to manufacture the viral spike protein *in vivo* at levels that may vary over a hundred-fold or more among vaccinees, and it is that very difference that has been overlooked when assessing the safety and pharmacokinetics of BNT162b2 and its components and derivatives. Individuals produce variable amounts of spike protein due to their genetics, age, hormonal, and nutritional status, which batch of vaccine they receive, and so on. Therefore, since the spike protein is not part of the BNT162b2 formulation but is in fact the active component of the vaccine, i.e., the actual immunogen, it should have been assessed as a gene therapy product.

11.3.1. Are modRNA Product Vaccines or Gene Therapies?

One might have thought that mRNA vaccines against infectious diseases would be regulated as gene therapy products, which they objectively are. When injecting nucleic acids, including mRNA, there are potential safety concerns specific to gene therapy products, such as genomic effects or immunological responses that may require additional regulatory assessment of safety risks for these products. However, nucleic acid vaccines have been subject to complex, contradictory, and unclear regulatory guidance such that no specific regulatory guidance for these products was available at the time the mRNA vaccines received their Interim Order from the Minister of Health in Canada on December 9, 2020.[13]

Of note, BioNTech and Moderna originally expected to see their products regulated as gene therapies. For example, Moderna's statement in their second quarter 2020 Securities and Exchange Commission (SEC) filing—"Currently, mRNA is considered a gene therapy product by the FDA"—is all the more curious given that Moderna had likely already filed an IND (Investigational New Drug) application to FDA to begin clinical trials.[14] The genome sequence for the SARS-CoV-2 virus only became available in mid-January 2020 a few months before.

In 2008, the EMA amended its definition of gene therapy products to state, "Gene therapy medicinal products (GTMPs) shall not include vaccines against infectious diseases."[15]As a result, the non-clinical requirements and controls as described in the EMA's Guidance for GTMPs would no longer apply, but no rationale was provided for this amendment. These controls include studies on biodistribution, dose response, potential targets of toxicity, identification of the target organ for biological activity, potential of integration into the genome and transmission in the germ line, toxicity related to the expression of structurally altered proteins, reproductive toxicity, tumorigenicity, repeated dose toxicity, and excretion into the environment.[16]

Similarly, in 2013, the FDA guidance on gene therapy products, without explanation, excluded from its scope vaccines for infectious disease: "This guidance does not apply to therapeutic vaccines for infectious disease indications that are typically reviewed in CBER/Office of Vaccines Research and Review (OVRR)."[17]

This exclusion serves only regulatory purposes. It does not change the FDA biological definition of gene therapy products, which remains as: "Gene therapy products are all products that mediate their effects by transcription and/or translation of transferred genetic material and/or by integrating into the host genome and that are administered as nucleic acids, viruses, or genetically engineered microorganisms."[18]

It is the 2005 WHO Guidelines that grants nucleic acid vaccines, including mRNA vaccines, the status of a vaccine: antigens produced *in vivo* in the vaccinated host following administration of a live vector such as an adenovirus or nucleic acid or antigens produced by chemical synthesis *in vitro* that must comply with this international regulation concerning GMP (Good Manufacturing Practices), including demonstration of the purity and quality of the starting material.[19] The WHO Expert Committee on Biological Standardization provided guidelines specifically for mRNA vaccines in April 2022, updated from the draft guidance document of 2020.[20] These advisory guidelines updated the information and regulatory considerations for modRNA and self-amplifying mRNA vaccine products, addressed development, manufacturing, and control of the vaccine, and clarified the requirements for non-clinical evaluation. However, modRNA vaccines remain regulated as vaccine products and not as gene therapeutic products, whereas therapeutic vaccines for non-infectious diseases such as cancer are, even though many of the same safety concerns apply.

11.3.2. Long-Term Follow-up after Administration of Gene Therapy Products

Despite the exclusion of vaccines against infectious diseases from gene therapy guidance, the FDA has active programs in infectious diseases within its Office of Tissues and Advanced Therapies, including laboratory research on replication deficient (adenovirus) and replication competent viral vector (measles, vaccinia).[21] Health Canada does not have specific guidelines or regulations relating to gene therapies; these products are regarded as biological drugs, as are vaccines.[22] However, the FDA provides guidance on the long-term follow-up of gene therapy products, such as viral vectors, which requires the manufacturers to systematically record delayed adverse events.[23] Specifically, the emergence of new clinical conditions such as "a new malignancy, new incidence or exacerbation of a pre-existing neurological disorder, a new incidence or exacerbation of a prior rheumatological or autoimmune disorder, a new incidence of a hematological disorder and new infections especially those potentially product-related" are to be recorded annually for a minimum of five years, followed by up to ten years of observation. However, these requirements are not imposed on biological or nucleic acid products reviewed under vaccine guidance.

Questions remain regarding the regulatory approval process for mRNA vaccines, specifically those regarding the pharmacological, pharmacodynamic characteristics, and safety risks unique to nucleic acid medicinal products, which are further reviewed by Banoun (2023).[24]

11.3.3. Manufacturing and Quality

Chemistry, manufacturing, and control (CMC) are processes to make sure that quality manufacturing standards have been established for the finished product. This is to ensure consistency in identity, safety, quality, stability, and strength between the product used in the clinical trials and individual lots produced for commercial purposes. For modRNA commercial vaccines, this would include creation of master and working cell banks, test method development and stability testing, process development, qualification, and validations, as well as quality assurance processes and techniques.[25] However, the modRNA platform was a novel manufacturing platform requiring novel control and analytical technology, and thus knowledge from prior platforms for similar products/vaccines were limited and could not be leveraged for quality control.

11.3.4. BNT162b2 modRNA Structure

In the Pfizer/BioNTech vaccine, the modRNA has been altered from the mRNA sequence of the spike protein of the SARS-CoV-2 coronavirus by: (a) including mutations to replace two adjacent lysine and valine amino acids with two prolines instead, to produce a more antigenically optimal pre-fusion conformation; (b) replacing all uridine bases with N1-methylpseudouridine to evade defenses against foreign RNA;[26] (c) including human-derived 5 prime and 3 prime UTRs (untranslated regions) and a poly-adenine (A) tail with a thirty A segment, a linker, and a seventy A segment, to enhance translation by ribosomes; and (d) optimizing codon use by selecting synonymous codons that will optimize expression (i.e., replacement of adenine and thymidine nucleotide bases with cytidine and guanidine nucleotide bases in the RNA, while still retaining the final spike protein amino acid sequence) (Figure 11.2, found in the insert). The design of the sequence can be facilitated by *in silico* methods; a published algorithm was used for the development of BNT162b2 used clinically.[27] Since this mRNA is bioengineered, its non-proprietary name is tozinameran, and Comirnaty is the proprietary name for the Pfizer/BioNTech product. BNT162b2 was the laboratory identifier used to describe the modRNA during its development and testing.

On October 2, 2023, the Nobel Prize Assembly at the Karolinska Institute announced the awarding of the prize for Physiology or Medicine to Drs. Katalin Karikó and Drew Weissman "for their discoveries concerning nucleoside base modifications that enabled the development of effective mRNA against COVID-19."[28] This is for work done by the Nobel Prize recipients that was published from 2005 to 2010.

In a seminal article written in 2014 by BioNTech founders Drs. Ugur Sahin and Özlem Türeci, along with Dr. Katalin Karikó, they noted that *in vitro* transcribed mRNA represents a new class of drugs to deliver genetic information into cells.[29] The complex pharmacology of mRNA and issues with delivery to achieve sufficient levels of encoded protein and to reach a high number of cells were discussed. Safety considerations of mRNA-mediated activation of immune mechanisms, potential mitochondrial toxicities associated with non-natural nucleotides and prolonged treatment, dosing, and tissue targeting were also identified. Finally, Sahin et al. (2014) noted that the development of an mRNA platform as a biopharmaceutical requires an "industry-compatible process" that was proposed to be less challenging than those required for cell therapies.[30]

11.3.5. modRNA Effects in Human Cells

While this genetic engineering of the viral mRNA results in high levels of spike protein production, it is now known that this modRNA can persist for days, weeks, and possibly months in humans,[31] as can the spike protein itself.[32]

The genetic engineering of the mRNA may result in aberrant protein production. The various modifications made to the mRNA may be prone to errors when translated in cells, and this may generate variations in the resulting spike proteins when compared to the Wuhan spike protein. For instance, differences in folding of the spike protein[33] and generation of other antibodies with unknown effects may occur.[34] Abnormal spike protein and fragments following vaccination have been documented.[35, 36] Interestingly, when the BNT162b2 was used to transfect cells in culture, the resultant spike protein was observed to be larger than predicted by its amino acid sequence, and this was assumed to be due to the attachment of complex polymers of sugar molecules (i.e., glycosylation) of the protein, but never confirmed experimentally. This was originally flagged by the EMA as one of its initial concerns and assigned as Specific Obligation-1 (SO1) for Pfizer to address.[37] As it stands, it is still unclear if these mutant spike proteins may be associated with unwanted and adverse events as has been demonstrated with other codon-optimized proteins.

The exact features of the spike protein produced by the synthetic mRNA are unclear, especially with the newer bivalent Wuhan/Omicron BA.4/5 and monovalent XBB1.5 COVID-19 vaccines. It is not known how the spike protein translated from the modified mRNA fully compares to the original Wuhan virus version. It was assumed the genetic engineering of the nucleotide sequence as undertaken with the COVID-19 vaccines would not alter the spike protein amino acid sequence. However, variations in the location where the spike protein is produced might give rise to different compositions in this highly sugar-coated protein.

There is a lack of clarity regarding the spike protein characterization despite several requests for such data from the EMA. A full comparison of the spike protein made by the mRNA in the vaccine to the natural virus has not been performed to date. Although the amino acid sequence of the spike protein produced by the engineered mRNA in the COVID-19 vaccines is currently unknown, thousands of distinct gene sequences for the spike protein are publicly available from direct gene sequencing of the SARS-CoV-2 virus and its variants. These concerns are further compounded for the bivalent modified mRNA injectable formulations released in Fall 2022 that encoded two distinct spike proteins, namely the original ancestral Wuhan strain and a combination of BA.4/BA.5 Omicron subvariants. This allowed for possible formation of unnatural trimeric complexes with novel mixes of spike proteins from both versions of the SARS-CoV-2 virus.

On December 6, 2021, at a meeting held by the WHO,[38] vaccinologist Professor Florian Krammer anticipated heterotrimer formation with bivalent vaccines, questioning whether this could "lead to problems in protein folding?"[39] Presumably this concern was raised because protein-folding differences could alter the safety and efficacy profile of the vaccine. However, if heterotrimer formation leads to an improved immunological response as Moderna claimed in its submission to the FDA at the CDC meeting on September 1, 2022,[40] it is reasonable to ask if there are also different toxicological or immunological responses that are currently unknown. This issue is less problematic with the more recently released monovalent COVID-19 vaccine with only the XBB.1.5 Omicron subvariant.

11.3.6. modRNA Production: Process 1 vs. Process 2

The manufacturing process of the modRNA was changed substantially for the commercial scale-up lots (Process 2) from the pilot-scale process used to produce the BNT162b2 vaccine candidate for the clinical trials (Process 1). This had implications for GMP, risked marketing authorization, and has implications clinically.

The modRNA drug substance in BNT162b2 is produced by *in vitro* transcription from a DNA template. The DNA template defines the sequence of the modRNA, but it is not supposed to be part of the final product.

Process 1 was used to produce modRNA evaluated in the clinical trials. Using a cell-free method, linear DNA was amplified using the polymerase chain reaction (PCR). This results in a linear template including the open reading frame (ORF) for the S1/S2 protein, and the 5 prime and 3 prime UTRs. The five-prime cap was added enzymatically as was the poly(A) tail at the 3 prime end.[41] However, this technique does not produce sufficient modRNA for billions of doses in the timeframe and fidelity required, as is possible from a plasmid DNA.[42]

Process 2 was used for commercial scale production of BNT162b2 vaccine. Using genetic engineering techniques, DNA containing a sequence for direct binding of translated RNA to ribosomes (called a Kozak sequence), untranslated regions (UTRs), viral spike protein sequence, and a poly(A) tail (to protect the translated RNA from degradation and aid in transcription termination), was inserted into a plasmid, which is a circular piece of DNA. In this case, plasmid pST4–1525 was used (Figure 13.3), which has 7,824 base pairs including a promoter for the T7 RNA polymerase, the recognition sequence for the endonuclease used for linearization of the DNA, a kanamycin resistance gene, and an origin of replication (ORI). The plasmid was taken into E. coli bacterial cells. As the E. coli cells grow and multiply in the presence of kanamycin, the plasmid multiplies along with them. Inclusion of the antibiotic kanamycin ensures that only those E. coli that received the plasmid to produce the spike RNA can survive and proliferate. The bacteria is then harvested and chemically lysed to recover the plasmid DNA, which is then further purified. Subsequently, the circular plasmid DNA is linearized by cutting it using a restriction endonuclease enzyme (Eam1104I) and purified by ultrafiltration and diafiltration (UFDF), similar to dialysis.[43]

The DNA template in both processes is then used as the starting material for the modRNA production. *In vitro* translation (IVT) transcription is an enzymatic reaction requiring an RNA polymerase, nucleotide triphosphate substrates (substituting N1-methylpseudouridine for uridine), the polymerase cofactor magnesium chloride ($MgCl_2$), and a pH buffer containing polyamide and antioxidants. Like Moderna, Pfizer/BioNTech used the T7 RNA polymerase (derived from the T7 bacteriophage), which binds to a cognate *promoter* sequence likewise derived from T7 that has also been engineered into the

DNA plasmid upstream of the gene for the spike protein. Only a few hours are needed to produce the modRNA, and the process can be standardized.[44] The 5 prime cap is also added during the IVT reaction for both processes. Rather than adding the poly(A) tail enzymatically as in Process 1, in Process 2 it is already encoded for in the plasmid.

At the completion of IVT using plasmid DNA as used in Process 2, several impurities may be present, notably host cell genomic DNA from E. coli, RNA, proteins, endotoxins (bacterial cell wall components from the E. coli cells) and plasmid isoforms for the plasmid DNA.[45, 46] These were quantified routinely. The steps in purification for both processes are presented in Table 11.1.

Table 11.1. Selected attributes of Process 1 and Process 2 lots derived from EMA's Rolling Review.[47]

	Process 1 (Clinical trial batches)	**Process 2** (Commercial batches)	**Comments**
DNA template	PCR amplified	Linearized plasmid DNA template	Information on control and analytical methods for the linearized DNA plasmid was pending at time of conditional marketing approval.
	Sequencing of DNA template for verification of RNA sequence performed	Sequencing of DNA template for RNA sequence no longer required	Stability of the linear DNA and filtered circular plasmid DNA intermediate should be addressed.
BNT162b2 characterization (modRNA)	HPLC-UV and LC/MS/MS—oligonucleotide mapping		Fragments corresponding to 90.5 percent of BNT162b2 sequence detected.
	Illumina MiSeq Next Generation Sequencing (NGS) of modRNA performed		"Process 1 and 2 were comparable."
	Circular dichroism spectroscopy to confirm higher order structure		No method for determining intact RNA included.

	Process 1 (Clinical trial batches)	Process 2 (Commercial batches)	Comments
BNT162b2 Purification Steps	*In vitro* transcription followed by:	*In vitro* transcription followed by:	Magnetic bead purification not scalable and replaced with protein K digestion and then filtration.
	1. DNase I digestion	1. DNase I digestion	
	2. Not applicable	2. Protein K digestion	
	3. Magnetic bead purification	3. Ultrafiltration/ Diafiltration	
	4. Final filtration and dispense	4. Final filtration and dispense	
Scale	0.35–0.72 liters	37.6 liters	Only limited data available for commercial scale batches at time of authorization.
RNA integrity (percent)	78.1–82.8 percent	59.70 percent	See main text for comments.
In vitro expression of BNT162b2	Consistent/ expected size	Consistent/ expected size	
5 prime cap by LC-UV/MS (percent)	56–67 percent	83 percent	Slightly higher capping levels in Process 2 were considered acceptable.
Poly(A) tail (percent)	116–127 percent	93–104 percent	Significant differences found with poly(A) tail pattern.
Poly(A) tail length and distribution (RP-HPLC-UV)	A30: 28–34A A70: narrow range	A30: 28–34A. A70: longer tails	
dsRNA (pg/µg RNA)	<80 to<120	Not more than 240	Higher levels with Process 2 noted.
Residual DNA template (ng/mg RNA)	1-<200; 873 in one batch due to incomplete DNA digestion	17–211	Increased levels seen in latest commercial batch.

A=adenosine; CMA=Conditional Marketing Authorization; dsRNA=double stranded RNA; LC/MS/MS=liquid chromatography/mass spectrometry; LC-UV=liquid chromatography-ultraviolet; RP-HPLC-UV=reverse phase high performance liquid chromatography ultraviolet

Manufacturers of biotechnological and biological products including vaccines often make changes to the manufacturing process, including increasing the scale of production, product stability, and any changes imposed by regulatory authorities, both during development and post-approval. The manufacturers must demonstrate that the relevant quality attributes do not adversely impact safety or efficacy of these changes. Although there are no specific guidelines for changes in manufacturing processes specific to nucleic acid products, the International Council on Harmonization Q5E[48] did anticipate that the "principles outlined in this document might also apply to other product types such as proteins and polypeptides isolated from tissues and body fluids," which would therefore include nucleic acids.

In particular, requirements for clinical comparative efficacy and safety studies are dependent on the stage of development and the type of change involved. If changes are made after the confirmatory clinical trials, as was done with the Pfizer/BioNTech vaccine, a thorough comparability assessment is generally required including: ". . . physicochemical and biological in vitro studies, and may include clinical pharmacokinetic and/or pharmacodynamic comparability studies. If this comparability exercise cannot rule out an impact on the efficacy and safety profile of the drug, additional clinical study (ies) may have to be performed."[49]

In its rolling review in November 2020, the EMA noted there was a decrease in the purity of the mRNA. In the clinical trial batches, the intact mRNA was 78–83 percent pure, which was much higher than in the commercial batches at 60 percent (Table 13.1).[50] Side-to-side comparisons based on analytical testing and biological assays demonstrated significant differences in the purity and amount of intact mRNA with the Process 2 batches. This may indicate notable physical, chemical, and biological differences, warranting further comparative clinical studies. Emails from the EMA leak/hack showed that the EMA's head of Pharmaceutical Quality, Dr. Jekerle Veronika, discussed the "differences in the level of mRNA integrity" between clinical and commercial material. It was hoped that an approval by the end of 2020 could be possible *if* the mRNA integrity issue (and two other major objections) were resolved.[51]

A protocol amendment to the pivotal trial was therefore added,[52] which required 252 patients receiving Process 2 lots to be compared to patients in the clinical trials receiving Process 1 lots for comparable safety and efficacy. To date, these data are unavailable.[53]

Recently, a Freedom of Information (FOIA) request to the UK Regulator (Medicines and Healthcare Products Regulatory Agency) obtained by the *Daily Skeptic* revealed, "This exploratory objective was removed and documented in protocol amendment 20 in September 2022 due to the extensive usage of vaccines manufactured via 'Process 2.' Thus, this process comparison was not conducted as part of the formal documentation within the protocol amendment."[54] Therefore, clinical comparability between these two manufacturing processes cannot be assumed and thus the approved version represents a new biological product that is not equivalent to the product used in the clinical trials.[55] In essence, the UK regulator used real-world evidence to support compatibility of the two processes, in contradiction to the original accepted method of a small, randomized trial.

11.3.7. Impurities Identified in Process 2 Batches

11.3.7.1. Truncated and Fragmented modRNA

As discussed previously, impurities in Process 2 lots including fragmented mRNA is considered a critical quality attribute, but it is not yet known what effects these smaller mRNA fragments (impurities) have in the body. These shorter spike protein fragments may be released more readily into the circulation from vaccine transfected cells. Such truncated fragments may lack the transmembrane domain and attached palmitate fatty acids at the back end of the spike protein, which would normally anchor them to the cell membrane. At the time of conditional approval, the allowable limits for fragmented mRNA were up to 45 percent in the final product.[56] Despite alteration of the sequence in the spike protein with two amino acid residues replaced by two proline residues from mutation of the mRNA sequence, which locks the spike protein in a prefusion state, the spike protein should still be able to engage angiotensin-converting enzyme 2 (ACE2) and other spike receptors that are expressed on cells of the body. ACE2 is important for reducing blood pressure through its ability to degrade the hormone angiotensin 2. The spike protein binds to ACE2,[57] TMEM16F,[58] and CD42b receptors on platelets and stimulates their activation and aggregation,[59] which contributes to thrombosis (blood clotting) and thrombocytopenia (reduction of production of platelets), known risks associated with COVID-19 vaccines.[60]

There was also little data on whether these fragmented mRNA pieces result in harmful proteins or peptides (small proteins) or whether they induce autoimmunity (cause the body to attack itself). For example, there can be as much as a 30 percent amino acid similarity between the spike protein and a human protein called Syncytin-1. Although cross-reactivity of anti-spike antibodies with Syncytin-1 in vaccinated individuals has not yet been reported,[61, 62, 63] autoimmunity often takes years before its manifests overtly in people.

11.3.7.2. Double-stranded RNA (dsRNA)

Other impurities in the BNT162b2 included dsRNA, which occurs secondarily to the *in vitro* transcription process that can generate dsRNA by-products.[64] dsRNA can induce pro-inflammatory cytokines such as type 1 interferon, trigger Toll-like receptor 3, and separately affect expression/translation of spike protein.[65] Removal of dsRNA is at best, 90 percent, which indicates that short segments of dsRNA may remain; this has been hypothesized to contribute to inflammatory reactions like myocarditis.[66] When present in LNPs, dsRNA will also be transfected into macrophages and dendritic cells.[67] Dendritic cells trigger immune responses in lymphoid tissues upon early sensing of infectious pathogens and communicate with immature dendritic cells present in peripheral tissues such as the myocardium, which may result in an autoimmune attack such as in myocarditis.

It is worth noting that gene editing to optimize a high cytidine and guanidine content in the spike proteins of both the Pfizer/BioNTech and Moderna COVID-19 vaccines produces tighter binding and stability of the dsRNA. This may facilitate more prolonged stimulation of cellular responses to perceived viral infection of cells, since dsRNA is not normally produced in healthy cells.

11.3.7.3. Endotoxin

The bacterial toxin endotoxin can be introduced into the modRNA drug substance, primarily from the E. coli used in the DNA template production but also from contaminated raw materials in the large-volume buffers used to make the mRNA vaccines.[68] Endotoxin is difficult to remove due to its ubiquity, high heat stability, and hydrophobic properties.[69] Lipopolysaccharides (LPS) from endotoxin can bind both the S1 and S2 subunits of the spike protein, which may result in enhanced inflammatory responses.[70] Endotoxin is a very potent stimulus of macrophages and monocytes even at picogram levels (a picogram is a trillionth of a gram).[71] Some researchers have suggested spike protein is only inflammatory in the presence of endotoxin or when it lacks glycosylation.[72] LNPs with or without modRNA can induce exacerbated inflammation in the presence of pre-existing inflammation due to endotoxin,[73] and concerns have been raised that the unrecognized contamination of nanoparticles with endotoxin may be associated with toxicity.[74] In view of the high level of DNA plasmid in the BNT162b2 vaccine as discussed in the next subsection, it is feasible that endotoxin levels may also exceed current regulatory limits.[75]

11.3.7.4. Plasmid Vector DNA

As mentioned above, to produce the mRNA that is encapsulated in LNPs that are used as COVID-19 vaccines, both Pfizer/BioNTech and Moderna utilize DNA copies of the spike gene that are incorporated into plasmids. These plasmids or vectors were used to transfect E. coli bacterial cells for high production of modRNA copies, which were subsequently purified from lysed bacteria. The purification protocols should have removed the plasmid DNA along with bacterial endotoxins and LPS. However, several laboratories have independently confirmed that as much as 35 percent or more of the nucleic acid in the COVID-19 mRNA vaccines is DNA.[76, 77, 78, 79, 80] The contamination appears to be higher in the Moderna vaccine than the Pfizer/BioNTech product, but most of the DNA fragments are much smaller, comprising fewer than two hundred base pairs in size.

A preprint by Canadian Citizens Care Alliance scientists and others showed that around 1.9–3.7 μg/dose of DNA by a fluorometry method appears to be typically found in vials of BNT162b2b that are supposed to contain 30 μg of Spike RNA, and 3.3 to 5.1 μg/dose for the Moderna product.[81] This would correspond to around a hundred billion or more DNA molecules in each injection and represent contamination levels that exceed 3.33 μg/mg of RNA. However, the DNA contamination in these COVID-19 vaccines still meets the European Medicines Agency (EMA) 0.33 μg/mg threshold[82] and the FDA's 0.010 μg/dose threshold using specifically the qPCR method for quantitation.[83] The large differences in residual DNA levels found between fluorometry and qPCR measurements may be due to the fact that qPCR cannot quantitate molecules smaller than the size of the amplicon (105–114 bp). Therefore, qPCR underestimates the total DNA in each vaccine, and this raises questions about the analytical methods recommended by regulatory agencies for modRNA vaccines. Health Canada, the FDA, and the European Medicines Agency have acknowledged the high degree of DNA contamination in the Pfizer/BioNTech and Moderna vaccines but have dismissed it and still consider the vaccines to be safe.[84, 85, 86, 87, 88] In the recent testing of twenty-seven mRNA Pfizer/BioNTech and Moderna vaccine vials obtained in Canada, "all vaccines exceeded the guidelines for residual DNA set by the FDA and WHO of [0.010 μg]/dose by 188–509-fold."[89] However, the transfection of these plasmid DNA contaminants using LNPs warrants reconsideration of the current regulatory limits, since these limits are based on injecting naked DNA into plasma where it may be rapidly destroyed before it enters into cells.

Residual DNA can result in type 1 interferon responses and poses a risk of genomic integration. One of the mechanisms that Pfizer/BioNTech took to reduce the amount of plasmid spike DNA was to digest it into smaller pieces with enzymes called nucleases. The consequence of this may be to further increase the probability of a piece of the DNA integrating into and disrupting the genomes of cells that take up the LNPs, as explained by South Carolina University professor Dr. Philip Buckhaults when he gave a speech to a South Carolina Senate Medical Affairs Ad-Hoc Committee.[90] This situation can lead to "insertional oncogenesis," which is when foreign DNA gets integrated next to critical growth-control genes, known as oncogenes or tumor-suppressor genes, and interferes with their normal regulation, thereby driving cancer cell proliferation. When DNA is circularized, as it is in an intact plasmid, it is less likely to integrate into the genome. When it is cut into linear fragments with nucleases, the probability of integration into host cell DNA increases.[91] Even fragments of DNA as little as seven base pairs have been shown to have disruptive rates of DNA integration or recombination.[92] Some LNPs have been developed to further improve on the delivery of DNA contents into the nuclei of cells, where the genome is normally present.[93]

One of the original scientists that noted the significant contamination of the mRNA vaccines with DNA is Kevin McKernan. In preliminary studies, he and his team have detected spike DNA integrated on at least two separate occasions into human chromosomes 9 as well as 12 in cancer cell lines that took up the COVID-19 vaccine mRNA.[94] One of the sites of integration on chromosome 12 was the FAIM2 gene, which is involved in programmed cell death, which facilitates cancer cell survival.

Another problematic aspect of the Pfizer/BioNTech vaccine is that the DNA plasmid includes an SV40 promoter/enhancer/origin of replication (*ori*) element, which is the portion of SV40 virus genome that drives the production of flanking genes. This inclusion was not originally disclosed to the EMA, nor to Health Canada, raising questions of adulteration and intention to deceive the regulatory agencies.[95, 96] Health Canada has recently confirmed the presence of the SV40 promoter/enhancer in the Pfizer/BioNTech vaccine after this was brought to their attention, but they have concluded that the risk/benefit profile continues to support the use of the Pfizer/BioNTech vaccine.[97]

This SV40 promoter might have been originally included to increase the rate of spike RNA production from the DNA plasmid during the production phase, although the AmpR promoter that was also present should have achieved this. However, if portions of the contaminating plasmid integrate into a cell's genome, this could result in increased rates of mRNA production of genes next to the SV40 virus promoter/enhancer elements, which again can potentially contribute to cancer. Moreover, the SV40 virus promoter/enhancer features a DNA nuclear-targeting sequence.[98] The SV40 virus was a common contaminant in inactivated polio vaccines that were offered from 1955 to 1963, so a substantial portion of the population over sixty years of age may have persistent SV40 infections.[99] The Large T antigen produced from the SV40 virus, which may be present in 10–20 percent of the population, can bind to SV40 virus promoter/enhancer elements, which could lead to even higher mRNA production of cellular genes at sites of genome integration. However, the risk of this is unclear at this time. The DNA plasmid used to manufacture the RNA in the Moderna COVID-19 vaccine did not include an SV40 promoter.[100]

Finally, it should also be appreciated that the RNA in the COVID-19 vaccines may also be converted back into a DNA copy through the action of RNA reverse transcriptase in host cells such as LINE-1.[101] Such a conversion of spike RNA into stable DNA in the nucleus of a liver cell line by LINE-1 was independently confirmed.[102] Liver is one of the major organs that accumulates the Pfizer/BioNTech vaccine LNPs,[103] and it is feasible that the DNA copy may permit more sustained production of spike RNA molecules and spike proteins.

11.3.8. Lipid Nanoparticles in COVID-19 RNA Vaccines

The application of lipid nanoparticles in vaccines is a novel use in humans, and its safety has not been rigorously assessed. The LNPs are semi-spheres made of fat (lipids) that protect the mRNA from degrading and also carry it into cells. They contain PEGylated lipid (ALC-0159) and the cationic lipid (ALC-0315), *neither of which have been used in humans before*. PEGylation refers to the addition of polyethylene glycol as a component of a lipid or a protein; in the case of LNPs, it reduces the rate of their clearance by organs such as the kidneys. PEGylated nanoparticles are often extensively covered with complement protein, which can result in potentially life-threatening reactions.[104] Physicochemical properties such as surface charge, aggregation, particle size, presence of lipids, and possible endotoxin contamination associated with CARPA (complement activation-related pseudoallergy) are all present on these innoculations.[105] This risk is normally identified for PEGylated nanoparticles, but a full independent review for pharmacology and toxicity for these novel excipients was not performed and is incomplete. PEGylated nanoparticles can also cause significant allergic reactions.[106] Cationic (positively-charged) lipids improve the escape of LNPs from endosomes and the transfection efficiency for the delivered mRNA. However, the release of mRNA from endosomes is the rate limiting step for spike protein expression, and LNPs may remain in lysosomes leading to cytotoxic effects.[107] These lipids are known to cause inflammation (both with and without mRNA cargo inside them) and can be directly toxic to cells.[108] There is limited data both on the metabolism and distribution of these lipids, and it is not known how much ends up in each organ. There is no formal, controlled clinical data to support the safety of repeated exposures to the LNPs in humans beyond two inoculations.

LNPs also contain cholesterol, which provides flexibility and enhances fusion with cell membranes, and other helper lipids that impart structural integrity and improve the encapsulation efficiency for mRNA. Bitounis et al. (2024) have written an extensive review on the strategies taken to reduce the risks of mRNA drug and vaccine reactivity with the immune system and toxicity.[109]

11.3.9. Analytical Procedures for modRNA Vaccine Quality

Due to the rapid development and newness of the mRNA platform, compendial standards were lacking. These are official quality standards contained in a pharmaceutical compendium such as the United Stated Pharmacopeia-National Formulary (USP-NF) or the European Pharmacopoeia (Ph Eur). The Ph. Eur standards for the assays used for the pro-vaccines are currently being developed, which will include mRNA-LNP medicinal products as well as the DNA template used for the preparation of the mRNA transcript.[110] The USP-NF has developed a second draft of their analytical procedures for modRNA vaccine quality.[111]

It is important to note that compendial standards define a common set of methods to determine mRNA vaccine quality but do not enforce those standards or determine the acceptance criteria for quality and purity, which is under the purview of regulatory agencies. The updated WHO 2022 guidelines for mRNA vaccines also noted that "detailed production and control procedures, controls were not yet standardized," and certain details are not in the public domain and may be considered proprietary and confidential.[112] No specific numerical limit for dsRNA, DNA, plasmid purity, and other process-related impurities were stated in the WHO 2022 guidelines. The WHO guidelines also stated testing for process or product-related impurities "may be reduced or discontinued once production consistency has been demonstrated," if the national regulatory agency is in agreement.

The United States Pharmacopoeia (USP) Draft Guidelines recommends more sensitive methods for analysis of the modRNA than was used by the manufacturer for Process 2 lots. Further, more in-depth analysis of purity of the modRNA drug substance such as nucleoside and residual T7 polymerase are additional proposed quality attributes. These are both welcome additions to detect and quantify these impurities since oxidized nucleotides are associated with age-related, especially neurodegenerative diseases.[113]

As noted earlier, residual dsRNA is a major contaminant of the modRNA drug substance secondary to the IVT process. dsRNA byproducts such as run-off transcripts or an antisense RNA molecule similar in size to the desired mRNA can occur but require various analytical procedures for determining purity and quality. Immunoblot or ELISA analysis used by the manufacturer may not detect these types of dsRNA contamination and are difficult to quantify.[114] Analytical tools such as native and gel electrophoresis were not included to determine these critical quality attributes by the manufacturer or in the draft USP Guidelines.

Finally, RNA sequencing for confirming the expected mRNA sequence in addition to RT-PCR, and a full plethora of DNA plasmid testing including sequencing, is also proposed by USP.[115] These proposed compendial standards provide a more sensitive and thorough analysis for purity and safety than were used for either Process 1 or Process 2 lots, raising questions about safety and purity of both the early and current vaccine product. In particular, the sequencing of the DNA starting material that identifies the mRNA sequence performed for Process 1 lots was replaced with qPCR of the RNA for Process 2 lots,[116] a less sensitive method. This raises troubling questions about the fidelity of transcription during IVT and risks for aberrant protein production that were not identified in safety or analytical testing.

Specifications for quality attributes and testing for the final vaccine product includes LNPs and their lipid contents, appearance, sterility, and selected attributes, which are included in the requirements for final vaccine product lot testing. However, the quality of the vaccine is ultimately reflected in its ability to induce a protective immune response without eliciting undesirable adverse reactions.

Importantly, subdivisible particles were noted in the Process 2 lots but were not described for Process 1 lots. These particles represent impurities and may have toxicological and clinical implications.[117] These impurities may have occurred due to instability of the buffer used in the initial Process 2 lots and were likely due to the fact that Process 1 lots had not been previously frozen and were in fact flown to the clinical sites by private jets as needed.[118] On October 29, 2021, the FDA authorized two presentations representing a major manufacturing change from the phosphate-saline/sucrose buffer to a Tris/sucrose buffer for increased stability, simpler storage requirements and a ready-to-use formulation.[119] Prior to this, the Pfizer/BioNTech vaccine required storage at -80° Celsius (-112° Fahrenheit) prior to its use. This may be viewed as a tacit admission that the stability of the initial lots of the Process 2 batches were suboptimal with unknown safety and efficacy effects.

11.3.10. Additional Issues

A high degree of variability in biodistribution of the COVID-19 vaccines can result from how they are inoculated into the deltoid muscles of recipients. A standard protocol of aspiration during intramuscular injection of COVID-19 vaccines was generally abandoned, since it can slightly increase the risk of pain during administration.[120] As a consequence, about 2 percent or more of the vaccinations almost certainly delivered the COVID-19 vaccine LNPs or adenoviruses directly into the bloodstream. This could account in part for why a small portion of vaccine recipients have much more severe adverse effects than most others.[121]

No one knows the potency, quantity, or duration of the spike protein produced in different organs or the endothelium (i.e., lining of blood vessel walls) given widespread biodistribution. There is no way to control the amount of spike protein produced or the duration of production. Tens of trillions of LNPs are injected with each vaccination. It is not known how age, sex, weight, or other characteristics affect the potency of the vaccine, nor is it known how much spike protein is made in each organ in humans that takes up the synthetic mRNA. Evidence appears to indicate that small amounts of LNPs may result in large amounts of spike protein being produced in particular organs.[122]

Mulroney et al. (2023)[123] recently noted that N1-methylpseudouridylation of mRNA occasionally causes +1 ribosomal frameshifting in mice and humans with the Pfizer/BioNTech COVID-19 vaccine. This results in production of "off-target" spike proteins that can feature different amino acid sequences after the frameshift, with the potential for eliciting off-target immune responses.[124] The degree to which such novel chimeric proteins are created in COVID-19 RNA-vaccinated individuals remains unclear as do the consequences of antibodies that may be produced against the novel sequences and their reactivities with human proteins.

Basic pharmacological data of the optimal dose, its range, and upper toxicity thresholds are lacking. By not performing pharmacokinetic and distribution studies of the encoded spike protein, which was already known to be toxic and bioactive (off-target effects), the regulatory submissions for the COVID-19 genetic vaccines were incomplete. From the very start, the nonclinical safety studies were designed to provide data that would put the manufacturers' products in a "good light." The critical flaw here was that the guidance documents used by Health Canada were only applicable to traditional vaccines and not vaccines using gene therapy technology.

Overall, mRNA vaccine quality has been questionable and variable. There appear to be substantial differences in the mRNA vaccines between batches and even between vials. This may be due to variations in handling, freezing/thawing/dilution requirements, and manufacturing variability. Stainless steel particles were even seen with the naked eye in some Moderna vials in particular lots.[125] A broad range of limits for purity and quality was permitted in the commercial production of the vaccines. Large manufacturing variability between batches plus patient-to-patient variability likely resulted in different levels of spike production and response to the vaccine product.[126]

There has been significant variability in the severity of adverse events, including lethality, with other COVID-19 vaccines by vaccine maker and batch number. For example, in the United Kingdom, a freedom of information request about adverse reactions with COVID-19 vaccines revealed that for the ten most reported batches up to April 24, 2022, the number of Yellow Card vaccine injury reports varied from one to seven reports per a thousand doses; this included 45,320 reports for the AstraZeneca, 32,766 reports for the Pfizer/BioNTech, and 12,550 reports for the Moderna vaccines.[127] Contamination has also been an issue, for example, with the AstraZeneca vaccines (which although manufactured by Emergent Biosolutions in Baltimore in the United States, were never approved for use by the FDA, but were exported to Canada and Mexico).[128] More than half of Canada's supply of the AstraZeneca came from the Baltimore plant until these vaccines were pulled on May 11, 2021, from the Canadian market.[129] Some of the problem involved cross-contamination with the Johnston & Johnson COVID-19 adenovirus vaccine. Likewise, there was a major issue with batches of the Moderna COVID-19 vaccines in Japan.[130] Two Japanese men died after receipt of the second dose of the same batch of a Moderna COVID-19 vaccine, and subsequent testing found black substances of a few millimeters in size in forty vials of a different batch of the Moderna vaccine. About half a million people in Japan were inoculated with three batches of the Moderna vaccine before 1.63 million doses were recalled by Moderna Inc, Takeda Pharmaceuticals Co Ltd, and the Japanese authorities.

Another retrospective study of 66,587 suspected adverse effects (SAE) across fifty-two specific batches of Pfizer/BioNTech BNT162b2 administered to 4,026,575 people in Denmark between December 27, 2020, and January 11, 2022, revealed large variations in the reported SAE.[131] The SAE rates were lower in the larger vaccine batches, and there were batch-dependent differences in the seriousness of the SAE. Certain smaller batches (representing 4.2 percent of all the vaccine doses) were associated with 71 percent of all SAEs, 27.5 percent of all serious SAEs, and 47 percent of all SAE-related deaths in the Danish study.

11.3.11. WHO Guidelines on Vaccine Evaluation

With regard to Health Canada's approval of the Pfizer COVID-19 vaccines, both Pfizer and Health Canada followed the internationally accepted guidelines from the WHO for vaccine evaluation stating that the "Pharmacokinetic studies (e.g., determining serum or tissue concentrations of vaccine components) are normally not needed."[132] With respect to scope, a WHO 2005 document states, "For the purposes of this document, vaccines are considered to be a heterogeneous class of medicinal products containing immunogenic substances capable of inducing specific, active and protective host immunity against infectious disease.[133]

The WHO 2014 Annex 2 guidelines states when it comes to scope, "This document addresses regulatory considerations related to the nonclinical and initial clinical evaluation of adjuvanted vaccines."[134] BNT162b2 does not contain an adjuvant, although the LNPs do cause inflammation. Essentially, the WHO publications are only applicable to traditional vaccines, and not vaccines using gene therapy technology.[135]

In a December 2020 draft document on regulatory evaluation,[136] WHO admitted that detailed information was not available for the production of the COVID-19 mRNA vaccines. The WHO confirmed that controls for safety and efficacy of gene-based mRNA vaccine biologic products were not standardized. Certain details of vaccine components remain proprietary and were not publicly disclosed. In light of these unknowns, the WHO conceded that it was not feasible to develop specific international regulatory guidelines or recommendations, and strict adherence to normal regulatory guidance may not be possible.

It appears that there is insufficient evidence that these vaccine products meet the quality required of pharmaceutical products, raising concerns about their safety and efficacy. Regulatory assessment using current vaccine guidance is likely inadequate to determine safety and efficacy for a genetic product.[137] Assessment using a comprehensive gene therapy guidance may have been more appropriate given the nature of transfection with a nucleic acid, but currently is *not required* if the *use* of the product is for prevention of infectious diseases such as a vaccine.[138]

11.4. Concluding Remarks

Based on the regulatory assessment of the mRNA vaccines, the following can be reasonably concluded:

1. These products are essentially genetic therapy products that were not fully assessed by regulatory authorities under the guidance and controls required for such products. Although they are indicated for the prevention of an infectious disease and are used as vaccines, under new definitions by the CDC and WHO, the mode of action of these products is based on transfection of a nucleic acid containing genetic information, but the appropriate regulatory controls and long-term safety studies were not performed.[139]
2. These products are mislabeled and adulterated. The label does not specify these are bioengineered nucleic acid mRNA, nor state the nano format of the LNPs which may act as an adjuvant and provide for biodistribution throughout the body. These products are contaminated with small amounts of endotoxin, dsRNA, and significant contamination with plasmid DNA from the template produced by E. coli. Residual dsDNA poses particular oncological infectious risks.[140] Furthermore, the frameshifting in the reading of

N1-methylpseudouridylated spike mRNA by ribosomes generates highly mutated forms of the spike protein that may interfere with the formation of the spike trimers in cells.

One of the main mechanisms to consider with the dsDNA is insertional mutagenesis, although this is not a prerequisite for limiting dsDNA in medicinal products approved for human use. Firstly, DNA and RNA can enter spermatozoa and be transmitted to the next generation, along with the traits they encode for, without chromosomal integration.[141]

Secondly, a related phenomenon is that of episomal expression, which has been used in the development of gene therapy to achieve genetic modification without altering the chromosomal DNA. Other aspects of how DNA limits were to be assessed, such as those found in FDA guidelines, were not addressed.[142]

3. The FDA proposed that any DNA contaminants smaller than about two hundred base pairs are unlikely to act as functional gene sequences, but specific types of contaminating sequences require particular scrutiny, including the SV40 promoter/enhancer sequence containing two seventy-two base pair repeats, as this sequence is a known nuclear localization sequence that can ferry DNA into the nucleus of cells.[143] The commercial product was produced with a sufficiently different manufacturing process (Process 2) requiring verification of clinical comparability for efficacy and safety. This data does not appear to be available. This is not a theoretical concern since a similar issue arose from the 1976 swine flu inoculations, where the original influenza vaccine had been field tested, but upon the declaration of a pandemic, the updated influenza vaccines were made without any confirmatory comparability testing.[144]
4. Several cases of Guillain-Barré syndrome (see chapter 13.9.1) were associated with the COVID-19 genetic vaccines, and issues with manufacturing such as endotoxin contamination were considered a potential cause.[145]

Real-world data falsifies the original claim that mRNA-based COVID-19 biologics function as an authentic vaccine for preventing viral infection and transmission rather than as a short-term gene-based therapeutic agent that might alleviate, at best, symptom severity. With this in mind, the authorization of these products should be suspended until the concerns raised in this and the next two chapters have been resolved and publicly verified by the regulatory authorities.

CHAPTER 12

Effectiveness of COVID-19 Vaccines

Steven Pelech

"However beautiful the strategy, you should look occasionally at the results."

—Winston Churchill

12.1. Approved COVID-19 Vaccines in Canada under Interim Order

Four COVID-19 vaccines, all targeting the spike protein on the surface of the SARS-CoV-2 virus, were approved for use in Canada in 2021 under Interim Order: Pfizer-BioNTech BNT162b2 (later named Comirnaty and tozinameran) and Moderna mRNA-1273 (later named Spikevax and elasomeran), which are both vaccines that deliver mRNA for production of the spike protein; and AstraZeneca's Vaxzevria and Janssen's Jcovden (Johnson & Johnson [J&J]) vaccines, which are both adenovirus preparations that contain DNA that provide for mRNA production to then permit the biosynthesis of the spike protein. In 2022, Novavax's Nuvaxovid and Medicago's Corifenz were also approved by Health Canada. These latter vaccines used preparations of spike protein that were purified from genetically engineered caterpillar cells and tobacco leaf cells, respectively, and delivered in a lipid nanoparticle along with a novel, untested adjuvant to stimulate an immune reaction; each Nuvaxovid vaccine dose contains about five microgram (μg) of spike protein, and Corifenz vaccine dose uses about 3.75 μg of a lipid membrane-encapsulated virus-like particle that is enriched in spike protein. (One μg is one millionth of a gram.)

The first two doses for those over twelve years of age of the Moderna vaccine each had 100 μg of the RNA for the spike protein, compared to 30 μg of the RNA for the same protein in each of the first two adult doses of the Pfizer-BioNTech vaccine. After six months, booster shots were recommended by health regulatory agencies for those twelve years of age or older with the Pfizer-BioNTech vaccine (30 μg/dose) and for those over eighteen years of age with the Moderna vaccine (50 μg/dose).[1]

For the COVID-19 vaccination of children six months and older, only the Pfizer-BioNTech and Moderna RNA vaccines were approved by Health Canada.[2] The Moderna product was approved for six month- to five-year-olds with a two-dose regimen (25 μg/dose one month apart), whereas the Pfizer product was approved with a three-dose regiment) (3 μg/dose at an interval of three weeks between the first and second doses, with eight weeks between the second and third dose). For five- to eleven-year-olds, the Pfizer-BioNTech vaccine was used at a dosage that was one third of the teen and adult dose (10 μg/dose),[3] whereas the Moderna vaccine was used at half the adult dose (50 μg/dose) for five- to eleven-year-olds,[4] and a quarter of the adult dose for six-month- to four-year-old children (25 μg/dose). Therefore, a five-year-old child received five-times higher levels of the spike protein mRNA with the pediatric dose of the Moderna vaccine when compared to the Pfizer-BioNTech product. A six-month-old child received an eight-times-higher level of the spike protein mRNA with the pediatric dose of the Moderna vaccine when compared to the Pfizer-BioNTech product. Normally, a dose of a vaccine would roughly be related to body weight, but it is quite evident that this was largely ignored with the dispensing of the COVID-19 vaccines.

Based on the doses of spike protein mRNA that have been used in these vaccines, it can be estimated that a single 100 μg inoculation may contain over ten trillion lipid nanoparticles that typically feature around five to ten copies of the spike protein gene. The whole SARS-CoV-2 RNA is close to thirty thousand nucleotides long and is single-stranded, but the spike gene is only around four thousand nucleotides. It is calculated that the human genome, with 2.9 billion nucleotides per strand weighs about 0.855 picogram per strand. (A pictogram is a trillionth of a gram.) Therefore, four thousand nucleotides would weigh around 0.00000118 picograms or 0.00000000000118 μg per four thousand nucleotide RNA molecules. With 100 μg of RNA in one vaccine inoculation, this works out to about eighty-five trillion RNA molecules by this calculation. (As discussed in chapter 11.3.7.4., there is also some contaminating plasmid DNA with the RNA, so the final number of RNA molecules may be slightly less.) From each genetically modified RNA molecule, it is feasible that hundreds of copies of the spike protein can be produced.

Traditional vaccines with attenuated, weakened strains of a pathogenic virus typically range from as low as fifty to a few thousand virus particles in an inoculation, with each virus having only one copy of each viral gene. Consequently, the COVID-19 genetic vaccines permit the generation of spike proteins in vaccine recipients that are at levels that could never be achieved with previous vaccines or a natural infection without causing severe disease or death. This incredible capacity of these RNA and adenovirus vaccines to produce such high levels of spike protein accounts for their ability to elicit strong immune responses, but also their higher potential for vaccine injury.

As mentioned, the four COVID-19 genetic vaccines that were offered in Canada were RNA-based using lipid nanoparticle carriers (i.e., Pfizer-BioNTech and Moderna) or DNA-based using adenovirus carriers (i.e., AstraZeneca and J&J). In each case, these particular vaccines deliver genetic instructions for the production of the spike protein of the SARS-CoV-2 virus inside of the host cells that take up these vaccines (initially at the site of the injection in the deltoid muscle region of the arm). The spike protein is then presented on the surface of these cells to elicit an inflammatory immune response that culminates in the stimulation and proliferation of T cells and B cells, the latter producing antibodies that specifically target epitopes on the spike protein. However, to produce the activation of T cells and B cells, this necessitates the damage and likely destruction of the spike-presenting transfected cells. This is particularly problematic for neurons and cardiac muscle cells (cardiomyocytes), which do not regenerate in adults.

Lipid nanoparticles and adenoviruses have been used previously to deliver drugs and toxins into animals for therapeutic purposes, and even to elicit immune responses.[5] Lipid nanoparticles or genetically engineered adenoviruses normally present the antigen of the pathogen on their surfaces for these vaccines. However, the combination of the lipid nanoparticles to get production of a target pathogen's protein on the surface of the body's own cells to elicit an immune response against that target remains experimental, especially since new information continues to accrue about the unexpected consequences of this novel method of antibody production.

In a sense, the genetic vaccines are "pro-drugs," which require further processing to produce active ingredients. Unfortunately, the production of the spike protein is very host cell-dependent, and this processing is influenced by many different factors, including vaccine dose to body size ratio, the cell type taking up the vaccine, health, nutritional, hormonal, and pharmacological status.[6] Consequently, the levels of spike protein could potentially vary by up to two orders of magnitude (i.e., a hundred-fold) or more. This can lead to marked variations in vaccine efficacy and injury from person to person.

Prior to the approvals of these vaccine formulations for human use by the FDA and Health Canada at the end of 2020, no such lipid nanoparticles or adenoviruses had ever been approved for any RNA- or DNA-based vaccine to produce immunity against a pathogen's proteins by specifying their production within the body's own cells. It should be noted that the European Medicines Agency did approve Johnson and Johnson's Zabdeno, an adenovirus-based vaccine for prevention of Ebola virus disease, under Emergency Use Authorization in 2020. However, this vaccine was only about 50 percent effective in tested animals, and its efficacy in humans still remains to be determined in a formal clinical trial, since ethically it would be wrong to test such vaccines in healthy volunteers.[7] Zabdeno was not marketed in Canada or the United States.

To counteract the COVID-19 pandemic crisis, the four COVID-19 genetic vaccines were first released for general use in the Canadian population starting in mid-December 2020 under an Interim Order. In the United States, only three of these vaccines (AstraZeneca's adenovirus vaccine was not approved) were authorized for general use through Emergency Use Authorization (EUA). It is noteworthy that EUA approval is normally granted only if there are no alternative treatments for a disease, although technically dexamethasone had already been shown to effectively treat many cases of hospitalized COVID-19 patients that require supplemental oxygen.[8]

In Canada, the United States, and elsewhere, these vaccines were still technically in Phase 3 clinical trials in early 2023. For example, the Pfizer-BioNTech COVID-19 vaccine, which is the most widely used, was in Phase 3 trials that were not scheduled to be completed until July 30, 2023.[9] The approvals provided by Health Canada and the FDA remain contingent on active and passive monitoring of the efficacy and safety of these non-traditional vaccines. Consequently, these COVID-19 vaccines are still regarded by many as highly experimental in nature. The fact that billions of people have been inoculated with these vaccines does not mean that they are not still experimental, as their efficacy and safety remain topics of intense biomedical research with ongoing publications in scientific journals.

As mentioned in chapter 10, the testing of drugs and vaccines by manufacturers normally requires pre-clinical trials in at least two different animal models to provide initial efficacy and safety data. Phase 1 trials are performed on healthy volunteers to evaluate initial safety concerns. Phase 2 trials are then undertaken with the main targeted participants (i.e., those most vulnerable to a disease) with different concentrations of the drug or vaccine to establish an optimum dose to elicit a desired therapeutic or immune response as appropriate. Phase 3 trials are subsequently conducted on usually thousands of targeted participants in multiple centers to investigate the longer-term efficacy and safety of the tested drug or vaccine at an optimal dose.

The importance of continuing Phase 3 studies with COVID-19 vaccines has been prompted by several factors, including an unprecedented shortening of the typical testing period (five to ten years) of a vaccine before approval for general release to under a single year with "Operation Warp Speed" in the United States. This was achieved by reducing the number of many cell and animal preclinical trials with the vaccines that are normally undertaken over one to three years down to a couple of months and running them in parallel with Phase 1 and 2 human trials. Of particular concern, many of the safety studies were performed in rats or mice, which is problematic, because these rodents do not feature ACE2 receptors that bind to the original Wuhan SARS-CoV-2 spike protein. Phase 2 and 3 trials—which instead of being conducted over the usual three to five years, were combined, and based on just two months of testing—were approved for dissemination to the general population with an Interim Order in Canada and an Emergency Use Authorization in the United States. For example, the Phase 3 clinical studies with the Pfizer-BioNTech vaccine commenced on July 27, 2020, and the vaccine was approved for general use for those over eighteen years of age by early December 2020. Ultimately, these novel genetic vaccines were approved for wide-spread use in about a tenth of the time as compared to traditional vaccines.

It should be appreciated that the RNA- and adenovirus-based genetic vaccines did not satisfy the CDC's original definition of a "vaccine," which was previously described as "a product that stimulates a person's immune system to produce immunity to a specific disease, protecting the person from that disease."[10] Later, on September 1, 2021, the definition of vaccine was simplified to "a preparation that is used to stimulate the body's immune response against diseases." This new definition of "immunity" was also problematic with "protection from an infectious disease." The CDC states that if "you are immune to a disease, you can be exposed to it without becoming infected."[11] Obviously, this must be false, because the actual infection with the virus still proceeds, but ideally, the immune system is able to eradicate the virus before it can evoke the symptoms of disease. It is amply clear that one can still become infected with SARS-CoV-2 after vaccination, but the claims were later adjusted to suggest that protection is provided to reduce the severity of the illness, but not necessarily to prevent infection. This means that one can still become infected and still transmit the pathogen.

The COVID-19 RNA and adenovirus "vaccines" are more like genetic therapy, because they do not contain the actual immunogen to elicit an antibody response but rather provide genetic instructions for the body to produce the immunogen. Normally, the use of genetic therapy products commands a much higher level of testing than traditional drugs or vaccines. It is also noteworthy that vaccines do not carry the same degree of liability to manufacturers for injury from these products in the United States compared with other drugs.[12]

As mentioned earlier, all COVID-19 vaccines were approved under Interim Order in Canada, and under Emergency Use Authorization in the United States. Most people would be surprised to learn that the efficacy and safety requirements for approval of a medication or device under Interim Order are minimal and, contrary to popular belief, even among health professionals, vaccines and drugs can be approved with little or even no evidence of efficacy and safety under Interim Order, as stipulated in Section 30.1 of the Food and Drugs Act,

R.S.C., 1985, c. F-27.[13] This is apparently what happened with Health Canada's approval of the COVID-19 genetic vaccines starting in December 2020. This does not mean that these experimental COVID-19 vaccines were known to be efficacious and safe at the time of their approval. As noted in Shawn Buckley's discussion publication:

> For COVID-19 vaccines, there were the following major legal changes to deliberately circumvent the normal protections in our drug approval law:
>
> a) The normal drug approval process requires objective proof of:
>
> i. safety;
>
> ii. efficacy; and
>
> iii. benefit outweighing risk.
>
> COVID-19 vaccines were exempted from this normal drug approval process.
>
> COVID-19 vaccines were approved under a subjective test which mandated that approval must be granted if the argument could be made that the benefits outweighed the risk. No actual proof of safety, efficacy or benefit outweighing risk was required;
>
> b) the law was changed so that the approval of a COVID-19 vaccine could not be revoked:
>
> i. due to evidence the vaccine was unsafe or not-effective;
>
> ii. due to assessments the benefits did not outweigh the risks.
>
> These legal changes were in force from September 16, 2020 to:
>
> i. September 15, 2021, for the Pfizer and Moderna vaccines;
>
> ii. November 18, 2021, for the AstraZeneca vaccine, and
>
> iii. November 22, 2021 for the Johnson and Johnson vaccine, and
>
> c) a classic conflict of interest was created where the Government was allowed to purchase and import unapproved vaccines while the Government waited for itself to approve the vaccines.[14]

12.2. Relative and Absolute Risk Reduction with COVID-19 Vaccines

As outlined in chapter 10, drugs and vaccines are "normally" expected to undergo a rigorous testing process, first in animals and then in people. This is not what happened with the COVID-19 vaccines. Animal trials, when actually performed, were conducted in parallel with human trials, and the Phase 3 human trials were predominantly carried out on healthy people or those who had only one co-morbidity and were mainly working-age adults. Normally, Phase 3 trials are carried out on those that would most benefit from a treatment.

Before reviewing the Phase 3 clinical trials with COVID-19 vaccines that were used to justify the Interim Order approval in Canada and equivalent approvals by regulatory agencies in other countries, it is instructive to understand the difference between "relative risk reduction" (RRR) and "absolute risk reduction" (ARR) in monitoring the effectiveness of a medical treatment. The ARR is the absolute difference in rates of an event (e.g., infection) between the experimental group and the control group. It is calculated by subtracting the experimental group event rate (ER) from the control group event rate (CR) and is usually expressed as a percentage. In contrast, the relative risk reduction (RRR), or vaccine efficacy (VE), represents the relative decrease in the risk of an adverse event in the experimental group compared to the control group. It is calculated as the relative risk of the rate of the experimental group event rate (ER) minus the rate of the control group (CR) divided by rate of the control group (CR), and, as with the ARR, is usually expressed as a percentage.

To illustrate this, consider a trial with two hundred participants (one hundred allocated to the experimental group and one hundred allocated to the control group); if one of the experimental participants becomes ill (rate 1/100 = 0.01), compared with two in the control group (rate 2/100 = 0.02) who become ill, the RRR of the vaccine is 50 percent (= (0.01–0.02)/0.02) x 100 percent), a potentially attractive reduction likely to persuade users to accept the treatment. In contrast, the ARR is merely 1 percent (= (0.02—0.01) x 100 percent), which means that most of the individuals who did not take the "vaccine" are still likely to remain free from the "disease" 98 percent of the time, as opposed to 99 percent of the time if they took the vaccine. This may give pause to patients and health professionals when considering the desirability of accepting a new treatment, especially considering the scant safety data.[15] Of note, while the RRR of the first Pfizer-BioNTech trial was 95 percent, the ARR was only 0.8 percent, which was calculated by independent investigators but not reported in the original peer-reviewed publication (although the raw data was available in the supplemental section to permit such calculations).[16]

Because communicating relative risk can be so misleading, not only to the public but also to health professionals, in a 2011 report entitled "Communicating Risks and Benefits: A User's Guide," the FDA instructed investigators to "provide absolute risks, not just relative risks," noting (on page 60) that patients "are unduly influenced when risk information is presented using a relative risk approach; this can result in suboptimal decisions. Thus, an absolute risk format should be used."[17] To put this into perspective, based on the COVID-19 RNA vaccine Phase 3 trial data in a six-month period (the duration of the clinical study to generate this data), vaccinating everyone in the vaccine group only reduced COVID-19 incidence by less than 1 percent compared to no vaccination, despite the RRR of 95 percent.[18] This was because the overall risks of getting symptomatic COVID-19 that was confirmed by PCR testing in the unvaccinated group during the six-months period was only about 4 percent.

12.3. Distinguishing Between the Unvaccinated and Vaccinated in Clinical Studies

It should be appreciated that vaccine efficacy estimates that have been published in clinical trial reports of Phase 3 clinical trials with COVID-19 vaccines and highly quoted by public health officials have been RRR and not ARR values. In the Phase 3 clinical trials to ascertain whether the COVID-19 vaccines reduced the actual occurrence of SARS-CoV-2 infection and COVID-19 symptoms, there have been numerous deficiencies in the haste to get these vaccines to market. These clinical trials did not assess whether the vaccines reduced transmission, severity, hospitalizations, or deaths. Moreover, they poorly evaluated whether COVID-19 vaccines reduced occurrence of the disease in segments of the population that are at greatest risk, namely the very elderly, obese, or those with comorbidities.

The preclinical, Phase 1, Phase 2, and Phase 3 trials were all accelerated for these vaccines, and the formal Phase 3 clinical trials never tested end points such as protection from COVID-19–induced death or transmissibility of the virus. Nor were biochemical studies of blood samples performed, such as D-dimer analyses to detect potential blood clotting, C-reactive protein for inflammation, and troponin for heart damage. In the absence of properly matched placebo controls, these deficiencies may not be clear from the post-marketing safety studies of the COVID-19 vaccines following their release to the public. Instead, the post-marketing, Phase 4 studies were relied upon to learn more about the benefits, limitations, and risks of the COVID-19 vaccines, for example, on pregnancy outcomes. For all intents and purposes, these novel RNA and adenovirus vaccines still remain "experimental" as more problematic issues have become identified over time. Ironically, as data accumulate regarding their clinical outcomes, regulations governing their use are constantly being refined. As highlighted in the next few paragraphs, the term "unvaccinated" is very problematic, and can cause significant misrepresentation of the COVID-19 data on public health websites.

In consideration of all the epidemiological studies that benchmark the risk reduction of acquiring COVID-19 with the vaccines relative to "unvaccinated" individuals, irrespective of whether such comparisons are made in the clinical trials or the post-approval release of these vaccines, the following points are significant and common issues that must be appreciated:

A. A higher testing bias by PCR or rapid antigen testing of unvaccinated people occurred, especially since the adoption of vaccine passports, where workplace testing was usually focused, or even restricted to those that were unvaccinated;

B. Very frail and elderly people, who are also at greatest risk of requiring hospitalization due to their fragile condition, were often not vaccinated in some places like Quebec for fear of vaccine-induced injury from mounting overly strong immune responses;
C. The definition of the "vaccinated" included only those who were two- to three-weeks after their vaccination (depending on the province in Canada). Hence, for statistical purposes, patients who were actually vaccinated but developed COVID-19 within the first two- to three-weeks post vaccination were categorized as unvaccinated. This is particularly problematic, because vaccination appeared to initially increase the risk of acquiring COVID-19, especially when this was performed during a wave of COVID-19 cases;
D. The over-reporting of hospital cases, ICU admissions, and deaths of individuals with COVID-19 under circumstances where the original hospitalizations were due to other reasons independent of having a SARS-CoV-2 infection, i.e., the individuals had an existing comorbidity or death from other causes but happened to test positive for SARS-CoV-2 at the time of admission or during their stay in hospital. By April 2022, only 46 percent of recorded COVID-19 cases in Ontario hospitals had COVID-19 symptoms at the time of admittance.[19] Likewise in British Columbia by the end of January 2022, only about 40 percent of all of the COVID-19 cases were symptomatic at admission;[20] and
E. Many of the "vaccinated" and "unvaccinated" cases already had immunity from natural infection with SARS-CoV-2. This was especially evident in children, most of whom were asymptomatic for COVID-19.

With respect to Point B, data from Scotland revealed that at the time of triple vaccination of the elderly, there were increased COVID-19 case numbers in the elderly as shown in a report provide by Public Health Scotland.[21] This was attributed to vaccination "and the prioritisation of the booster/third dose to the clinically extremely vulnerable at the beginning of the booster programme." However, as will be further explained, due to the extremely high production of spike protein with each vaccination, the capacity of the highly mobile immune system may be overwhelmed initially with appearance of spike protein on body cells and is unable to also deal with SARS-CoV-2 virus particles that enter into the respiratory system. Facing less resistance in the upper airways and lungs, these viruses can propagate sufficiently to then produce illness. This is why vaccination during a COVID-19 wave with increased cases is not advised, because it may actually increase the spread of the disease.

With respect to Point C, one of the reasons why the aggregation of COVID-19 cases diagnosed within two weeks of injection together with the unvaccinated is very problematic becomes apparent upon the analyses of epidemiological data that was provided by the Alberta Health website.[22] Data in tabular and graphic forms were provided for the occurrence of COVID-19 in vaccinated individuals as a function of time following vaccination that was available between August 11, 2021 and January 11, 2022 online. One of these figures (Figure 4 on the website) showed the timing of COVID-19 infections in people that were vaccinated only once. Note that this data must be recovered using the Way Back Machine website[23] as it was removed on January 11, 2022. This figure revealed a dramatic rise in COVID-19 cases in the first seven days post-inoculation. After about nine days, the number of COVID-19 cases started to decline. It is clear that vaccination actually increased the chances of getting COVID-19 during the first two weeks. If it did not, then the rate of COVID-19 should have remained unchanged for about a week, and then it should have dropped with the development of immunity. In view of this vaccine-induced increase in COVID-19 cases within the first two weeks of the first vaccination, it is highly inappropriate to include these cases with the unvaccinated cases, which was routinely done by public health authorities. It renders case counts, hospital admissions, and deaths higher than they should be for the unvaccinated and makes the single vaccinated data look more favorable for vaccine-induced protection from SARS-CoV-2 infection and COVID-19 disease with vaccines. The high levels of spike production during this initial period places a burden on the immune system that may divert it from an effective response to an actual SARS-CoV-2 infection in the airways. Antibodies and T cells that could recognize the spike protein, rather than targeting incoming SARS-CoV-2 virus particles, are instead preoccupied with attacking the vaccinated cells that are actively producing the spike protein throughout the entire body.

An increased risk of getting COVID-19 immediately following a second COVID-19 vaccine inoculation was also evident in Figure 5 from the same Alberta Health website.[24] There was also a rise in COVID-19 cases in the first seven days. Considering that these individuals would have been vaccinated typically about four weeks to six weeks before, and should still have had peak immunity, it was surprising to see an increase in COVID-19 case counts immediately following the second shot. This likely explains why, for some people, the vaccine appeared to increase susceptibility to infection with SARS-CoV-2, which is a phenomenon also consistent with antibody-dependent enhancement. The data shown in Figure 5 of the Alberta Health website indicated that the peak number of the COVID-19 vaccine breakthrough cases up to November 29, 2021 (just prior to the Omicron wave) occurred at around three months after the second shot. This indicated that the window of protection offered from COVID-19 by the COVID-19 vaccines for the SARS-CoV-2 Delta variant for many people was only about three months rather than the six months that was commonly stated by public health authorities. The Alberta Health website was one of the few such public health websites that presented such data, but it was removed without explanation in January 2022.

12.4. The Pfizer-BioNTech BNT162b2 Phase 3 Studies

The Pfizer-BioNTech BNT162b2 Phase 3 clinical studies exemplify many of the deficiencies in the general testing of the COVID-19 genetic vaccines. This vaccine was approved under Interim Order in Canada and Emergency Use Authorization in the United States after just two months of human Phase 3 clinical data had been collected.[25] A 95.1 percent Relative Risk Reduction among the vaccinated cohort (30 μg of spike RNA in the initial inoculation followed by a second 30 μg of spike RNA shot three weeks later) relative to the unvaccinated participants was reported in the *New England Journal of Medicine* (*NEJM*). The clinical trial participants were all sixteen years or older, 22 percent were sixty-five years or older, but only 4.5 percent were seventy-five years or older. Those with more than one co-morbidity were excluded, and only 21 percent had a co-existing condition. A confirmed COVID-19 diagnosis was based on FDA criteria "as the presence of at least one of the following symptoms: fever, new or increased cough, new or increased shortness of breath, chills, new or increased muscle pain, new loss of taste or smell, sore throat, diarrhea, or vomiting, combined with a respiratory specimen obtained during the symptomatic period or within 4 days before or after it that was [PCR] positive for SARS-CoV-2."[26] There were eight out of 21,720 vaccinated participants (0.036 percent) that got symptomatic COVID-19, which was confirmed by a PCR test, seven days to two months after their vaccination, compared to 162 out of 21,728 unvaccinated participants (0.7456 percent). This worked out to a ((0.007456–0.00036) x 100 percent =) 0.71 percent Absolute Risk Reduction of symptomatic COVID-19 and a Relative Risk Reduction of ((0.007456–0.00036)/0.007456) x 100 percent =) 95.2 percent. Following dose 1, but before dose 2, the RRR was 52.4 percent. In the COVID-19 vaccinated group, one out of eight participants (12.5 percent) had severe COVID-19, compared with nine out of 162 (5.6 percent) in the unvaccinated group. The trial did not assess whether the COVID-19 vaccine prevented asymptomatic COVID-19 nor transmission of SARS-CoV-2. In this study, the authors did not observe an increased rate of COVID-19 in the vaccinated group compared to the unvaccinated group in the first twelve days following the first inoculation, which contrasts with the Alberta Health data.

For the six-months stage of the same clinical Phase 3 study, Thomas et al. (2021) updated their clinical findings in *NEJM*, and also included data for twelve- to fifteen-year-olds of age that were vaccinated.[27] There were eighty-one out of 22,166 vaccinated participants (0.365 percent) that got symptomatic COVID-19 confirmed by PCR seven days to six months after their vaccination, compared to 873 out of 21,689 unvaccinated participants (4.025 percent). This worked out to a ((0.04025–0.00365) x 100 percent =) 3.66 percent ARR and a 90.7 percent RRR of symptomatic COVID-19. The incidence of COVID-19 apparently increased in the unvaccinated group from eighty-one symptomatic cases per month in the first two months of the Phase 3 study to 145.5 cases per month in the next four months of trial. However, in the double vaccinated group, the number of symptomatic COVID-19 breakthrough cases per month increased from four to 20.3 in the first two months compared to the next four months. This indicated a trend toward reduced efficacy of the COVID-19 vaccine over time. Between four and six months after the second inoculation with the vaccine, the RRR with the vaccine was reduced to 83.7 percent. These data indicate that for a portion of the vaccinated participants, there appeared to be an increased risk of getting COVID-19.

Some of the issues associated with the Thomas et al. (2021) study related to the potentially biased testing of the trial participants, since the study was unblinded to the study subjects and the researchers after two months into the Phase 3 trial.[28] This unblinding revealed to both the participants and the researchers who in the trial was actually inoculated and who was not with the BNT162b2 vaccine, which compromised the study and allowed the introduction of bias. The physician researchers in the study decided which participants were to be further tested by PCR to confirm COVID-19 cases. Less than 10 percent of the trial participants with COVID-19 symptoms were actually tested by PCR. When the suspected and confirmed cases of COVID-19 together were compared in the vaccinated (1,602/22,166 participants) and non-vaccinated (1,978/21,689 participants) populations in the six-month Pfizer study, the RRR was actually only 19 percent. One has to wonder what was causing the COVID-19-like symptoms of most of the people in the vaccinated group, since the incidence of RSV and influenza in the general population had plummeted during the same period? Moreover, about 89 percent of the unvaccinated participants later opted to receive the COVID-19 vaccine, which effectively ended longer term evaluations of safety and efficacy with the experimental vaccines.

The six-months Pfizer-BioNTech clinical study was performed at 153 sites worldwide, with 130 of the testing sites in the United States. According to the *British Medical Journal* (*BMJ*), a former regional director Brook Jackson, who worked at one of sites that was operated by the Ventavia Research Group, alleged that "the company falsified data, unblinded patients, employed inadequately trained vaccinators, and was slow to follow up on adverse events reported in Pfizer's pivotal phase III trial."[29] After repeatedly notifying Ventavia of these problems, Ms. Jackson emailed a complaint to the FDA, and Ventavia fired her later the same day. In August 2021, after granting full approval of the Pfizer-BioNTech vaccine, the FDA reported that it had previously performed inspections at nine of the trial's 153 sites, which excluded the three Ventavia sites, but it had not undertaken any new inspections in the eight months following the FDA's Emergency Use Authorization in December 2020.[30]

Following the release of the COVID-19 vaccines to those that were eighteen years and older, Pfizer conducted an additional series of Phase 3 studies to permit the marketing of their vaccine to toddlers through to teenagers. This was based on the concept that while these age groups were at extremely low risk of severe COVID-19, they could still acquire SARS-CoV-2 infections and be highly transmissible. These were much smaller-sized Phase 3 studies, and their endpoints were primarily to demonstrate that the vaccines successfully boosted anti-spike antibody levels. Very few of the participants, even in the unvaccinated groups, were sick with COVID-19. The number of trial participants was insufficient to identify serious safety risks that may have occurred in less than one in a few thousand people.

In the first two very small immune-bridging trials conducted by Pfizer, fewer than 2,500 participants were enrolled. Each study was designed to establish the presence of effective neutralizing antibody concentrations in the blood of a small subset of twelve- to fifteen-year-old (n=190) and five- to eleven-year-old (n=264) children compared to young adults, and provided only preliminary descriptive outcomes for clinical efficacy and safety of the Pfizer-BioNTech vaccine compared to placebo controls.[31, 32] The Phase 2/3 clinical results from testing the Pfizer-BioNTech vaccine in 1,517 children from five- to eleven-year-olds with two vaccine doses (10 μg RNA in each dose) spaced one month apart and followed for 2.3 months was compared to 751 that were treated with a placebo.[33] The mean age of the participants was 8.2 years; 20 percent of children had coexisting conditions (including 12 percent with obesity and approximately 8 percent with asthma), and at least 9 percent previously had SARS-CoV-2. The authors reported a RRR of 90.7 percent for acquiring COVID-19. However, there were only three presumed COVID-19 cases in total in the vaccinated group and sixteen in the unvaccinated group. None of the COVID-19 cases were severe. The ARR was a mere 2 percent for both age groups, which were at little to no risk of developing severe COVID-19. Based on this, Health Canada authorized use of Pfizer-BioNTech COVID-19 vaccine in children twelve to fifteen years of age on May 5, 2021, and this was followed by approval for use of this RNA vaccine (at a third of the adult dosage) for five- to eleven-year-olds on November 19, 2021.[34] Thereafter, Health Canada approved on March 17, 2022, the Moderna Spikevax COVID-19 vaccine (two doses, 50 μg RNA in each dose, four weeks apart) for six- to eleven-year-olds.[35] It should be appreciated that the amount of spike RNA in Moderna COVID-19 vaccine for this age group of children was 67 percent higher than the adult dose of Spike RNA in the Pfizer-BioNTech vaccine.

On June 15, 2022, the FDA authorized the Pfizer-BioNTech for children six months or older[36] and then similarly authorized the Moderna vaccine on July 14, 2022; in Canada, the Pfizer-BioNTech vaccine for this age group was approved on September 9, 2022, following a review by the National Advisory Committee on Immunization (NACI).[37, 38] Like the earlier Pfizer COVID-19 mRNA vaccination trials in five- to eleven-year-olds and twelve- to fifteen-year-olds, the studies with two- to four-year-olds and six- to twenty-three-month-olds were also very small immuno-bridging trials, enrolling fewer than three thousand participants in each cohort. They were "not designed to establish the superiority of vaccination compared to naturally acquired immunity," but only the non-inferiority of "neutralizing" antibody concentrations in the blood of a small number of two- to four-year-olds (*n*=143), and six- to twenty-three-month-olds (*n*=82) participants compared to children that were five- to eleven-years old (*n*=264). Because antibody titers in the blood are not a clinically validated measure of efficacy for mucosal infections of the respiratory tract, any study claims regarding efficacy are actually speculative. Moreover, in these studies, assessment of "neutralizing" antibodies only focused on those antibodies that block the binding of the original Wuhan strain of SARS-CoV-2 to the ACE2 protein and entry into test cells. Many of the mutations in the first Omicron variants occurred within the receptor binding domain of the spike protein. Furthermore, over 95 percent of antibody responses to the SARS-CoV-2 spike protein in both vaccinated and SARS-CoV-2-infected individuals are directed toward other regions of the spike protein, and most of the immune protective responses are not measured by "neutralizing" antibody tests.

From seven days to three months post-vaccination for those less than five years of age, the aforementioned studies provided descriptive RRR values in symptomatic cases of COVID-19 of 82 and 76 percent, respectively, for children aged two- to four-years-old and six- to twenty-three-months-old. Moreover, when outcomes were analyzed to reflect the net benefit of the vaccinations in these groups, the ARR in mild symptomatic COVID-19 was a mere 2 percent or lower for all groups following COVID-19 vaccination. In addition, the vaccines did not demonstrate an ability to reduce severe COVID-19 or halt transmission, rendering any claims regarding protection in the majority of children dubious. The trial was originally planned to investigate the vaccinal efficacy of two doses. Of great concern, however, were findings in the two- to four-year-olds cohort that showed that following the first dose, the vaccine was associated with a 199 percent relative risk increase in severe COVID-19 and a 149 percent relative risk increase in multiple COVID-19 infections compared to the placebo control subjects.[39] Astonishingly, the 76 percent RRR noted for six- to twenty-three-month-old infants was based on just three participants in this age group who tested positive for SARS-CoV-2 (one vaccinated versus two placebo); the 82 percent RRR was based on just seven participants in the older two- to four-year-olds (two vaccinated versus five placebo) and was only after triple vaccination of these children.

The pivotal child vaccination studies were much too short (i.e., three months) to establish vaccinal efficacy and did not control for natural immunity. Natural immunity was only assessed by the detection of antibodies against the nucleocapsid protein of SARS-CoV-2, which often fails to be measurable in people that have recovered from COVID-19. Moreover, the child vaccine trials were designed to test vaccines developed against the original Wuhan strain of SARS-CoV-2, which had not been in circulation for over two years. While this probably did not make much difference with respect to the overall immune response to Omicron variants, this does make a difference if the serological tests narrowly rely on detection of antibodies that are "neutralizing" and just targeted the ACE2 receptor binding domain of the spike protein.

Pregnant women were originally excluded from the earlier Pfizer-BioNTech clinical trials for their monovalent COVID-19 vaccine based on the Wuhan spike RNA sequence. On February 18, 2021, Pfizer-BioNTech commenced a four thousand-person Phase 2/3 study to evaluate the efficacy and safety of their vaccine on pregnant women.[40] As of August 2024, there have been no published reports from this specific trial.

It is noteworthy that Pfizer originally recommended that the second dose of the BNT2b2 vaccine should be administered about twenty-eight days after the first inoculation. They had observed declines in anti-spike antibody levels in especially the elderly after twenty-eight days in their original clinical study.[41] However, Almeida et al. (2024) have noted about 31 percent higher production of anti-spike antibodies with a three-month rather than one-month interval between the doses.[42]

12.5. Post-Marketing Performance of COVID-19 Vaccines

With the rollout of COVID-19 vaccines starting in December 2020, in Canada, the initial priority was to vaccinate hospital workers and those at high risk, in particular the very elderly in nursing homes, Indigenous people living on reservations, and those with comorbidities. A shortage of COVID-19 vaccine supply in Canada meant that most people had to wait several months after their initial vaccination to receive their second shot. This was much longer than the manufacturers' recommended three- to four-week interval, which was used in the Phase 3 clinical studies.

The National Advisory Committee on Immunization (NACI) and the Canadian federal government felt that people in Indigenous communities were particularly at risk from COVID-19 and should be prioritized. This had nothing to do with any genetic differences between Indigenous and non-Indigenous people, but was because these communities had fared more poorly in past pandemics and diseases. This decision was largely political.[43] Consequently, Indigenous adults as young as eighteen years old were prioritized for vaccination before non-Indigenous seventy-year-old people in Canadian provinces like Ontario and British Columbia. A cynical observer might wonder why the First Nations communities would be among the first to receive experimental, poorly tested vaccines considering the historical experimentation on these populations in North America in the past for much less altruistic reasons.

Despite the availability of COVID-19 vaccines for everyone by the summer of 2021, Canada continued to experience successive waves of COVID-19, in part from the emergence of new, more infectious variants of SARS-CoV-2. Much ado was initially expressed from health officials that it was primarily unvaccinated people who were filling the hospitals and ICUs and dying from COVID-19. Often in the late summer of 2021, provincial public health officials would state that "since the vaccination program began in December 2020, the vast majority of hospital cases and deaths were unvaccinated." Even US president Joe Biden famously claimed during a town hall in Cincinnati, Ohio on July 21, 2021 that "Ten thousand people have recently died; 9,950 of them, thereabouts, are people who hadn't been vaccinated."[44] President Biden's comment was based on a July 1, 2021, statement by Dr. Rochelle Walensky, then the director of the CDC, that during the prior six months, 99.5 percent of COVID-19 deaths occurred in the unvaccinated.[45] The problem with such comments is that the vast majority of COVID-19 deaths in the previous six months occurred in the first couple of months of 2021 when most people were unvaccinated. One of the largest waves of COVID-19 deaths spiked in January 2021, with a smaller peak of deaths in April and May of 2021.[46] By April 3, 2021, only 13.3 percent of Canadians were COVID-19 vaccinated once and 1.9 percent vaccinated twice. By July 31, 2021, 59.2 percent of Canadians had been doubly vaccinated and 10.9 percent vaccinated only once.[47] In July 2021, with the fifth major wave of COVID-19, the number of cases and deaths slowly began to increase again.

With the initial COVID-19 vaccinations applied so close to the resurgence of COVID-19 cases in the late summer and fall of 2021, these vaccinations were likely effective in temporarily reducing the incidence of COVID-19 hospitalization and deaths during a limited period of three to six months. However, it soon became apparent that high rates of COVID-19 vaccination in Canada, the United States, and elsewhere did not prevent an individual from getting COVID-19 or transmitting SARS-CoV-2 if they did become infected.

Eventually, real-world, in-the-field data started to reveal that these COVID-19 vaccines had limited effectiveness. At a time when vaccination should have reduced the incidence of hospitalizations and deaths from COVID-19, these actually increased in Canada and the United States when compared to the pre-vaccination period in 2020.

The RNA and adenovirus COVID-19 vaccines appeared to be initially effective at inducing a strong immune response and conferring protection from infection by SARS-CoV-2 within the first few months following an initial inoculation and a booster shot (dose 2) a month later. It appeared that COVID-19 vaccination pre-Omicron may have at least temporarily reduced the severity of hospitalized patients with COVID-19. For example, Mercadé-Besora et al. (2024) undertook a major study of aggregated data from 10.17 million vaccinated and 10.39 million unvaccinated people collected primarily in 2021 in citizens from the United Kingdom, Spain, and Estonia and examined the effect of up to two doses of COVID-19 vaccines on the risk of post-COVID-19 cardiac and thromboembolic complications.[48] Their analyses indicated a vaccine-associated reduction of risk (45–81 percent) for thromboembolic and cardiac events in the acute phase of COVID-19 disease. The risks for post-acute COVID-19 venous thromboembolism, arterial thrombosis/thromboembolism, and heart failure were reduced to a lesser degree (24–58 percent), whereas a reduced risk for post-COVID-19 myocarditis/myopericarditis and ventricular arrhythmia/cardiac arrest in vaccinated people was evident only in the acute phase.

However, these COVID-19 vaccines clearly had waning efficacy to lower than 50 percent relative risk reduction by six months after double vaccination. This period of protection continued to decline with further boosting and started to produce negative efficacy in preventing COVID-19.

This trend was already evident in 2021. For example, one of the largest studies indicating that the effectiveness of COVID-19-injections waned over time was conducted on more than 780,225 of the US Veteran Health Administration (VA) patients.[49] The study indicated that in a time span of around nine months from February 1 to October 1, 2021, the ability of COVID-19 vaccines to protect from infection declined from 86.9 percent to 43.3 percent for the Pfizer/BioNTech product, from 89.2 percent to 58 percent for the Moderna product, and from 86.4 percent to 13.1 percent for the Janssen product. For those aged sixty-five and older, the ability of COVID-19 vaccines to protect from death was 70.1 percent for the Pfizer/BioNTech product, 75.5 percent for the Moderna product, and 52.2 percent for the Janssen product.[50] It should be appreciated that this was a passive reporting study and included an elderly population with a high risk of death, as well as US veterans that have a higher rate of lifetime injury (following military duty) and co-morbidities than the general population. The poorer performance of these vaccines in the elderly was not surprising. In the original Pfizer/BioNTec six-month Phase 3 trial with the BNT162b2 mRNA COVID-19 vaccine, although 58 percent of the people at risk from death from COVID-19 were seventy years years of age, only 4 percent of the trial participants were in this age group.[51]

With respect to the ability of the COVID-19 vaccines to reduce the acquisition and spread of COVID-19, these vaccines clearly failed. Early on, one study in Dane County, Wisconsin, which had among the highest vaccination rates in the United States at the time, indicated equally high viral loads in the vaccinated (84 percent) and the unvaccinated (83 percent)—in other words, an equal capacity of both to spread infection.[52] It is now widely accepted that COVID-19 double vaccinated individuals can still become infected with SARS-CoV-2, develop sickness, and transmit the virus with equal viral loads as unvaccinated individuals.[53] This has been clearly expressed by Dr. Anthony Fauci, who was, until the end of 2022, the director of the US National Institute for Allergy and Infectious Diseases (NIAID).[54]

One study with Delta and Omicron variants showed that COVID-19 vaccine boosted individuals were slightly more likely to transmit active SARS-CoV-2.[55] In this study, 38.5 percent of boosted people still carried live, culturable virus at ten days after the beginning of the infection. This contrasted with unvaccinated and double vaccinated people with COVID-19, of whom, respectively, 31 percent and 22 percent of the participants were still contagious at day ten of the same study. In the same study, by fifteen days after initial infection, 31 percent, 38 percent, and 23 percent, respectively, unvaccinated, double-vaccinated, and further-boosted participants still shed PCR-detectable, but mostly inactive viral RNA.

British Columbia was one of the provinces in Canada that provided regular breakdowns for the incidence of COVID-19 hospitalization, ICU admissions, and deaths, which was posted on the British Columbia Centre for Disease Control (BCCDC) website. From April to June, 2022, hospitalizations and critical care cases per a hundred thousand persons were at best two-fold higher for unvaccinated as compared to double or triple vaccinated individuals.[56] Moreover, during this period, the rates of COVID-19–related deaths were fairly comparable in the vaccinated versus the unvaccinated group. This is despite the fact that deaths included all individuals with a COVID-19-positive laboratory result who had died from any cause (COVID-19 or non-COVID-19, as recorded in Vital Statistic, BC Ministry of Health, within thirty days of their first laboratory positive result date). In considering such data, it is important to also recognize the caveats presented earlier (chapter 12.3). Such comparative data was no longer provided on the BCCDC website after June 23, 2022, possibly because such data no longer supported the public health agency's narrative.

A survey of 5,372 health workers in Canada, conducted from May 8 to August 14, 2023, revealed that of the 92 percent that were fully COVID-19 vaccinated, 76 percent of health-care professionals, 71 percent of allied health works, and 58 percent of auxiliary health workers still subsequently contracted COVID-19.[57]

The phenomena of increased rates of COVID-19 cases numbers, hospitalizations, and deaths in vaccinated compared to unvaccinated persons in other countries also become quite apparent in 2022 as different Omicron variants successively predominated over each other. For example, in the March 27, 2022 report of the UK Health Security Agency, using data from the Office of National Statistics, as presented in Table 13 of the report for the period of February 20 to March 13, 2022, the incidence rates of COVID-19 cases were typically three-fold or greater for those who were at least triple vaccinated than they were for those who were unvaccinated per hundred thousand persons.[58] For those who were hospitalized or died with COVID-19, the differences in the rates between the at-least-triple vaccinated and unvaccinated groups for those under fifty years of age was very similar. For those over fifty years of age, there appeared to be a reduction in hospitalizations and deaths of up to three-fold with three or more vaccinations, but it was likely that these individuals were just recently vaccinated and did experience some temporary protection. Interestingly, no data were provided on the COVID-19 cases numbers, hospitalizations, or deaths for those who had only one or two doses of a COVID-19 vaccine in Table 13 of the same report. These can be calculated based on the data presented in the earlier Tables 10, 11, and 12 in the same report. In these tables, the numbers of COVID-19 cases, hospitalization, and deaths were either higher or comparable in the population over eighteen years of age who received only two vaccine doses compared to those that were not vaccinated. A footnote was added to Table 14 of the report that stated "Comparing case rates among vaccinated and unvaccinated populations should not be used to estimate vaccine effectiveness against COVID-19 infection."[59] However, such data was quick to be used when it appeared to support COVID-19 vaccination campaigns earlier on. The surveillance reports stopped providing this information after March 2022. Collection of such information after April 1, 2022, became limited as free COVID-19 testing was suspended by the UK government. It would seem that the epidemiology data no longer supported the UK Health Security Agency's narrative of COVID-19 vaccine efficacy and was no longer presented.

Careful analysis of studies claiming vaccine efficacy against hospitalization and death from COVID-19 have indicated that they are systemically flawed and biased.[60] Responses to FOIs requesting hospitalization rated by vaccination status data inevitably reveal disproportionately higher rates among the vaccinated. For example, Public Health Wales confirmed that in the first two weeks of October 2021, 2.5 percent of hospitalized patients aged sixty-plus years were unvaccinated compared with 96 percent that were double vaccinated.[61] This would be during the period in which the Delta variant of SARS-CoV-2 predominated, prior to the prevalence of Omicron variants. Consequently, reduced immune recognition of Omicron variants does not explain why so many COVID-19 vaccinated people were hospitalized.

With so many breakthrough infections with SARS-CoV-2 with Omicron variants in highly vaccinated individuals, it became possible to compare the immune protection afforded by the hybrid immunity as compared to from COVID-19 vaccination alone. In a study by Nantel et al. (2024), it was found that cell-mediated immune responses in those individuals that previously received two doses of a COVID-19 vaccine and then got infected with SARS-CoV-2 were comparable to those that received a third intramuscular vaccine dose.[62] However, the hybrid immunity was superior with respect to higher salivary IgG and IgA antibody levels, which recognized the ancestral Wuhan spike protein and Omicron variants as well as the SARS-CoV-1 spike protein, and greater detectable serum neutralizing antibody levels against the Wuhan spike protein and Omicron variant.

Large scale studies of COVID-19 vaccination in children have shown extremely poor efficacy for the RNA vaccines. In one study of 74,208 children and adolescents aged five to eleven years at 6,897 sites across the United States, the estimated vaccine effectiveness (VE) to reduce COVID-19 incidence was only 60.1 percent one month after the second dose and 28.9 percent after two months.[63]

In another study conducted in New York State with 365,502 fully vaccinated children five- to eleven-years old after the emergence of Omicron BA.1, VE was only 12 percent effective after five weeks of inoculation.[64]

12.6. Keeping up with "Variants of Concern"

It has been commonly suggested that inoculation with COVID-19 vaccines based on the structure of the original Wuhan strain of SARS-CoV-2 renders the antibodies that are produced much less effective against the Omicron variants. This appears to be incorrect based on several points:

a. The overall difference in amino acid structure between the spike proteins of the Wuhan and Omicron strains is only 3 percent (i.e., approximately thirty-four mutated amino acids out of 1273 amino acids in the whole protein). As shown in Figure 8.1 in the insert, recovered COVID-19 survivors each generate antibodies against scores of different parts of the spike protein;

b. The actual regions in which most people tend to make antibodies against the spike protein are largely distinct from where the Omicron mutations occur, as also shown in Figure 8.1;
c. The vaccines that are produced with the Wuhan spike protein RNA are still effective, at least initially for reducing Omicron infections in vaccinated people, so the antibodies that are produced must still recognize the Omicron variants;
d. RNA vaccines that are based on the Omicron spike protein, when tested in monkeys and other animals, gave no better immune protection against COVID-19 than RNA vaccines based on the Wuhan spike protein amino acid sequence.[65, 66, 67, 68] Note that some studies observed a decline in "neutralizing" antibodies that specifically target the ACE2 receptor binding domain of the spike protein.[69, 70] However, most protective antibodies can still permit the tagging of virus and bacteria for their efficient recognition by immune cells and the complement system, which leads to their destruction; and
e. The fact that previously infected people get milder symptoms with Omicron variants and are able to more quickly recover from these variants clearly shows the capacity of the immune system of these individuals to recognize and neutralize the Omicron variants.

In a large study with the Moderna mRNA-1273 COVID-19 vaccine, the VE of booster shots against Omicron variants was assessed.[71] The study included 30,809 SARS-CoV-2-positive and 92,427 SARS-CoV-2-negative individuals aged eighteen years and older, tested during the January 1 to June 30, 2022 period. While three-dose VE against BA.1 infection was high and waned slowly, VE against BA.2, BA.2.12.1, BA.4, and BA.5 infection was initially moderate to high (61.0–90.6 percent fourteen to thirty days post third dose) and waned rapidly. The four-dose VE's against infection with BA.2, BA.2.12.1, and BA.4 ranged between 64.3–75.7 percent, was low (30.8 percent) against BA.5 fourteen to thirty days post fourth dose, and was lost beyond ninety days for all subvariants. The three-dose VEs against hospitalization for BA.1, BA.2, and BA.4/BA.5 was 97.5 percent, 82.0 percent, and 72.4 percent, respectively; four-dose VE against hospitalization for BA.4/BA.5 was 88.5 percent. In analyses of three-dose VE (versus unvaccinated) against infection with Omicron subvariants by time since vaccination, the three-dose VEs against BA.1 ranged from 85.8 percent in the fourteen to thirty days after the third dose to 54.9 percent greater than 150 days after the third dose. VEs for these two different time intervals, respectively, were 61.0 percent and −24.9 percent for BA.2, 82.7 percent and −26.8 percent for BA.2.12.1; 72.6 percent and −16.4 percent for BA.4; and 90.6 percent and −17.9 percent for BA.5. In summary, there was a clear trend to negative efficacy by five months after the third dose for the various Omicron variants that followed BA.1. That is, the vaccination appeared to increase the chances of getting COVID-19 over time relative to that of an unvaccinated person.

Adisesh et al. (2024) similarly described declines in anti-spike RBD antibodies after each vaccination with either the Pfizer or Moderna COVID-19 vaccines after initial increases, and the reductions in antibody titers were most rapid after the third dose. Adverse vaccine side-effects were also highest in those that had the strongest anti-spike RBD antibodies responses.[72]

With the predominance of Omicron variants of SARS-CoV-2 in late 2021, there were large numbers of breakthrough cases of COVID-19 in those who were double vaccinated, which exceeded the total numbers of unvaccinated persons with COVID-19. To offset the relative loss of efficacy of the original COVID-19 vaccines with the Omicron variants, new bivalent COVID-19 vaccines were tested in clinical studies that use a combination of mRNA for the original Wuhan spike protein and the Omicron BA.1 variant spike protein.[73] This was despite the fact that the Wuhan SARS-CoV-2 virus and even the Omicron BA.1 variant were already supplanted worldwide by the Omicron BA.4 and BA.5 variants. On August 31, 2022, bivalent COVID-19 vaccines from Moderna and Pfizer/BioNTech that include mRNA for the Wuhan spike protein and a variant that features the mutations in the BA.4 and BA.5 lineages of Omicron were approved by the FDA based only on pre-clinical studies in mice.[74] At the same time, monovalent vaccines based on the original Wuhan spike protein were no longer authorized as booster doses for individuals twelve years of age and older. It is noteworthy that the Pfizer bivalent COVID-19 vaccine was approved based on studies with only eight mice for their efficacy in producing "neutralizing" antibodies that blocked Omicron BA.4 and BA.5 spike protein binding to ACE2.[75] From a safety standpoint, the Wuhan SARS-CoV-2 spike protein is not capable of binding to mouse or rat ACE2, so evaluation of spike protein toxicity was highly compromised in these laboratory animal models.[76] Data from no other animal model or humans was presented to the FDA by these manufacturers for these particular bivalent vaccines prior to their approval.[77]

More recent studies have continued to reveal negative efficacy associated with the booster vaccines. From COVID-19 surveillance data from January to July 2023 across thirty-three California state prisons, primarily a male population of 96,201 individuals, the incidence rate of new COVID-19 infections among COVID-19-bivalent-vaccinated and entirely unvaccinated groups (those not having received either the bivalent or monovalent vaccine) was compared.[78] The authors noted the infection rates in the bivalent-vaccinated and entirely unvaccinated groups were 3.24 percent and 2.72 percent, respectively, with an absolute risk difference of only 0.52 percent. Among those aged sixty-five and above, the infection rates were 6.45 percent and 4.5 percent, respectively, with an absolute risk difference of 1.95 percent. The bivalent-vaccinated group had a slightly, but statistically significant, higher infection rate than the unvaccinated group in the statewide category and for those aged fifty years and above.

In another study performed in Japan with 19,998 adults aged sixty-five or older, bivalent COVID-19 mRNA vaccination between October 1 and December 31, 2022, with a bivalent COVID-19 booster shot after at least two prior monovalent COVID-19 vaccinations was only 33.6 percent more effective at reducing the risk of a SARS-CoV-2 infection than being unvaccinated, and only 18 percent more effective in recipients that had already received two or more monovalent COVID-19 vaccinations.[79] This effectiveness peaked within fourteen to twenty days after inoculation with the bivalent vaccine, and thereafter gradually declined. There was no evidence of a benefit from administration of a bivalent COVID-19 vaccine to someone that was previously unvaccinated but had recovered from COVID-19.[80]

One of the most devastating studies that challenged the wisdom of booster COVID-19 vaccines for reducing COVID-19 was performed on 51,017 employees of the Cleveland Clinic who were tracked for VE of the bivalent COVID-19 vaccines over a six-month period that started September 12, 2022.[81] The bivalent-vaccines were associated with a VE of 29 percent of COVID-19 during the BA.4/5-dominant phase, a VE of 20 percent in the BQ-dominant phase, and a VE of 4 percent during the XBB-dominant phase. What was particularly striking from the study was that the risk of getting COVID-19 increased successively with each vaccination up to four COVID-19 vaccine doses, with the lowest risk for COVID-19 by far in the unvaccinated employees (shown in Figure 12.1, which can be found in the insert). More recently, in a follow-up study with 47,561 Cleveland Clinic employees, the 2023–2024 COVID-19 vaccine formulations were found to have an efficacy of only 23 percent against the predominating JN.1 SARS-CoV-2 variant, and "a higher number of prior vaccine doses was associated with a higher risk of COVID-19."[82]

On June 15, 2023, the FDA's Vaccines and Related Biological Products Advisory Committee met to discuss their recommendations for the next COVID-19 booster vaccine for Fall 2023.[83] Presentations from Pfizer, Moderna, Novavax, the National Institutes of Health (NIH), and the FDA all documented that the bivalent Wuhan/BA.4/5 vaccines failed to produce neutralizing antibodies that would block the binding of the spike protein of Omicron XBB variants to ACE2. Ultimately, the Committee recommended that these companies should focus on development of a monovalent vaccine that targeted the spike protein of the XXB.1.5 variant. As discussed in chapter 5.5, the XXB.1.5 variant was largely supplanted by newer variants such as EG.5 by the time the XXB.1.5 spike protein–based COVID-19 vaccines were launched in September

2023. The monovalent XXB.1.5-based COVID-19 vaccines were not any more effective against the newer SARS-CoV-2 variants. With the strong focus on neutralizing antibodies against the spike protein by industry and government agencies for assessing the effectiveness of vaccines, this undervalues the actual effectiveness of natural immunity and older COVID-19 vaccines against the earlier SARS-CoV-2 strains to prevent COVID-19 and reduce illness.

Collectively, all of these findings seriously call into question the wisdom of vaccination of youth and most working adults considering that they are already at such low risk of hospitalization and death from COVID-19, especially in view of the poor and even negative efficacy of these COVID-19 genetic vaccines, and their potential for vaccine injury in the short and long term as presented in the next chapter. In fact, from a Freedom of Information request in Israel, with a population of 9.4 million, it was determined that only 356 people between ages eighteen and forty-nine died with COVID-19 during the COVID-19 pandemic up to May 29, 2023.[84] Of the twenty-seven people for which full data was available, none of them died from COVID-19, but instead from other comorbidities.

12.7. Development of Tolerance

The apparent reduction in immune recognition following repeated large exposures to an immunogen is a classic response known as development of tolerance. It is the way in which the immune system learns to recognize self and common benign substances in the environment from new and potentially dangerous ones. Repeated booster injections over several years of large amounts of spike mRNA, for what is essentially a protein that is 97 percent identical, is a recipe for immune tolerance and can account for the waning efficacy of the COVID-19 vaccines. This likely explains why highly vaccinated individuals can still suffer frequent re-infections. They have essentially damaged their natural immunity against the SARS-CoV-2 virus and potentially other coronaviruses.

With natural infection with SARS-CoV-2, antibodies of the proinflammatory IgA, IgM, and IgG1 and IgG3 classes are produced, which provide broad immune protection in the air passages and blood circulation. With initial COVID-19 vaccinations, the primary response is the production of especially IgG1 class antibodies and to a lesser extent IgG3 class antibodies.[85] However, especially with more than two COVID-19 mRNA inoculations, there is a shift to the production of IgG2 and IgG4 class antibodies, which confer immune tolerance.[86, 87, 88, 89, 90] IgG4 antibody class switching can be induced by excessive antigen concentration and prolonged exposure to an antigen, repeated vaccination, and the type of vaccine used. Elevated IgG4 levels appear to have a protective role through prevention of immune over-activation. IgG4 has a more non-inflammatory character than IgG1 and IgG3, with reduced affinity to most FcγRs and C1q (see chapter 11.2 and Figure 11.1 [in the insert]), and much reduced potential for antibody-dependent cellular cytotoxicity (ADCC) and the C1q complement-mediated killing of cells that have antigen-antibody complexes on their surfaces. IgG4 antibodies also uniquely undergo structural changes that render them to be functionally monovalent and unable to form immune complexes. They also suppress the actions of other IgGs, further contributing to immunosuppression.[91] Immunosuppressive drugs have been shown to have a minor inhibitory effect on the production of IgG4 antibodies after a third COVID-19 mRNA vaccine inoculation, and the production of interleukins 4 and 13 as well as tumor necrosis factor have been implicated to have roles in IgG4 class switching.[92]

This switching to IgG4 antibodies with booster shots of the mRNA vaccines appears to result from the very high levels of spike protein production that they elicit. With more traditional vaccines, the spike protein is a component of the vaccine and presented at lower concentrations, more similar to a natural infection with a coronavirus, and the immune response is not as profound and less likely to revert to tolerance. For example, Kalkeri et al. (2024) found that in blood serum of recipients of three to four doses of the Novavax NVX-CoV2373 vaccine, the levels of anti-spike IgG3 antibodies were greater than ten-fold higher than in those with three to four doses of a COVID-19 mRNA vaccine. By contrast, the levels of anti-spike IgG4 antibodies were found to be more than a hundred-times higher in the mRNA vaccine recipients than in NVX-CoV2373 immunized participants.[93] This conversion to immunotolerant IgG4 class antibody following more than two doses of the COVID-19 mRNA vaccines also occurred in immunocompromised recipients and raises the concern that further booster injections may render them even more vulnerable to future infections.

Repeated booster injections of vaccines have also been associated with immune suppression through T cell exhaustion, which is a condition in which CD8+ T cells have a progressive decline of cytokine production and cytotoxic potential.[94] Such a reduced T cell response against SARS-CoV-2 has been noted one month following the third and fourth doses of COVID-19 vaccines.[95] This could contribute to the observations of higher COVID-19 risk with increased COVID-19 vaccine boosters.[96, 97, 98] Vecchio et al. (2024) recently documented some differences in T cell receptor recognition of the spike protein between vaccinated and unvaccinated individuals with COVID-19.[99]

In a recent study by Adhikari et al. (2024) with 152 hospitalized adult patients with acute respiratory failure admitted to Ohio State University Hospital between May 2020 and November 2022, it was found that vaccinated patients had a significantly higher risk of mortality.[100] For those patients with COVID-19, mortality among vaccinated patients was 70 percent and with unvaccinated patients it was 37 percent. Higher levels of SARS-CoV-2 antibody levels were measured for the survivors, and there was a trend toward increased total IgG4 antibody levels in the vaccinated patients with COVID-19.

The accumulating evidence, in part provided in this chapter, has shown that the COVID-19 genetic vaccines have limited efficacy and, when used repeatedly, may actually damage the immune response toward negative efficacy. On this basis alone, the use of these products must be called into question. In the next chapter, the safety of these genetic vaccines is further investigated and also found to be problematic.

CHAPTER 13

Safety of COVID-19 Vaccines

Steven Pelech & Christopher A. Shaw

"You can die of the cure before you die of the illness."

—Michael Landon

"Sometimes no problem is a sign of a different problem."

—Mark Rosenthal

Ultimately, the decision to approve a drug or vaccine for general use is based on the level of the severity of the disease and on the safety and effectiveness of the treatment. As described in chapter 6, COVID-19 was a potentially life-threatening disease for especially the elderly and those with multiple comorbidities. However, as detailed in chapter 11, the production of COVID-19 genetic vaccines had major issues, and in chapter 12, these products were shown to have fleeting efficacy and, in the longer term, apparently negative efficacy. In this chapter, the issue of the safety of these vaccines is given closer scrutiny. The spike protein produced by the COVID-19 vaccines or SARS-CoV-2 is now well recognized to be pathogenic on its own.[1] Thus, high levels of spike production in the human body with the vaccines might be expected to have negative consequences *a priori*. This would be expected to generate inflammatory reactions, including immune cell attack, throughout the body against cells that express the spike protein following uptake of COVID-19 genetic vaccines.

As will become apparent throughout this chapter, vaccine-mediated disruption of the immune system could have profound negative side effects throughout the body. Something to bear in mind is that the inflammatory response induced by the COVID-19 genetic vaccine may be even more dramatic following the "education" of the adaptive immune system by prior infection with SARS-CoV-2 or previous COVID-19 vaccine inoculations. The magnitude of COVID-19 vaccine-induced injury has been linked to previous history of COVID-19, allergies, and being female, and increased with the second inoculation as compared to the first.[2]

13.1. Preclinical Safety Studies

With COVID-19 mRNA or DNA vaccinations, the genetic information to manufacture the spike protein of SARS-CoV-2 is initially injected into the deltoid muscle area. From there, the lipid nanoparticle or adenovirus carriers do not remain localized, but instead disseminate throughout the body and may result in spike production by various tissues and organs. Previous animal studies have highlighted the potential of lipid nanoparticle carriers to widely spread throughout the body, particularly as shown in earlier mice and rat studies with their accumulation in the ovaries.[3] While biodistribution data is lacking for the actual COVID-19 mRNA vaccines in animal and human studies, Pfizer did submit data to regulatory agencies in their bid for approval of their COVID-19 mRNA vaccine BNT162b2. This information first came to the attention of the public from translated documents recovered from the Japanese government regulatory bodies through the efforts of Dr. Byram Bridle of the Canadian Citizens Care Alliance.[4] The same data were later evident from Pfizer submissions to the European Medicines Agency (see page 47 of the EMA Assessment report for Comirnaty)[5] and most likely were available to the FDA and Health Canada. These biodistribution studies performed in rats using lipid nanoparticles with a similar formulation to those used in the Pfizer/BioNTech vaccine demonstrated that they travel practically throughout the entire body, with accumulation in many tissues and organs, especially the liver, spleen, adrenals and ovaries, over the forty-eight-hour study window, after which the experiments were terminated.[6] These lipid nanoparticles also traversed the blood-brain barrier.[7]

By not performing pharmacokinetic and distribution studies of the encoded spike protein, which was already known to be toxic and bioactive (off-target effects), the regulatory submissions of the mRNA vaccines were incomplete. It is also problematic that the rodent studies conducted to evaluate the toxicity of the spike protein, when it was produced, were compromised by the fact that the spike protein was based on the structure of the Wuhan version, and the receptor binding domain of the original strain of the SARS-CoV-2 poorly interacts with the ACE2 protein in laboratory rats and mice, although later variants of the SARS-CoV-2 virus developed the ability to infect these rodents.[8, 9] The Wuhan version of SARS-CoV-2 more readily infects Syrian golden hamsters, so this animal model would have been better suited for earlier testing for toxic effects of spike protein production from the COVID-19 vaccines.[10]

It would seem from the very start that the preclinical safety studies were designed to provide data that would put the mRNA COVID-19 vaccines in the best possible light. Another critical flaw was that the guidance documents used by Health Canada were only applicable to traditional vaccines and not vaccines using gene therapy technology.

13.2. Clinical Safety Studies

For efficiency, the pre-clinical studies on the COVID-19 genetic vaccines were often performed in parallel with human clinical trials, if done at all. As the Pfizer/BioNTech COVID-19 RNA vaccine was the most widely used of the COVID-19 vaccines in North America and Europe, this chapter will tend to focus on the BNT162b2 (Comirnaty) product. These initial clinical studies were all undertaken with more purified preparations of this vaccine developed with their Process 1 manufacturing method (see chapter 11.3.6). The Phase 3 clinical study with BNT162b2 has been more fully described with respect to efficacy in chapter 12.4. The initial results after two months were published in the *New England Journal of Medicine* (*NEJM*),[11] and this was used to justify the efficacy and safety concerns to the FDA, Health Canada, and other regulatory agencies in countries around the world to permit its conditional approval for those eighteen years and older. There were 21,720 people sixteen years of age or older in the vaccinated cohort, who received two doses of BNT162b2 a month apart, and 21,728 matched participants who were unvaccinated. In the *NEJM* publication, the authors reported that "the safety profile of BNT162b2 was characterized by short-term, mild-to-moderate pain at the injection site, fatigue, and headache. The incidence of serious adverse events was low and was similar in the vaccine and placebo groups."[12]

For the six-months stage of the same clinical Phase 3 study, Thomas et al. (2021) updated their clinical findings in *NEJM*, which also included data for twelve- to fifteen-year-olds who were vaccinated.[13] The vaccinated participants had 300 percent more total adverse events and 75 percent more severe adverse events than observed with the placebo-injected, control participants (considered unvaccinated). The authors noted, "new adverse events attributable to BNT162b2 that were not previously identified in earlier reports included decreased appetite, lethargy, asthenia [abnormal physical weakness or lack of energy], malaise, night sweats, and hyperhydrosis [excessive sweating not related to heat or exercise]." Around 5 percent of vaccinated recipients experienced severe adverse events from the inoculations. Moreover, there were more deaths in the vaccinated than in the unvaccinated control group (twenty-one versus seventeen deaths; and two of these deaths in the vaccinated group were previously unvaccinated but opted after two months to get vaccinated after unblinding of the trial). The vaccine-associated deaths had higher rates of cardiovascular disease including arteriosclerosis, cardiac arrest, congestive heart failure, and hypertensive heart disease.[14] It has been suggested that, due to the delay in inclusion of the death data in the original filings of BNT2b2, approval by the FDA and the European Medicines Agency was able to proceed more smoothly, since about 75 percent of the deaths in the vaccinated group were cardiac-related.

A re-analysis of the Pfizer six-month clinical study with BNT162b2 with respect to the thirty-eight deaths in vaccinated and unvaccinated participants was later performed by an independent group of researchers associated with the *Daily Clout*.[15] In their analysis, they noted:

> Surprisingly, a comparison of the number of subject deaths per week during the 33 weeks of this study found no significant difference between the number of deaths in the vaccinated versus placebo arms for the first 20 weeks of the trial, the placebo-controlled portion of the trial. After Week 20, as subjects in the Placebo were unblinded and vaccinated, deaths among this still unvaccinated cohort of this group slowed and eventually plateaued. Deaths in the BNT162b2 vaccinated subjects continued at the same rate. Our analysis revealed inconsistencies between the subject data listed in the 6-Month Interim Report and publications authored by Pfizer/BioNTech trial site administrators. Most importantly, we found evidence of an over 3.7-fold increase in number of deaths due to cardiovascular events in BNT162b2 vaccinated subjects compared to Placebo controls. This significant adverse event signal was not reported by Pfizer/BioNTech.[16]

Likewise, in a Substack article, Drs. Tore Gulbrandsen, Martin Neil, and Norman Fenton described anomalous behavior of the mortality data associated with the Pfizer six-month clinical study with BNT162b.[17] They concluded that "the only explanation compatible with all the non-random patterns is that the records of vaccine recipients suffering adverse events and death were changed, moving them to the placebo arm after the event."

In another secondary analysis of the six-month, placebo-controlled, Phase 3 randomized clinical trials of the Pfizer/BioNTech and Moderna mRNA COVID-19 vaccines in adults (NCT04368728 and NCT04470427), the authors calculated an excess risk of serious adverse events (AE) with vaccination of one in 990, and one in 662 over placebo baselines, respectively.[18] These AE were defined as an adverse event that results in any of the following conditions: death; life-threatening at the time of the event; inpatient hospitalization or prolongation of existing hospitalization; persistent or significant disability/incapacity; a congenital anomaly/birth defect; or a medically important event, based on medical judgment.

In further clinical studies with younger age BNT162b2-vaccinated participants in smaller trials, the studies were too underpowered to pick up adverse events that would occur in less than a thousand participants. However, it is noteworthy that one thirteen-year-old participant in the twelve- to fifteen-year-olds BNT162b2 trial conducted at the Cincinnati Children's Hospital, Maddie de Garay, within twenty-four hours of her second dose of the vaccine experienced severe adverse reactions. As described in an FDA submission by her parents:

> She received her first dose on 12/30/2[0] and had the expected side effects which were no cause for concern. She got her second dose on 1/20/21 and less than 12 hours later she experienced severe abdominal pain, painful electric shocks on her spine and neck, swollen extremities, ice-cold hands and feet, chest pain, tachycardia, pins and needles in her feet that eventually led to the loss of feeling from her waist down. She had blood in her urine from 7 tests over 3 months, mysterious rashes, peeling feet, reflux, gastroparesis, vomiting, and eventually the inability to swallow liquids or food, dizziness, passing out, convulsions, the inability to sweat, swollen lymph nodes in her armpits, urinary retention, heavy periods with clots of blood, decreased vision, tinnitus, memory loss, mixing up words, extreme fatigue, and sadly more. She spent 64 days in the hospital, had 3 hospital stays, and 9 trips to the ER. We are 9 months into this, we have no real answers.[19]

Maddie de Garay was referred to hospital for a full assessment and a doctor diagnosed her with a "functional disorder."[20] As described by Dr. Maryanne Demasi in her Substack, "this doctor decided she had a pre-disposition to hysteria, and she was referred to a mental health facility. Professor and psychiatrist David Healy subsequently conducted a thorough review of her medical records, including an interview with her family, and found no such history of pre-existing conditions or mental illness." While Maddie de Garay was acknowledged as a participant in a Pfizer Phase 3 study with an adverse event with BNT162b2, her condition was described in an official Pfizer report as merely abdominal pain. However, her case was not mentioned in the *NEJM* publication that published the results of this clinical study.[21] As of January 21, 2024, Maddie de Garay remained wheelchair-bound and had to be fed by a nasogastric tube, but started to regain feeling in her legs and the ability to hold up her neck.[22]

A glaring deficiency in all of the COVID-19 genetic vaccine Phase 3 trials has been the reluctance to perform biochemical tests to actively monitor potential injury from vaccination in all trial participants. For example, there were apparently no blood tests performed, such as D-dimer analyses to detect for potential blood clotting, C-reactive protein for inflammation, and troponin for heart damage.

On page 27 in section 2.5.3 of Pfizer's Overview of Clinical Overview document, it states: "Pharmacokinetic studies are not usually required for vaccines. Measurement of the plasma concentration of the vaccine over time is not feasible."[23] At the time that Pfizer's Nonclinical Overview was approved the definition of a vaccine was: "A product that stimulates a person's immune system to produce immunity to a specific disease, protecting the person from that disease." As this product did not meet the definition of a traditional vaccine, the pharmacokinetics of the encoded spike protein (i.e., the viral antigen) should really have been determined in an ascending dose Phase 1 clinical trial along with the appropriate biomarkers (as mentioned in the previous paragraph) associated with possible vaccine adverse effects. The other advantages for having a full pharmacokinetic profile would be to estimate the variability in levels of spike protein production between individuals, which so far had not been established, its persistence in the circulation, and its distribution out of the circulation and into tissues, as well as the efficiency of translation from mRNA. Also, adverse effects could then be collated with the spike protein concentration in the blood. These studies were never completed.

13.3. Post-marketing Safety Studies

Further concerns regarding the safety of the Pfizer/BioNTech vaccine were raised by the first release of Pfizer's originally confidential post marketing pharmacovigilance report to the FDA.[24] On November 17, 2021, the FDA released the first batch of what was predicted to be at least 451,000 pages of documents that they were ordered by a court to provide. This was to satisfy a Freedom of Information request by a group called Public Health and Medical Professionals for Transparency, who wanted access to the data used by the FDA to approve Pfizer/BioNTech's COVID-19 inoculations. The FDA originally asked in court to have fifty-five years to release the documents and then calculated it would take seventy-five years. It makes one wonder how the FDA was originally able to review the vaccine information within a couple of months to provide its continuing approval. With the first release that covered the period of up to February 28, 2021, there were 42,086 cases of adverse events, of which 11,361 (27 percent) had not recovered, and 1,223 deaths recorded.[25] In the nine pages of the appendix of this report, there were over 1,236 different diseases that were potentially linked with the Pfizer/BioNTech COVID-19 vaccine. By June 18, 2022, Pfizer had records with an accumulation of 4,964,106 total adverse events across 1,485,027 total cases.[26]

Since late 2022, Naomi Wolf and her War Room/*DailyClout* research team of over three thousand volunteers have pored through 1,875 Pfizer clinical trial documents (for ages sixteen years and older) and have published regular reports on the *Daily Clout* with their findings.[27] Some eighty-nine reports on the Pfizer Reports have been issued on the *Daily Clout* website as of October 16, 2023.[28] Their work has revealed numerous vaccine AE and cover-ups by Pfizer to minimize the extent of these vaccine injuries. The team expects to be reviewing another 101 Pfizer adolescent (ages twelve to fifteen years old) clinical trial documents and forty-six Moderna clinical trial documents throughout 2024 and 2025 (estimated to be about four million pages of documents).

Recently, Raethke et al. (2024) reported the results of a survey of 29,837 participants from nine European countries for adverse events from COVID-19 vaccines between February 2021 to February 2023.[29] About 74 percent of respondents experienced at least one AE, but only about 0.24 percent reported serious AEs after the first and second vaccination, and for those that had a third dose, about 0.26 percent had a serious AE. The people that had recovered from COVID-19 were 2.6-times more likely to experience an AE after a first dose of COVID-19 vaccine, and 1.25-times likely to have an AE after a second dose than someone who had not previously had COVID-19.

13.4. Vaccine Adverse Event Reporting Databases

As discussed in chapter 10.2, several government agencies have established public reporting sites for recording adverse events related to specific drugs and vaccines post approval of these products. These websites warn that reports of injury from drugs or vaccines do not necessarily infer a causal relationship, as many of the same illnesses can arise from other causes in the general population. Reports of AE and especially death from COVID-19 vaccines are typically described by public health officials "as very rare, and when such deaths are reported, they do not necessarily mean that the vaccine caused the death." However, it is notable that there are more reports of severe injury and deaths from the four COVID-19 vaccines in the last three years in the FDA Vaccine Adverse Effects Reporting System (VAERS) than in the previous thirty-three years for all other vaccines combined since VAERS was established in 1990.[30] As of February 23, 2024, there were 2,588,225 AE reports posted on VAERS since its inception, and 1,630,913 (63 percent) were related to COVID-19 vaccines. Of the total of 47,458 deaths associated with all vaccines in VAERS since its inception, 37,231 (78.5 percent) were specifically linked to COVID-19 vaccines. Of the COVID-19 vaccine-related deaths, 90 percent occurred between December 2019 and December 2022, and only 10 percent in 2023, in parallel with the large decline in COVID-19 vaccination uptake in 2023. In 2020, there were only 420 reports of deaths associated with any vaccine.[31]

It should be appreciated that most VAERS reports are made by doctors and other health professionals, and the system is supposed to be closely monitored for the quality of the reports. Table 13.1 shows the number of reports filed on VAERS following the release of the COVID-19 vaccines to the public around mid-December 2020.[32] Moreover, these numbers underreport the true extent of AEs after injection of the COVID-19 vaccines by an underreporting factor (URF) from a hundred-times[33] to forty-one-times.[34] If the number of deaths reported in the United States up to December 29, 2023 in VAERS is multiplied by the most conservative URF, this would approximate to over 180,000 deaths in the United States from the COVID-19 vaccines. About half of the 1,148,691 deaths with COVID-19 in the United States up to October 14, 2023 are thought to actually be from co-morbidities, in part due to the federal government offering strong financial incentives in the United States to attribute any death to COVID-19.[35] This really calls into question the benefits of lives saved by COVID-19 vaccination versus injury and deaths from the administration of COVID-19 vaccines.

Table 13.1. Number of filed reports in VAERS related to COVID-19 vaccinations worldwide and in the United States from December 2020 to December 2023. Data was recovered from Open VAERS.[36]

	Mar. 5, 2021	Dec. 31, 2021	Dec. 30, 2022	Dec. 29, 2023	Dec. 29, 2023; US only
Adverse Reports	31,079	1,016,999	1,494,382	1,621,120	1,000,725
Hospitalizations	3,477	113,303	188,270	213,536	88,992
Urgent Care	5,806	110,785	143,153	153,718	118,073
Deaths	1,524	21,382	33,469	36,986	18,493
Anaphylaxis	292	8,765	10,315	10,737	2,480
Bell's Palsy	367	12,765	16,572	17,621	6,314
Thrombocytopenia/Low Platelet	103	5,102	8,386	9,076	3,638
Heart Attacks	332	10,863	18,115	21,335	9,241
Myocarditis/ Myopericarditis	NA	23,713	26,096	28,052	5,118
Severe Allergic Reaction	1,917	36,955	41,955	46,622	36,441
Miscarriages	66	3,511	4,643	5,086	2,048
Life Threatening	NA	24,344	35,788	39,216	14,922
Permanently Disabled	NA	36,758	61,764	69,316	17,774

In response to a federal court order in January 2024, the CDC has had to make public more of the findings of its V-safe system, which is a text-message system launched in December 2020 by the agency to monitor possible side-effects of COVID-19 vaccines.[37] Over ten million V-safe participants completed more than 150 million health surveys about their experiences following COVID-19 vaccination.[38] At least twenty CDC scientific publications from these data have advanced that serious adverse events from COVID-19 vaccination are rare, and the vast majority of adverse effects are mild and resolve quickly.[39] However, nearly 8 percent of the V-safe participants required medical attention or hospital care after vaccination, and about 25 percent had to miss school or work, or the vaccination impacted their other normal activities.[40]

Several other post-hoc passive surveillance systems also track COVID-19 vaccine injury, including the Canada Adverse Events Following Immunization Surveillance System (CAEFISS), the United Kingdom Yellow Card Scheme, the WHO VigiAccess website, and the European Medicines Agency EudraVigilance website. The data in these systems can be difficult to interpret. AEs are widely underreported, and those that are filed are vetted with strict criteria.[41] Nevertheless, numerous AEs have been attributed to the current COVID-19 vaccines in all of these databases. As of April 1, 2024, reported AEs worldwide with COVID-19 vaccines had surpassed 5.3 million in the WHO reporting system VigiAccess.[42] Table 13.2 shows how vaccine injury reports with the COVID-19 genetic vaccines compare with the other most commonly applied vaccines. It is evident that the COVID-19 vaccines have fifty-six-times more reports of vaccine AEs than influenza vaccines during the same period, which are also widely used. This clearly shows that the COVID-19 genetic vaccines incur more adverse vaccine injuries than reported from any of the traditional vaccines in the past.

Table 13.2. VigiAccess listing of vaccine adverse events (AEs) associated with the most commonly used vaccines. Sourced on April 8, 2024 and searched with "COVID-19" and other terms shown in the first column.[43]

Disease Targeted	Number of Total Adverse Events	Since First Year of Reporting	Number of Adverse Events since 2021	Rate Compared to Diphtheria since 2021
COVID-19	5,315,891	2021	5,315,891	31,822X
Influenza	327,179	1968	94,685	567X
Polio	141,965	1982	31,483	189X
Hepatitis B	113,273	1985	12,888	77X
BCG for TB	41,461	1973	7,957	48X
Measles	11,260	1968	5,638	34X
Tetanus	16,960	1968	2,763	17X
Diphtheria	1,974	1979	158	1X

Despite the high levels of COVID-19 vaccine injuries that have been reported with the VAERS, VigiAccess, EudraVigilance, and UK Yellow Card vaccine injury reporting systems, relatively few adverse events reports are posted for the COVID-19 vaccines in Canada's CAEFISS.[44] This is possibly due to the long time it takes (over twenty minutes) for a doctor or nurse to file a vaccine injury report to local public health units, the strict criteria applied to local acceptance of an injury report with significant rejection rates, and the further scrutiny subsequently applied at the level of the Public Health Agency of Canada, which manages the CAEFISS database. Physicians have been reprimanded by professional colleges for filing COVID-19 vaccine injury reports, such as exemplified in disciplinary proceedings that were taken by the Ontario College of Physicians and Surgeons against Dr. Patrick Phillips.[45] Dr. Phillips submitted six COVID-19 vaccine injury reports to CAEFISS, and all but one were rejected, with his patients being advised to get further vaccinations for COVID-19.

About 72.5 percent of all AE reports to CAEFISS were from women, which is also a phenomenon observed in VAERS, Yellow Card, and VigiAccess.[46] This has been attributed to differences in health-care-seeking behavior, as well as biological differences between females and males.[47]

As of January 5, 2024, the last report issued on Government of Canada website, there were 58,712 reported adverse events for Canadians on CAEFISS following administration of 105 million COVID-19 vaccine doses, which corresponds to about 5.6 out of ten thousand people that were vaccinated.[48] Of all of the reports, 11,702 were deemed to be serious. For 9,948,907 bivalent COVID-19 vaccines given to Canadians, there were 1,044 AEs, of which 261 AEs were considered serious (three out of a hundred thousand vaccinations). For 5,694,993 monovalent XBB1.5 COVID-19 vaccines given to Canadians, there were 278 AEs, of which twenty-seven AEs were considered serious (0.5 out of a hundred thousand vaccinations). Of 488 reports of death associated with the COVID-19 vaccines in Canada, only four were deemed to be causally associated with the vaccinations, although there were 244 deaths that were unclassifiable or indeterminate due to insufficient information.[49]

Anaphylaxis was evident in about one report for every hundred thousand COVID-19 vaccine doses administered in CAEFISS. The two safety signals for COVID-19 vaccines that were acknowledged as confirmed on CAEFISS were thrombosis (blood clotting) with thrombocytopenia syndrome (low platelet count in blood) and myocarditis/myopericarditis.

13.5. Blood Abnormalities

13.5.1. Thrombosis and Thrombocytopenia

An increased risk of thrombosis was one of the earlier risks associated with COVID-19 vaccines. This concern was raised in Canada when Dr. Charles Hoffe, a family physician in Lytton, British Columbia discovered that about 62 percent of his recently Moderna COVID-19-vaccinated patients had evidence of elevated D-dimer levels. He reported this in an open letter on April 5, 2021 to Dr. Bonnie Henry, the chief medical officer in British Columbia.[50] D-dimer is a breakdown product of blood clots, and Dr. Hoffe thought that these might be arising from microclots induced by the COVID-19 vaccines. He also noted that there had been numerous allergic reactions, including two cases of anaphylaxis, three cases of people with "ongoing and disabling" neurological deficits, and what appeared to be a vaccine-related death among his practice of about nine hundred patients of primarily Indigenous background. Elevation of D-dimer levels have since been confirmed in COVID-19 vaccinated individuals (in nine of twenty published reports), along with thrombosis, thrombocytopenia, elevated anti-platelet factor 4 antibodies, and myocardial infarctions (heart attacks) in a systematic literature review.[51]

Due to issues of blood clotting and vaccine-induced immune thrombotic thrombocytopenia (VIIT) following injection with the AstraZeneca COVID-19 adenovirus vaccine Vaxzevria/COVISHIELD, the National Advisory Committee on Immunization (NACI) in Canada recommended a pause for using this vaccine in people under fifty years of age.[52] Ontario Public Health suspended offering the AstraZeneca vaccine on May 11, 2021 out of caution due to the increased risk of blood clots of one in 55,000 that were vaccinated,[53] although it continued to be offered in other provinces such as British Columbia until December 19, 2023. Health Canada never approved AstraZeneca's COVID-19 vaccine for those under eighteen years of age, based on continuing increased safety concerns for this age group.[54] Ultimately, Vaxzevria/COVISHIELD along with the Jcovden COVID-19 vaccine (Ad26.COV2.S) from Janssen Inc. were withdrawn from the market in Canada by the manufacturers.

It should be appreciated that the COVID-19 RNA vaccines have also been linked with elevated D-dimer and VITT as exemplified in cases studies of individuals that were vaccinated with either the Pfizer/BioNTech or Moderna vaccines for COVID-19.[55, 56] In a systematic review of the literature,[57] Tan et al. (2023) reported:

> Studies included in this review included 10 cohort studies and 57 case report or case series. A total of over 24,000 thrombotic events have been reported, the majority of which have been associated with adenoviral vector-based vaccine, particularly AstraZeneca (5 in 100,000 up to 6 in 1000), followed by Janssen (8–30 in 1,000,000 doses), Pfizer (6 in 1,000,000 up to 1 in 1000 doses) and Moderna (4 in 10,000,000).[58]

13.5.2 Post-mortem Blood Clots

With the introduction of the COVID-19 vaccines, there have been a number of morticians that have noted an increased frequency of blood clots during the embalming of cadavers, and in particular white, fibrous, "calamari-like" clots that are shaped like blood vessels. The Canadian Citizens Care Alliance interviewed UK funeral director John O'Looney and US embalmer Richard Hirschman about these abnormal blood clots that they found during the embalming process of the deceased.[59] Hirschman presented images of abnormal clots retrieved from deceased individuals. Other embalmers as well as US pathologist Dr. Ryan Cole have also reported a rise in these irregular, hardened blood clots.[60, 61] Their findings have been confirmed in a survey that was prepared by Tom Haviland and Laura Kasner, which was sent to thirty state funeral director/embalmer associations and eight hundred funeral homes primarily in the United States to determine if they were seeing unusual blood clots in corpses.[62] From 128 respondents: 68.75 percent had observed large whitish "fibrous" structures/clots in the corpses embalmed. Traditional "grape jelly" clots were reported by 66.4 percent of the respondents, especially in 2020, 2021, and 2022. In 2022, about 68.7 percent of the respondents observed large whitish, "fibrous" structures/clots, with 44 percent of the respondents finding these in cadavers 20 percent or more of the time. These clots were primarily found in the neck and legs. At the Canadian NCI Hearings on COVID-19, Laura Jeffrey noted that in her twenty-seven years of experience as a funeral director, she observed these unusual clots starting in the spring of 2021 and had not seen these before in all of her years in the industry.[63]

In view of the frequency and large size of these abnormal blood clots, the question arises: why have they not been observed in living people? Surely individuals with such occlusions would be extremely sick and easily diagnosed. It seems more likely that they are a post-mortem artefact that is generated after death by a process involving aggregation of fibrin possibly induced by the SARS-CoV-2 spike protein.[64, 65, 66, 67] With the termination of blood flow after death and cooling of the body temperature, especially with refrigeration, the aggregation of microclots might accumulate over time and the compression of these clots as the embalming fluid is forced into the cadaver might account for the large size and shape of the clots observed by many morticians.

Since the spread of COVID-19 vaccine lipid nanoparticles occurs throughout the body and endothelial cells that line blood vessels are likely to have high spike protein expression, it is feasible this might contribute to the formation of microclots that in some people could develop into more serious blood clots. More research is required to establish the frequency of the abnormal blood clots identified by several morticians, and the underlying mechanisms that produce them. Throughout the COVID-19 pandemic, autopsies were discouraged and rarely performed.

13.5.3. Menstrual Cycles and Bleeding

Soon after the COVID-19 genetic vaccines were introduced into the general population, there were many anecdotal reports that vaccinated women were experiencing prolonged menstrual cycles and heavier menstrual bleeding, even including in some post-menopausal women.[68] A Facebook group featured over twenty thousand testimonials regarding abnormalities in menstrual cycles before it was deleted in an act of censorship. Since then, other organizations such as My Cycle Story emerged to record such experiences.[69] Initially these claims were largely dismissed by health officials. However, this has been investigated in several prospective studies, almost all of which support the finding of abnormal menstrual periods with COVID-19 vaccination, although to different degrees of severity.

One published report by Wong et al. (2022) was based on responses collected between December 14, 2020 and January 9, 2022 from an open-ended survey submitted by 63,815 out of 5,975,363 female participants in the V-safe system eighteen years and older.[70] While these women were not specifically queried about menstrual irregularities or vaginal bleeding associated with COVID-19 vaccines, unsolicited they described such changes. The authors noted that "Several types of menstrual symptoms were reported, with most being related to disruptions in menstrual timing (83.6%) or increased severity of menstrual symptoms (67.0%), such as bleeding or pain. Some respondents also described symptoms related to perimenopausal and postmenopausal bleeding (4,0%), and resumption of menses after a long period of no menses (2.8%)." These symptoms became more evident after their second vaccine dose when compared with their first vaccine dose.

In the Pregnancy Study Online (PRESTO) with 1,137 participants from the United States and Canada, who were trying to conceive without fertility treatment, it was noted that the women "had 1.1 day longer menstrual cycles after receiving the first dose of COVID-19 vaccine and 1.3 day longer cycles after receiving the second dose."[71] The authors "did not observe strong associations between COVID-19 vaccination and cycle regularity, bleed length, heaviness of bleed, or menstrual pain." The participants were followed over five menstrual cycles and of the 437 that were vaccinated at least once, 93 percent of them received a COVID-19 RNA vaccine (60 percent Pfizer/BioNTech vaccine and 32.9 percent Moderna vaccine). Another larger US prospective study with 3,959 participants also noted a slight increase in the length of the menstrual cycle, but no change in the duration of the menses period.[72]

Another prospective study, the Nurses' Health Study 3, with 3,858 premenopausal American and Canadian female nurses that were not taking hormonal contraceptive medications, similarly found a change to longer menstrual cycles within the first six months after COVID-19 vaccination.[73] This was particularly evident among women who took the COVID-19 adenovirus vaccines and whose cycles were short, long, or irregular before vaccination; by contrast SARS-CoV-2 infection did not produce any changes in menstrual cycle characteristics.

The delay in menstrual periods in recently vaccinated women was found to be reduced if they were taking hormonal contraceptive medications. In a study with 1,273 British and French women, the study authors speculated "that menstrual changes following vaccination may be mediated by perturbations to ovarian hormones."[74] In this study, for participants with "progesterone-only contraception," their periods post-vaccination were significantly heavier than usual. Heavier menstrual bleed was also more evident in older women following vaccination.

Other studies have also described heavier and/or more prolonged bleeding during menses in women after COVID-19 vaccination. A Norwegian study of 3,972 women between eighteen and thirty years of age found that while menstrual disturbances were common regardless of vaccination status, "increased risks of prolonged bleeding, shorter interval between menstruations, and stronger pain during menstruation were also observed after both doses" of COVID-19 vaccines.[75] This research group also tracked unexpected vaginal bleeding and COVID-19 vaccination in non-menstruating women comparing three months before and then after SARS-CoV-2 mRNA BNT162b2 vaccination.[76] The authors noted:

> Among 7,725 postmenopausal women, 7,148 perimenopausal women, and 7,052 premenopausal women, 3.3, 14.1, and 13.1% experienced unexpected vaginal bleeding during a period of 8 to 9 months, respectively. In postmenopausal women, the risk of unexpected vaginal bleeding (*i.e.*, postmenopausal bleeding) in the 4 weeks after COVID-19 vaccination was increased two- to three-fold, compared to a prevaccination period. The corresponding risk of unexpected vaginal bleeding after vaccination was increased three- to five-fold in both nonmenstruating peri- and premenopausal women. [77]

Another study included women aged eighteen to fifty years without known gynecologic comorbidities who regularly monitor their menstruation through electronic calendars. A total of 219 women in this study met the inclusion criteria. Of these, fifty-one (23.3 percent) experienced irregular bleeding following the vaccine. Almost 40 percent (n = 83) of study participants reported a menstrual change following vaccination with the BNT162b2 SARS-CoV-2 mRNA vaccine.[78]

Likewise, in a cross-sectional European study with 14,153 women, who were double COVID-19 vaccinated at least three months before, 78 percent of them (many of them older or smokers) reported premenstrual symptoms including "increased fatigue (43%), abdominal bloating (37%), irritability (29%), sadness (28%), and headaches (28%)" and the predominant changes were "more menstrual bleeding (43%), more menstrual pain (41%), delayed menstruation (38%), fewer days of menstrual bleeding (34.5%), and shorter cycle length (32%)."[79]

In a large US study with 39,129 participants who were followed for three months after receiving two doses of a COVID-19 vaccine and had not contracted COVID-19, the authors reported:

> 42% of people with regular menstrual cycles bled more heavily than usual, while 44% reported no change after being vaccinated. Among respondents who typically do not menstruate, 71% of people on long-acting reversible contraceptives, 39% of people on gender-affirming hormones, and 66% of postmenopausal people reported breakthrough bleeding. We found that increased/breakthrough bleeding was significantly associated with age, systemic vaccine side effects (fever and/or fatigue), history of pregnancy or birth, and ethnicity.[80]

As mentioned earlier, hormonal changes induced by the COVID-19 vaccines appeared to partly underlie the menstrual changes observed with vaccination. Since the Pfizer COVID-19 vaccine lipid nanoparticles have been shown to accumulate in the ovaries, it is possible that this might contribute to the abnormal menstrual cycles in some fertile women following vaccination. The hypothalamus and pituitary glands in the brain and the ovaries hormonally control the menstrual cycle, so damage to the ovaries from an inflammatory attack might contribute to this effect, as well as platelet depletion following blood clotting induced by the COVID-19 vaccines.

It is important to appreciate that a female is born with all of the oocytes that she will have in her lifetime, and once she becomes fertile after puberty, she will have approximately four hundred periods in which one (and sometimes more) oocyte is converted to a fertilizable egg by the process of meiosis. The vast majority of oocytes die off without undergoing meiosis during a woman's fertile life. Menopause occurs in women when they deplete their supply of oocytes. Inflammatory damage to the ovaries can endanger the overall supply of oocytes and could lead to an earlier onset of menopause. In working women, there is a trend to delay having children, so if the ovaries are damaged by COVID-19 vaccine injury, there could possibly be a much shorter window in which they will be able to conceive. While this is a hypothetical risk, it is serious enough to warrant caution when weighing the risks and the benefits of the COVID-19 genetic vaccines.

13.6. Female and Male Fertility

13.6.1. Birth Rates

Although menstruation changes with COVID-19 vaccination appear to be reversible, there has been a reduction in the overall birth rates in Canada and other countries since the introduction of the COVID-19 vaccines. This decrease in birth rates may be over and above a steady decline in sperm counts in men that has been tracked since at least the early 1970s.[81] There may be significant differences in how males and females respond to the COVID-19 mRNA vaccines, particularly based on the biodistribution studies of the lipid nanoparticles used, which become enriched in the ovaries and testes.[82]

From 2019 to 2020, the Canadian fertility rate declined by 4.1 percent from 1.47 children per woman in 2019 to 1.41.[83] In 2021, it slightly increased by 2.1 percent to 1.44 children per woman, but then dropped by 7.6 percent to 1.33 in 2022.[84] The highest decline in birthrate was in women twenty to twenty-four years with a 37.5 percent decline, followed by 34 percent in fifteen- to nineteen-year-olds, 17 percent in twenty-five- to twenty-nine-year-olds, then dropping to 7.6 percent in thirty- to thirty-four-year-olds, and leveling off after that for thirty-five- to forty-nine-year-olds.[85] From 2019 to 2022 in Canada, the crude birth rate decline was 8.6 percent; total fertility rate decline was 12 percent.

By contrast in the United States, there has been a steady rise in the fertility rates of 0.06 percent to 0.11 percent per year from 2019 through to 2023, which is currently around 1.78 births per woman.[86] US birthrates declined by 1.6 percent in this period, but these data were not broken down by age.[87]

Reductions in fertility rates of women have also been noted in England and Wales, where the number of live births declined by 3.1 percent in 2022 compared to 2021.[88] There was a 2.0 percent increase in births in England and Wales from 2020 to 2021, but the number of births had previously declined by 4.2 percent from 2019 to 2020, and followed a downward trend since 2012. In the European Union, the total number of live births also declined by 2.4 percent from 2019 to 2020, was unchanged from 2020 to 2021, and then further decreased by another 4.4 percent from 2021 to 2022.[89]

Worldwide, the decline in fertility during the pandemic period of 2019 to 2023 in fertility has continued, but includes both countries with high mRNA vaccine uptake, as well as those with very low rates. It should be appreciated that birthrates have declined yearly by approximately 4 percent per annum since the 1950s in most nations.[90]

The median age of new US mothers increased from twenty-seven years in 1990 to thirty years in 2019. Women that have not been pregnant have double the odds of reaching menopause before forty years of age, and are

30 percent are more likely to begin menopause between forty and forty-four years of age.[91] Perimenopause is the period of about ten years that precedes menopause and is accompanied by a decline in estrogen levels. In 2011, the average age for a woman to begin perimenopause was forty-five years, but this since advanced to earlier average ages for the onset of primenopause.[92] The reduction in birthrates from the beginning of the COVID-19 pandemic to the later introduction of mRNA and other COVID-19 vaccines may arise from a number of possibilities such as the influence of COVID-19 or the COVID-19 genetic vaccines on fertility, the overall decline in male sperm levels, increased economic hardship, and social impacts of the pandemic, as well as concerns about having children given the current world situation. In Canada, conscious decisions not to have children during the current uncertain period and the lack of available housing in addition to these other factors have contributed to the lower birth rate during the COVID-19 crisis.[93] Thus, while it may be tempting to attribute the decline in birthrates at least in part to COVID-19 vaccines, it is premature to attribute this to SARS-CoV-2 infections or COVID-19 vaccination.

13.6.2. Sperm Counts and Motility

A possible factor that may have also contributed to the reduction in birth rates may be a temporary reduction in the production of sperm in men following COVID-19 vaccination. Gat et al. (2022) reported that inoculation with two doses of the Pfizer/BioNTech BNT162b2 COVID-19 vaccine in thirty-seven Israeli males (median age of twenty-eight years) was associated with a 15.4 and 22.1 percent temporary decline, respectively, in total spermatozoa concentration in semen and in their motility seventy-five to 125 days after the second inoculation, which was largely recovered by 145 days later.[94] Abd et al. (2022) tested sixty Iraqi males (eighteen to fifty years of age) and found that their sperm concentrations and sperm motility were reduced by 6 percent, at least ninety days after a second vaccination with a COVID-19 vaccine as compared to any prior vaccination.[95]

In a meta-analysis of seven publications (which excluded the study by Gat et al. mentioned above but included the Abd et al. report) where investigators examined sperm concentration and quality, the authors noted that most studies failed to observe differences in total sperm count, semen volume, sperm concentration, total sperm motility, and morphological changes with COVID-19 vaccination after two doses.[96] Gonzalez et al. (2021) actually reported increases in sperm counts and motility about seventy days after double vaccination in their study of forty-five men (median age of twenty-eight years).[97] Likewise, Barda et al. (2022) reported slight increases in sperm counts and total motility counts in thirty-three sperm donors (median age of twenty-seven years) seventy-two days or later after a second dose of the Pfizer/BioNTech BNT162b2 vaccine.[98] Safrai et al. (2022) failed to observe any significant changes in sperm volume, counts, and motility in their study of seventy-two men (median age of 35.7 years) about fifty days after their second dose of the BNT162b2 vaccine, but there were large differences in these parameters within each pre- and post-vaccination subgroup (as much as sixteen-fold for sperm motility).[99] In 106 men (older than eighteen years) undergoing assisted reproduction technology, a pairwise comparison between the first (while unvaccinated) and second attempt (median of seventy-five days after COVID-19 vaccination) did not reveal any changes in the sperm quality or successful fertilization rates.[100] Olano et al. (2022) also did not find any changes in sperm counts or motility in forty-seven males (median age of twenty-nine years) tested seventy days after a second inoculation with BNT162b2.[101] Examination of sperm production and quality in seventy-five Israeli men (younger than forty-five years) one to two months after a second dose of the BNT162b2 vaccine only showed one participant that had reduced sperm motility and another participant with a sperm concentration that was below the normal expected range.[102] However, in this study the sperm counts and motility of the participants were not determined prior to vaccination. In a study performed by Xia et al. (2022) with the Sinovac and Sinopharm chemically-inactivated whole virus vaccines, vaccination of 105 men (median of thirty-three to thirty-four years of age) did not appear to significantly affect semen volume, sperm count, and motility.[103] The difference in time between vaccination and sperm acquisition for testing was a median of 80.6 days.

In most of the aforementioned studies, sperm samples were typically taken about seventy-five days or less after the participants' second vaccination, whereas the reduction of sperm numbers and motility in the Gat et al. (2022)[104] study were between seventy-five and 125 days later. Most of the male participants in all studies were under forty years of age and often excluded those with low sperm counts to begin with. The vast differences in parameters from these studies in men who were vaccinated or not make it difficult to determine if alteration in sperm concentration and mobility may be vaccine-induced.[105] At the very least, any reductions in sperm counts and motility with the COVID-19 vaccines appear to be reversible.

It would be remiss not to mention that SARS-CoV-2 infection is strongly associated with a temporary reduction in sperm levels and motility as reviewed by Pourmasumi et al. (2022).[106] In many of these studies of the effects of COVID-19 on sperm concentration and quality, the COVID-19 vaccination status of the participants was not defined.

13.7. Impact of COVID-19 Vaccines on Pregnancy and Postnatal Development

13.7.1. Efficacy and Safety for Pregnant Women

This section primarily examines the evidence for the efficacy and safety of the mRNA vaccines against COVID-19 that were administered to women before or during pregnancy. To do so effectively requires consideration of the following aspects where some, often very limited, data may be available for evaluation:

a. The efficacy and safety of the mRNA vaccines in non-pregnant women in general, mostly based on the initial phase trials of the mRNA manufacturers, and some later studies in the scientific literature;
b. The impact of these vaccines on fertility, which was discussed in the previous section;
c. The impact of these vaccines on pregnancy during the various trimesters, including any changes in rates of spontaneous abortions and miscarriages;
d. Health outcomes for infants born to mothers vaccinated against COVID-19; and
e. Finally, the evidence, if any, that the vaccines may induce developmental disorders, particularly of the nervous system, in some children.

Taking these in order, what does the existing literature show about efficacy or safety for women in general following vaccination with any of the COVID-19 mRNA vaccines? The efficacy of any intervention in health is typically assessed by the use of a double-blind, randomized clinical trial (RCT), as described in chapter 10. This level of evaluation was never done for pregnant or potentially future pregnant women before the deployment and recommendation of the COVID-19 vaccines to the entire population. In fact, pregnant women were excluded from the initial Phase 3 studies, although some women did get pregnant during these clinical trials. Remarkably, this omission did not stop medical authorities in various countries from recommending COVID-19 vaccination for women before or during any trimester of pregnancy on the assumption, never tested, that infection with COVID-19 *might* be more serious for the mother and potentially harmful to the fetus. The same authorities then opted to measure effectiveness (real world data) in place of efficacy. Note that efficacy can only be determined prospectively in the context of an RCT. To do so, often unblinded data was frequently used (mostly from registries), often retrospectively, using different definitions of what a COVID-19 case was (typically positive PCR testing exclusively), from symptomatic COVID-19 diagnoses, to hospitalizations based on PCR tests, etc. More importantly, studies determining effectiveness almost never investigated adverse events in the same populations, so a risk/benefit analysis in the pregnant population is non-existent when it should be the basis of any rational consideration of whether COVID-19 vaccination during pregnancy is indeed "safe and effective."

After more than four years since the COVID-19 crisis started, there has been more than enough time to undertake a double blind RCT in pregnant women with a large enough sample to be able to extrapolate results to the general pregnant population. However, the latest results from Pfizer, published in the US Clinical Trials.gov website,[107] regarding a Phase 2–3 placebo-controlled, randomized, observer-blind trial in pregnant women managed to recruit only 174 women in each group (i.e., a total of 348 women), which is statistically insufficient to detect all potential poor outcomes, and makes extrapolation to the full population of pregnant women impossible. Comparatively, the retrospective design studies with statistical corrections that allegedly equalize the differences across groups (e.g., the study of Fell et al. [2022])[108] have managed to compare 43,099 vaccinated women versus 42,063 non-vaccinated women. So, the question that needs to be answered is why are there no larger RCTs underway given how important the issue is?

It should also be noted that the cited Pfizer study did not administer the vaccine before week twenty-four or twenty-seven of gestational age, so there is little to no data related to miscarriages (defined as terminated pregnancy before twenty weeks), which has been one (or the main) point of debate regarding administering the mRNA injection to pregnant women.[109] Indeed, Table 6 of the Pfizer report may deliberately blend data across trimesters, which gives the impression that vaccinated and non-vaccinated have the same level of miscarriages when Pfizer's own data may support the opposite conclusion. These concerns render the pregnancy data far less than evidence-based. Sadly, the data for fertility, lactation, and postpartum adverse events are even less acceptable. In conclusion, the data presented in support of COVID-19 vaccination during pregnancy fails to make a successful case that the vaccines are safe or effective.

Almost all the studies supposedly designed to evaluate the safety of mother and baby were determined retrospectively in case control studies, using registry data, which did not match groups of vaccinated and unvaccinated pregnant women, that is women with similar characteristics (i.e., demographic, ethnic, socioeconomic characteristics, substance consumption profile, comorbidities, etc.). Such matching is essential since these different characteristics (regardless of the vaccination status of the mother) may be responsible for differences in the outcome of the pregnancy and the overall health of the mother and the baby. Instead of attempting to match the groups, many researchers opted for complicated statistical corrections that tended to make the different characteristics across groups disappear, leading to a conclusion that the vaccinations were not responsible for any differences in outcomes. However, some of the most striking differences between the vaccinated versus the unvaccinated for COVID-19 were not separately considered. These variables, such as cigarette use, consumption of other substances, and socioeconomic income or poverty index known to negatively impact pregnancy were higher in the unvaccinated group.[110]

An important question to consider in relation to such data is how reliable are the statistical methods to erase differences between unvaccinated mothers who consumed cigarettes or other drugs and lived in more impoverished conditions (which generally entail worse overall health status and nutritional status) vs. vaccinated mothers who did not consume any substances and who benefited from a better socioeconomic status (which generally means better overall health baseline status)? Can one be certain that a lower number of adverse events in vaccinated pregnant women means that the vaccination is not associated with poorer outcomes (i.e., harms), or could it be that the harms in the healthier vaccinated population becomes like that of unvaccinated mothers dealing with worse overall health conditions, cigarette use, and/or other substance abuse issues, all of which are known to produce poorer outcomes during pregnancy? This is a key question that needs to be resolved, as based on the characteristics of the vaccinated and unvaccinated groups there may be a very real issue of "selection bias" in these studies.

The initial Phase 3 trials for mRNA vaccines, specifically those by Pfizer, did not separate the male and female participants such that women of reproductive age were not separately assessed. Additionally, any women who might be initially pregnant were excluded from the trials. Moderna's initial trials also assessed the efficacy and safety data for both sexes, without considering a separate analysis in woman of reproductive age.

Based on these evaluations of male and female efficacy and safety data, few sex-based conclusions about the impact of mRNA vaccines can be used as baseline values. Further, such data cannot really be used as a comparator to women during the various trimesters of pregnancy.

In place of this is a 2021 report by Pfizer/BioNtech on BNT162B2 entitled "Cumulative Analysis of Post-Authorization Adverse Event Reports of PF-07302048 (BNT162B2) Received Through 28-FEB-2021."[111] This analysis covered through to the end of February 2021. It evaluated 42,086 vaccine recipients, of whom 29,214 were female and 9,182 were male. A further 2,990 patients were listed as "No data," which may simply mean that the sex of some participants was not recorded, which is odd considering the importance of sex [not: gender] differences. The data were gathered from reports in twenty-six countries in which the trials were held.

In regard to safety as measured by adverse events in pregnant women, Tables 5 and 6 of the document are revealing. In Table 5, the report discusses "Vaccine-Associated Enhanced Disease" (VAED) or Vaccine-Associated Enhanced Respiratory Disease (VAERD). It lists 138 cases, including 317 "potentially relevant events." The authors write:

> Conclusion: VAED may present as severe or unusual clinical manifestations of COVID-19. Overall, there were 37 subjects with suspected COVID-19 and 101 subjects with confirmed COVID-19 following one or both doses of the vaccine; 75 of the 101 cases were severe, resulting in hospitalization, disability, life-threatening consequences or death. None of the 75 cases could be definitively considered as VAED/VAERD. In this review of subjects with COVID-19 following vaccination, based on the current evidence, VAED/VAERD remains a theoretical risk for the vaccine. Surveillance will continue.[112]

Whether these cases might represent antibody-dependent enhancement (ADE) as discussed in previous chapters was not clear, nor was it apparently evident to Pfizer, assuming they even acknowledge that ADE exists.

Table 6 in the report listed 413 adverse event cases, of which eighty-four were listed as "serious" and 329 as "non-serious."[113] How these descriptions were determined is not specified. Of these overall adverse events, in the presumably serious cases, twenty-three showed spontaneous abortions, two showed premature death with neonatal death, and two showed spontaneous abortion with intrauterine death (total twenty-seven). The adverse events during pregnancy listed as "non-serious" included those in the first trimester (fifteen), second trimester (seven), and third trimester (two).

In the next paragraph of the report, it listed 124 "mother cases," with forty-nine cases characterized as non-serious and seventy-five cases as serious.[114] Why the numbers varied was not clear. In this paragraph, spontaneous abortions included twenty-five of the cases. Taking the latter number and not being certain in which trimester the twenty-five spontaneous abortions occurred (although the first trimester would be most likely) would give a rate of 29.98 percent for "serious cases" (which one would have to conclude these cases were) or 7.6 percent of those deemed "non-serious." In comparison, US data for pregnancy in general shows the percentage of first trimester spontaneous abortions were highly dependent on the mother's age, with 15 percent occurring in those under thirty-five years, 20–35 percent in the thirty-five- to forty-five-age range, and 50 percent in the over forty-five age group.[115]

A clearer answer to the question of the potentially negative impacts of COVID-19 vaccines on pregnancy would be to look at stillbirth data, which is the death of fetuses over twenty weeks of gestational age. In the richer countries with advanced medical care, stillbirths are quite uncommon so it would be extremely concerning if the numbers of stillbirths in women taking the COVID-19 vaccines just before or during the pregnancy were higher. However, the Pfizer study did not appear to clearly distinguish spontaneous abortions from stillbirths. Some insights into this issue can be found in the last paragraph of page 12 in the report in the section on "Pregnancy cases."[116] Of the 270 adverse effects reported, four were described as "serious foetus/baby cases" of which two were "premature baby" and one death. Two of these are described as occurring in the first trimester.

Taking the numbers of spontaneous abortions in this report as accurate, the Pfizer mRNA vaccines would seem to have almost doubled the number of such cases for under thirty-five-year-olds, coming in at about the same in the thirty-five- to forty-five-year-old group, and showing lower numbers than in the over forty-five years and up age group. It should be stressed, however, that the overall numbers in the Pfizer data were small and will thus not have the same accuracy and statistical power to make valid conclusions or extrapolation of the data to the general pregnant population.

During the same time period as when the Pfizer report came out, a number of studies appeared in the peer-reviewed literature as referenced next. The main issues for these studies include concerns about study design, exclusion criteria, the use of PCR testing at too high thermal cycle thresholds (see chapter 8.2), and the fundamental differences between the use of relative efficacy and safety vs. absolute efficacy and safety values.

An article by Morgan et al. (2022) also demonstrated other study design issues, namely that non-vaccinated women were younger, belonged to the Hispanic or the African-American community, had a higher body mass index, and had a positive smoking status.[117] The authors attempted to deal with these issues by statistical correction. Additionally, Remdesivir had been taken by twenty women in the unvaccinated group compared to none in the vaccinated group, a variable that was not corrected for in this and other studies.[118, 119, 120, 121, 122]

In terms of effectiveness, the relative rate reported by these studies ranged from 71 percent to 88 percent; the absolute rate was between 0.1 and 5.6 percent. Effectiveness was also assessed in relation to specific severe forms of COVID-19, such as cases requiring hospitalization, with a relative risk reduction of 71.4 percent, but an absolute risk reduction of only 0.1 percent.[123] In one retrospective observational study, researchers from Israel and the United States carefully matched 15,060 pregnant women in Israel according to age, gestational age, residential area, population subgroup, parity, and influenza immunization status into vaccinated/unvaccinated pairs.[124] Their findings indicated that vaccination with BNT162b2 in pregnant women lowered the risk of SARS-CoV-2 infection, with a relative efficacy rate of 78 percent, but an absolute difference of only 1.31

percent. In both the vaccinated and non-vaccinated women that were infected with SARS-CoV-2, about 16 percent were asymptomatic. Of eighty-eight pregnant women who were symptomatic for COVID-19 in the vaccinated group, ten were hospitalized (11.4 percent), whereas twenty-three of the 149 non-vaccinated pregnant women were hospitalized (15.4 percent). Therefore, there appeared to be little difference with respect to the severity of COVID-19 once it was acquired in either vaccinated or unvaccinated women. The authors noted that "there were no notable differences between the vaccinated and unvaccinated groups regarding preeclampsia, intrauterine growth restriction, infant birth weight, abortions, stillbirth, maternal death, or pulmonary embolism." While sixty-eight of 7530 (0.9 percent) of the vaccinated women experienced vaccine-related adverse events, none of these were considered severe.[125]

Bookstein, Peretz et al. (2021) compared 390 pregnant Israeli women who were vaccinated with 260 non-pregnant women who were also vaccinated between January and February of 2021 and concluded that there were no significant differences in reported side-effects of Pfizer-BioNTech vaccinations after two doses associated with pregnancy.[126] However, in this retrospective study, the pregnant women had 21 percent lower serum SARS-CoV-2 IgG antibody levels compared to non-pregnant, vaccinated women ($p < 0.001$). This study had no comparable cohort of unvaccinated pregnant women with which to compare, and it did not evaluate whether vaccination reduced the incidence of COVID-19.

In several studies, most of the pregnant women who were admitted to the hospital that were positive for SARS-CoV-2 had no symptoms of COVID-19 at presentation. This amounted to 87.9 percent of thirty-three PCR-positive obstetrics patients at the New York–Presbyterian Allen Hospital and Columbia University Irving Medical Center,[127] 52.2 percent of twenty-three PCR-positive pregnant patients at an Indonesian hospital,[128] and in a meta-analysis of five studies, between 45 and 100 percent of 131 PCR-positive obstetric patients presenting to hospitals, of which 49 percent to 68 percent remained asymptomatic for COVID-19 during their hospital stay.[129]

Cumulatively, a summary of the existing data on vaccine effectiveness in vaccinated versus unvaccinated women during pregnancy shows major flaws in study design and interpretation, much like that which attended the Phase 3 trials cited in chapter 12. First, claims made that the COVID-19 genetic vaccines may be effective in pregnant women to prevent infection with SARS-CoV-2 are speculative, especially given the absolute efficacy numbers. Also, because a woman's immune system is distinctly different during pregnancy than in non-pregnant states, any statements about how well the COVID-19 mRNA vaccines work in pregnant women based on studies that excluded these women as in the original Phase trial data are largely conjecture. Also, of note, a key problem in most studies has been the short reporting time post vaccination and the small sample sizes. In some cases, they are simply based on surveys that are filled retrospectively by study participants, as exemplified in the Canadian COVERED study by McClymont et al. (2023).[130]

In the COVERED study with 4,528 respondents,[131] 99 percent were either vaccinated before, during, and/or after their pregnancy. Less than a percent remained unvaccinated. About 80 percent of the participants were white and only 3.4 percent had a maximum of a high school education or less. The extent of natural immunity in all of the study respondents from previous SARS-CoV-2 infections prior to pregnancy was not considered, although this would be difficult to ascertain without serological testing since about 41 percent of adults are asymptomatic for COVID-19 following infection with this virus.[132] About 27.4 percent of the vaccinated study participants tested positive for an active SARS-CoV-2 infection after vaccination. While none of these infected individuals experienced more than mild symptoms of COVID-19, the study was silent about the severity of COVID-19 cases in the unvaccinated group. However, the authors did note that the side-effects of COVID-19 vaccination (redness, pain, or swelling at the site of injection [in over 65 percent of vaccinated participants], tiredness, headache, muscle pain, chills, fever, and nausea) in the pregnant women were more commonly observed than evident in non-pregnant COVID-19 vaccinated women, and these were generally more pronounced after the second dose of a COVID-19 vaccine. Only 23.6 percent of the vaccinated group received one or two doses of a COVID-19 vaccine in the first trimester, which would be the most dangerous to the developing fetus as spike levels would be at their peak soon after vaccination. Since the study was underpowered in the number of participants, rarer adverse effects of the COVID-19 vaccinations would be harder to identify. Receiving a vaccination in the latter half of the second trimester (weeks thirteen through twenty-seven of pregnancy) or in the third trimester (weeks twenty-eight to forty) would not cause a spontaneous abortion (which by definition occurs before the twentieth week of pregnancy). Even so, the higher rate of spontaneous abortions in the vaccinated group (eighteen out of 2,868) as compared with the unvaccinated group (four out of 1,660) (i.e., 0.63 percent vs 0.24 percent) was dismissed on the basis that the survey was retrospective and the number of respondents between the two groups was unequal, even though the rates were adjusted for this by percentage. It was also evident that there were five stillbirths and three neonatal deaths in the COVID-19 vaccinated group and none in the unvaccinated group. While not statistically significant, there were seizures in nine babies born to vaccinated mothers (0.32 percent) compared to four babies with unvaccinated mothers (0.24 percent).[133]

The UK Yellow Card Vaccine Monitoring Group (YCVM) collected adverse event reporting data for COVID-19 vaccines from about thirty thousand registrants (some six hundred thousand people were invited), and issued an interim report in July 2021 that was presented for advice to the Pharmacovigilance Expert Advisory Group (PEAG) of the UK Medicines and Health products Regulatory Agency (MHRA).[134] This not-for-publication interim report was finally released following a freedom of information request by Cheryl Grainger, filed in April 13, 2023. This report was analyzed by Professor Norman Fenton in the School of Electronic Engineering and Computer Science at Queen Mary University of London, who is an expert on risk assessment and statistics with a focus on Bayesian probability. His report showed:

> An astonishing 53% of all those in the YCVM reported at least one ADR (adverse drug reaction). Of those receiving the AZ vaccine 59.2% reported at least one ADR, compared to 38.8% for Pfizer and 59.3% for Moderna. There were 1,366 pregnant women in the YCVM. Of those who received the AZ vaccine a whopping 66% (124 out of 203) reported at least one ADR; 38% of the Pfizer recipients and 61% of the Moderna recipients reported at least one ADR." This report was never issued to the public from the MHRA despite the fact that it was due in mid-2022.[135]

From data obtained from a Freedom of Information request by the Canadian Citizen Care Alliance for nine billing codes for payment by the Ontario Health Insurance Plan (OHIP) related to reproductive disorders from January 2015 through to December 2022, Amy Kelley of the *Daily Clout* noted striking increases in the filing of the associated diagnostic codes with the availability of COVID-19 vaccines.[136] Compared to 2015 to 2020 trends, there were 24 percent or more increases in 2021 and 2022 in the filings of OHIP diagnostic/billing codes for inflammation of testicles and the epididymis (code 604), male infertility due to low or no sperm counts (code 606), inflammation of the ovaries or fallopian tubes (code 614), menopause or post-menopausal bleeding (code 627), infertility (code 628), other disorders of female genital organs (code 629), missed miscarriage or spontaneous abortion from lack or defective fetal development (code 632), and incomplete or complete abortion (code 634).

Ultimately, to draw a meaningful conclusion regarding the effects of vaccines on pregnancy, the outcomes should be recorded from vaccination until birth. Moreover, a snapshot of seven days post-vaccination (as recorded in certain studies, such as that of Sadarangani et al. [2022]),[137] seems meaningless when the health authorities themselves consider people who received one dose of the vaccine less than fourteen or even twenty-one days prior as unvaccinated, and people with two doses were only considered fully vaccinated if more than seven days post-second dose. So, as per the definition of health authorities, when counting hospitalized vaccinated patients, these vaccinated pregnant women would have fallen in the category of unvaccinated for the one-dose recipients (unvaccinated and one dose less than fourteen days), and of one-dose patients (one dose greater than fourteen days) for the two-dose recipients. They would have never counted in the fully vaccinated hospitalized patients. Immune-mediated mechanisms (such as autoimmunity or molecular mimicry) typically take longer to manifest, as opposed to local reactions, general systemic reactions (like fever or malaise), and allergies.

Among other concerns is the lack of animal or Phase 1/2 studies in humans that addressed teratogenic/toxic effects of individual components of these vaccines; for example, lipids used in the nanoparticles and the spike protein and its potential truncated versions. Another issue is the low numbers of participants in the clinical trials, particularly in the first trimester when most miscarriages typically occur. In these studies, where there were claims of no increased risk of miscarriage, these statements were based on comparison to historic cohorts, where the frequency of miscarriages varies widely between 8 and 20 percent.

Finally, the data for adults using a non-vaccine immune population may be clinically irrelevant since at the time of the trial most people already had some level of immunity—either acquired naturally or vaccine-induced.

Despite all of the aforementioned caveats, it is still important to collectively review the data that is available despite its sparsity with respect to the maternal and neonatal outcomes of COVID-19 vaccination during pregnancy. Among the best available is a meta-analysis of thirty-seven published studies that together tracked maternal, neonatal, and immunological outcomes in 141,107 pregnant women (36.8 percent vaccinated) performed by Marchand et al. (2023).[138] The extent of SARS-CoV-2 infections in the vaccinated women was 13.1 percent and in the non-vaccinated women was 19.1 percent. Such a difference can easily be accounted for by extra testing in non-vaccinated women who were pregnant from strong encouragement from their potentially biased health-care providers. The meta-analysis revealed that vaccination for COVID-19 was associated with what was described as a reduced risk of premature delivery (Odds Ratio of 0.71; $p<0.00001$) by a day or so, and slightly increased risk for a Cesarean section delivery (Odds Ratio of 1.20; $p=0.007$) as compared to non-vaccinated pregnant women. (Odds Ratios provide a measure of the association of an exposure with an outcome. If the Odds Ratio is close to one, there is no association. A positive number supports a positive relationship, whereas a negative number supports an inverse relationship.) The authors described the delivery of the babies as occasionally slightly more premature in the non-vaccinated mothers. However, presumably the non-vaccinated mothers should be considered as the expected normal controls, especially since 80.9 percent of them were apparently not infected with the SARS-CoV-2 virus during their pregnancies. Thus, it is more appropriate to suggest that the vaccinated women may have a slight risk of a delay in their deliveries. Although not quite statistically significant in their analysis, there also appeared to be a small trend toward increased gestational diabetes in the vaccinated pregnant women (Odds Ratio of 1.28 based on two studies; 10.6 percent vs. 8.96 percent) and postpartum hemorrhage (Odds Ratio of 1.68 based on three studies; 3.9 percent vs. 3.4 percent; p=0.08).[139]

A recent retrospective cohort of 6,057 women by Dick et al. (2023) also found a slightly higher rate of gestational diabetes (47 percent increase; 12.2 percent versus 8.3 percent; p=0.02) among vaccinated pregnant women, and in triple vaccinated women as compared to non-vaccinated mothers slightly more Cesarean deliveries (12 percent increase; 18.6 percent versus 16.6 percent, p=0.52), as well as higher rates of postpartum hemorrhage (195 percent increase; 9.5 percent versus 3.21 percent; p<0.001).[140] Another meta-analysis of the literature by Pratama et al. (2023) based on thirteen observational studies with COVID-19 mRNA vaccines with 48,039 pregnant women failed to detect any differences between vaccinated and non-vaccinated women with respect to maternal, delivery, and neonatal outcomes.[141]

Kory and Pfeiffer (2024) have noted in a Substack article that the CDC reported 429 out of 1205 women who died during their pregnancy died with COVID-19 in 2021.[142] While this is tiny in view of the 3.6 million successful births that year, it represented a 321 percent increase in COVID-19-associated deaths during pregnancy recorded in 2020. When the deaths that were directly attributable to COVID-19 were examined, there was a 2,000 percent increase, from sixteen mothers who died in 2020 to 335 in 2021.[143] Thankfully, the number of maternal deaths with COVID-19 declined in 2022, but this begets the question of whether the introduction of the COVID-19 vaccines at the time of the predominance of Delta variants (more virulent and lethal than omicron variants) put pregnant women at greater or lesser risk.

13.7.2. Breastfeeding

In regard to lactation, there are limited studies, of which the work of Kachikis et al. (2022) may be the most representative.[144] One of the possible adverse effects reported by 355 of 10,278 (3.5 percent) lactating women included a decrease in their breast milk supply. However, all signs and symptoms were recorded during the first twenty-four hours post-vaccination and from a pre-determined list of options. When asked about other signs and symptoms post-vaccination, the participants were instructed to record them only if they thought they were related to vaccination, which makes the data collection subjective to the participants' own biases.

In the Pfizer analysis,[145] the authors considered 133 reports of breastfeeding in vaccinated mothers, where 116 were taken to be normal and seventeen cases included adverse events with three that were considered as "serious" and fourteen as "non-serious." The symptoms in the infants included: pyrexia (fever), rash, irritability, vomiting, diarrhea, insomnia, poor feeding, lethargy, abdominal discomfort, allergy to vaccine, increased appetite, anxiety, crying, poor sleep quality, belching (eructation) agitation, pain, and hives (uticaria).

Fu et al. (2022) conducted a meta-analysis of twenty-three studies that examined the immune response in pregnant and lactating individuals to COVID-19 vaccination.[146] They noted that these individuals experienced vaccine-related reactions at a similar rate to the general population. With respect to whether the levels of IgA anti-spike protein antibody in breast milk was higher following vaccination against COVID-19 or if it was higher in lactating mothers who had previously been infected with SARS-CoV-2, the authors noted that the findings in the literature were conflicting.

In addition to the previously mentioned problems with the published studies on the vaccination of pregnant women in general and with breastfeeding specifically, other issues included small sample sizes and lack of control groups, as well as short duration follow up of 4.6 to seventeen weeks.[147] A small sample size was also used by Blakeway et al. (2023),[148] none of whom were vaccinated during the first trimester with 85.7 percent vaccinated in the third trimester, thus limiting the ability to monitor stillbirths. Additionally, many of the reporting authors had conflicts of interest with relationships with COVID-19 vaccine companies.

Studies of breast milk have confirmed that mothers that have been vaccinated with either the Pfizer/BioNTech BNT162b2 or Moderna mRNA-1273 vaccines could have detectable spike mRNA for up to forty-eight hours.[149, 150]

13.7.3. *Impacts of mRNA Vaccines on Early Infant Health*

Much of the literature about this age range is based on the official reports from health agencies such as NIH, CDC, Health Canada, and others. These simply repeat the mantra that the mRNA vaccines are "safe and effective" without critical analysis. However, in the Pfizer report,[151] part of the list in Table 6 may provide some insight, primarily into what was not analyzed. In a section entitled "Use in Paediatric Individuals <12 years of Age," it listed thirty-four cases ranging from two months of age to nine years old. The following adverse effects are reported: vaccination site pain (three), upper abdominal pain (two), COVID-19 (two), facial paralysis (two), lymphadenopathy (disorder of the lymph nodes) (two), malaise (two), pruritus (itchy skin) and swelling (two). From this, the authors concluded that there was no significant difference compared to "the non-paediatric population."

13.7.4. Impacts of mRNA Vaccines on Neurological Development in Children

Finally, the question about whether children born to women vaccinated against COVID-19 have more developmental delays is a question that cannot yet be answered, especially for neural development. For example, autism spectrum disorder (ASD) remains a neurological disorder of unknown etiology. While claims have been made that ASD levels have risen in lockstep with the increase in pediatric vaccines that are recommended for children, clearly, correlation, even if suggestive, does not equal causation. Other environmental insults have also been proposed and there are indications that ASD has a genetic component, although one that likely involves at most selected nucleotide sequences, often in non-coding regions of DNA. (For references to these and other points, see Shaw, *Dispatches from the Vaccine Wars*, 2021.[152])

Due to the complexities of the development of the brain, it can take several years before diseases such as autism can clearly manifest in a toddler. According to the 2019 Canadian Health Survey on Children and Youth, about 2 percent of those between one and seventeen years of age were diagnosed with ASD, and "over two-thirds of these had another long-term health condition, with attention deficit disorder/attention deficit hyperactivity disorder, learning disability/disorder and anxiety disorder being the most common."[153] ASD symptoms include "impairments in speech, non-verbal communication and social interactions combined with restricted and repetitive behaviours, interests or activities." Most children are diagnosed with ASD before they turn five years old, but with a median of 3.7 years of age. This precludes an early answer to the question of mRNA vaccines in pregnancy and neural outcomes in postnatal life at this time. In addition, such a study would be highly complicated by the numerous other prenatal and postnatal events to which children might be exposed.

However, some recent studies have raised some concerns. In a recent study by Erdogan et al. (2024) the consequences of treatment of pregnant rats with COVID-19 mRNA BNT162b2 vaccine during gestation was investigated.[154] In particular, the authors noted:

> the male rats exhibited pronounced autism-like behaviors, characterized by a marked reduction in social interaction and repetitive patterns of behavior. Furthermore, there was a substantial decrease in neuronal counts in critical brain regions, indicating potential neurodegeneration or altered neurodevelopment. Male rats also demonstrated impaired motor performance, evidenced by reduced coordination and agility.[155]

These developmental changes were preceded by changes in the expression levels of brain-derived neurotrophic factor (BDNF) and other neurodevelopment markers that have been linked with autism. While the Erdogan study involved a small number of rats, it is worth bearing in mind that the ACE2 receptor of laboratory rats has a low affinity for SARS-CoV-2 spike protein, so it is possible that the effects of COVID-19 mRNA vaccination during pregnancy in humans may be even more profound. However, this will be hard to track due to the already high rates of ASD in human children.

Jaswa et al. (2024) have investigated whether maternal COVID-19 vaccination *in utero* was associated with a risk for neurodevelopmental impairment in 2,261 twelve- and 1,940 eighteen-month-old infants in the United States between May 2020 and August 2021.[156] Based on scoring with an Ages and Stages Questionnaire (ASQ) completed by the mothers, the researchers found more evidence of developmental delays in males compared to females, regardless of vaccination of their mothers. There was a trend toward statistically significant deleterious delay in twelve-month old-males with vaccination, but this was not evident in the eighteen-month-old males, although it was when compared to females at eighteen months from vaccinated mothers. The children from mothers that were vaccinated in the first trimester performed the worst, with less harm evident with children whose mothers were vaccinated in the second trimester, and little impact if their mothers were vaccinated in the third trimester. After performing adjustments for maternal age, race, ethnicity, education, income, maternal depression, and anxiety in multivariable mixed-effects logistic regression models, the authors claimed that vaccination during pregnancy had no statistical effect on ASQ scores, although the trend was still an increased risk in twelve-month-old males and a decrease in eighteen-month-old females. This makes the adjustments performed somewhat dubious. In any event, additional studies are warranted to assess the risk of *in utero* exposure of COVID-19 vaccines to the developing fetus. COVID-19 vaccine mRNA has been detected in placental and cord blood post vaccination of at least two pregnant women that have been examined, so it is evident that the vaccine lipid nanoparticles are able to penetrate the fetal-placental barrier and reach the intrauterine environment.[157]

13.7.5. Concluding Remarks on Vaccine Safety in Pregnant Mothers and Their Babies

The FDA's February 28, 2021 review of Pfizer's early pharmacovigilance safety database clearly showed that mRNA product (BNT162b2) injections may cause harm to mothers, pregnancy, lactation, and breastfeeding infants. This review makes clear that this database cannot be used to calculate incidence rates or test hypotheses, but that it should be used to detect potential indicators of harm or safety signals. This raises the question of how much harm is acceptable before halting use of these products. Despite a deficiency of safety data, these products continue to be declared as "safe" in pregnancy. Studies used to support these claims are generally of poor quality, consisting mainly of observational studies and voluntary registries. As such, they are only able to speculate that associations seen between suspected injuries and the mRNA product are not due to the COVID-19 mRNA products. The primary limitation of most of these studies is that they focus on short-term harms to the mother or only highly observable immediate harms such as miscarriage, stillbirth, preterm birth, or infant size at birth. None of the studies monitored the health of the mother and child carefully enough—or long enough—to detect subtle but significant changes to maternal or infant bodily systems, including but not limited to the reproductive, immune, or cardiovascular system. Additionally, these studies have significant statistical issues that further bring their findings into question. They lacked any reliable denominators in their calculations, standardization, stratification of significant variables, adequate tracking, and follow-up of participants, and they incorrectly interpreted what data were available. Recently meta-analyses of these same observational trials have been published and have failed to establish safety risks for these COVID-19 mRNA products in pregnant women. These analyses suffer from the same limitations as the observational trials and are no substitute for the robust and long-term RCT data that are required to prove product safety.

13.8. Myocarditis and Myopericarditis

13.8.1. Nature of Myocarditis and Incidence Pre-COVID-19

Myocarditis, also known as inflammatory cardiomyopathy, is a disease that results from infiltration of heart muscle with immune cells that attack, damage, and may kill cardiomyocytes. These are the contractile cells of the middle layer of the heart that permit it to beat and pump blood through the circulatory system. If the cardiomyocytes are killed, they are replaced by non-contractile scar tissue, and the surviving heart cells have to expand in size to maintain circulation and blood pressure, which results in enlargement of the heart. Myocarditis is the principal cause of about 20 percent of sudden cardiac death in people under forty years of age.[158] It can occur within an hour of symptoms, such as dizziness, chest pain, sudden loss of consciousness, lack of pulse, and no breathing. Continuing symptoms include feeling fatigued, shortness of breath, chest pains, and palpitations (sensation of heart racing). While the symptoms of myocarditis subside gradually, the actual physical damage to the heart may become permanent, although full recovery from symptoms is usually observed. Myopericarditis has a similar pathology to myocarditis and involves damage to the pericardium muscle tissue that envelopes and protects the heart. It tends to be less severe than myocarditis. Both myocarditis and myopericarditis can be triggered by a wide range of factors such as kidney failure, cancer, drugs, toxins, and many viruses, including SARS-CoV-2.[159] It can also be induced by COVID-19 vaccines.

Historically, the outcomes from myocarditis are usually favorable. However, since the damage from myocarditis can be irreversible and may be cumulative, it is inappropriate to suggest that a person can have a mild case of myocarditis based on symptoms. The acute observable effects may be experienced as mild, and apparently asymptomatic in most cases, but it may induce more serious heart issues in the longer term. Scarring that may result with myocarditis can cause life-threatening arrhythmia of the heart. While the long-term outcomes of COVID-19 vaccine-induced myocarditis are yet unknown, viral induced myocarditis causes death in about 20 percent of those afflicted within six years.[160] The lethality of myocarditis is also highlighted in *The Journal of Clinical Medicine* article "Occurrence, Trends, Management and Outcomes of Patients Hospitalized with Clinically Suspected Myocarditis—Ten-Year Perspectives from the MYO-PL Nationwide Database,"[161] which concluded that:

> Myocarditis has been shown in post-mortem studies to be a major cause (up to 42% of cases) of sudden and unexpected death in children and young adults. In contrast, a recently published study on autopsies reported that 6% of 14,294 sudden deaths were assigned as being caused by myocarditis. In patients with biopsy-proven myocarditis in long-term observation (the median follow up of 4.7 years), all-cause mortality was 19.2%, while sudden death occurred in 9.9% of cases.[162]

Another older report noted that:

> The Myocarditis Treatment Trial reported mortality rates for biopsy-verified myocarditis of 20% and 56% at 1 year and 4.3 years, respectively. These outcomes are similar to the Mayo Clinic's observational data of 5-year survival rates that approximate 50%. Survival with giant cell myocarditis is substantially lower, with <20% of patients surviving 5 years.[163]

The global incidence of myocarditis and deaths from this disease steadily climbed over thirty years between 1990 and 2019 by 62 and 65 percent, respectively, although the age-standardized death rate (ASDR) (about sixteen per hundred thousand) was stable during this period.[164] The age-standardized incidence rate (ASIR) in North America during this period for all ages and sexes was 18.2 per hundred thousand, and this serves as a useful bench mark for consideration of the expected background rates of myocarditis during the

COVID-19 pandemic. Worldwide in 2019, men were on average 35 percent more likely than women to get myocarditis. The risk of myocarditis increases with age; in 2019, 77.76 percent of cases were in those sixty-five years and older, 12.26 percent in forty- to sixty-four-year-olds, and 9.98 percent in those under forty years of age. The ASDR from myocarditis is less than one in hundred thousand for those under seventy years of age. In the fifteen- to twenty-four-years-old bracket, the ASIR were 12.3 in males and 7.3 in females per hundred thousand, and the ASDR were 0.13 in males and 0.07 in females per hundred thousand.[165] Due to the rarity of myocarditis in children and young adults, it is much easier to observe unusual incidence of this disease in these populations, including from COVID-19 and COVID-19 vaccines.

Another study by Nasreen et al. (2022) examined the historical rates in Ontario between 2015 and 2022 of myocarditis and myopericarditis along with a range of other diseases that have been linked to COVID-19 vaccine adverse events.[166] They noted:

> The average annual population was 14 million across all age groups with 51% female. The pre-pandemic mean annual rates per 100,000 population during 2015–2019 were 191 for acute myocardial infarction, 43.9 for idiopathic thrombocytopenia, 28.8 for anaphylaxis, 27.8 for Bell's palsy, 25.0 for febrile convulsions, 22.8 for acute disseminated encephalomyelitis, 11.3 for myocarditis/pericarditis, 8.7 for pericarditis, 2.9 for myocarditis, 2.0 for Kawasaki disease, 1.9 for Guillain-Barré syndrome, and 1.7 for transverse myelitis. Females had higher rates of acute disseminated encephalomyelitis, transverse myelitis, and anaphylaxis while males had higher rates of myocarditis, pericarditis, and Guillain-Barré syndrome. Bell's palsy, acute disseminated encephalomyelitis, and Guillain-Barré syndrome increased with age. The mean rates of myocarditis and/or pericarditis increased with age up to 79 years; males had higher rates than females: from 12 to 59 years for myocarditis and ≥12 years for pericarditis.[167]

13.8.2. Myocarditis from COVID-19

Early on in the COVID-19 pandemic, health officials widely proclaimed that a person who got COVID-19 was much more likely to get myocarditis than getting the disease from a COVID-19 vaccine. For example, as part of a resource guide produced by the Office of the Chief Medical Officer for Ontario, which was presented in information sessions to doctors, nurses, and pharmacists to encourage COVID-19 vaccination of children five to eleven years of age, in slide number 41, it is indicated that for those under sixteen years of age, the risk of hospitalized myocarditis was "133 per 100 thousand COVID-19 infections or 1 in almost every 750 infections."[168] The citation provided in the slide was

Boehmer et al. (2021),[169] which was based on the number of US children under sixteen years of age that showed up in hospitals and clinics, between March 2020 and January 2021, with COVID-19. This was not the total number of children who were actually infected with SARS-CoV-2, which should include those that were asymptomatic or mildly sick, or about a hundred-fold higher (see Table 6.1). The total number of children tracked in this age group was 3,735,660, of which only 1.7 percent were reported to be infected with SARS-CoV-2. The number of children under sixteen years of age presenting at hospitals with myocarditis was 132 with COVID-19 and 86 without COVID-19. The incidence of myocarditis in all age groups was only 42.3 percent higher in 2020 than in pre-pandemic 2019. When all age groups were considered in aggregate, there were 2,116 cases presenting at hospitals with symptomatic myocarditis with COVID-19 and 2,953 cases without COVID-19. Only about 4 percent of the total number of people tracked in this study (i.e., 36,005,294) had been diagnosed with COVID-19, but the actual number was likely substantially higher as only about 5.7 percent of known COVID-19 cases were likely hospitalized (see Table 6.1).

Interestingly, when Nasreen et al. (2022)[170] examined the prevalence rates of various diseases using the mean of incidence values from 2015 to 2019 and compared them with 2000, the first year of the pandemic in Ontario, there were no increases in the total incidence of myocarditis and pericarditis, and actually slight decreases of 15 and 2.5 percent, respectively. They also noted that the rates of Guillain-Barré syndrome also decreased by 28 percent and acute myocardial infarctions (heart attacks) by 11 percent. The authors ascribed the reduced myocarditis due to the effectiveness of lockdown measures and less influenza in 2020.

Another study by Singer et al. (2021) has been used to support the contention that the risk of myocarditis is substantially higher from COVID-19 than from COVID-19 vaccines for those under twenty years of age.[171] The authors used proprietary data for over sixty million people tracked by forty-eight US health-care organizations in aggregate to examine the general population of twelve- to nineteen-year-olds who were pre-screened to have had COVID-19. There were only six out of 6,846 reported COVID-19 cases (0.09 percent) for twelve- to seventeen-year-old males tracked from April 2020 to March 2021 who had symptomatic myocarditis, which is about a one in 1,141 rate. Apart from being a very low number of symptomatic myocarditis cases, it is clear that the total number of male teenagers in this age group in the database likely exceeded 1.5 million, which would indicate an infection rate of with SARS-CoV-2 of only around 0.45 percent, which is highly unlikely, and even the authors considered that about 9.2 percent of the twelve- to seventeen-year-olds were infected by this point. This and other dubious assumptions led the authors to suggest an adjusted rate for symptomatic myocarditis of forty-five per hundred thousand for males, and 21.3 per hundred thousand females following SARS-CoV-2 infection. Since about 99.5 percent of people with symptomatic myocarditis are typically admitted to a hospital, it is likely that total symptomatic myocarditis cases were captured in the study, but the number of SARS-CoV-2 infections was likely underestimated by more than ten times.

Yet another multicenter, retrospective study by Kamath et al. (2023) of the Hospital Corporation of America enterprise-wide database identified 8,162 patients eighteen years and older with SARS-CoV-2 infections from January 1, 2020 to May 14, 2020.[172] They reported that 929 (11.38 percent) of these patients met their diagnostic criteria for myocarditis, which was elevated blood troponin T (a marker of heart damage) and brain natriuretic peptide as proxies (as observed in other studies of COVID-19-induced myocarditis[173]). About 48 percent of the patients had European ethnicity, 26.3 percent had African ancestry and the rest were from other races, and most of them had pre-existing medical conditions, including over a quarter with heart disease. Of the COVID-19 patients with acute myocarditis, 37.9 percent required respiratory support via ventilation during their hospital stay and 29.8 percent died, compared to only 9 percent of COVID-19 patients without acute myocarditis that required ventilation and 5.8 percent that experienced in-hospital mortality.[174] These findings were similar to another earlier study that was performed with 187 patients with myocarditis in Wuhan, China from January 23, 2020 to February 23, 2020.[175] These studies indicate that COVID-19 can have very serious consequences for hospitalized patients with pre-existing conditions, but these rates of myocarditis with COVID-19 should not be taken as applicable to young, healthy individuals that become infected with SARS-CoV-2.

There have been very few studies that have accessed the incidence of myocarditis among otherwise healthy young adults who get COVID-19. For high performance athletes under twenty-four years who had COVID-19, the occurrence of clinical symptomatic myocarditis was shockingly estimated in one study to be about one in 177. This number was based on full testing with cardiac magnetic resonance imaging (MRI) of 1,597 COVID-19-recovered athletes (60.4 percent males) from thirteen US universities from March 1, 2020 through December 15, 2020 for myocarditis. Only nine participants were symptomatic for myocarditis, and another twenty-eight were subclinical and asymptomatic (twenty-seven of the thirty-eight were males).[176] Data on age and race were not collected, nor was the prevalence of myocarditis estimated in unvaccinated athletes who tested negative in serological tests for previous SARS-CoV-2 infection. The higher rates of COVID-19-associated myocarditis with this particular select group of athletes likely reflect the extreme physical exertions that come with practice from training and competition. It appeared that there were three times more asymptomatic myocarditis, but underlying heart damage was still evident based on cardiac MRI. It is reasonable that high performance athletes are much more likely to develop symptomatic myocarditis than the general public, as the intense exercise can precipitate symptomatic myocarditis. It is important to note that 2,461 athletes in this study were identified as COVID-19 cases based on PCR testing for SARS-CoV-2, but many asymptomatic individuals may not have been tested. Some nine thousand athletes would have been training in the thirteen universities at the time. A higher proportion of the athletes in the study were likely infected by the virus by the end of 2020, higher than 27 percent. Thus, the risks of SARS-CoV-2-induced myocarditis were likely lower than represented. These studies demonstrate that most people with asymptomatic myocarditis from SARS-CoV-2 infection are unaware of the damage to their hearts from the underlying inflammation. This would also be true with asymptomatic myocarditis and myopericarditis from COVID-19 vaccines.

It should be noted that myopericarditis is also a possible consequence of COVID-19. A study by Buckley et al. (2021) found that 1.5 percent of 718,365 COVID-19 patients developed new-onset myopericarditis.[177]

A significant advantage of these early studies is that COVID-19 vaccines were not yet available, so the impacts of vaccination on the rates of myocarditis and myopericarditis are not a confounding issue. However, previous exposure to SARS-CoV-2 might have a significant impact on COVID-19 vaccine-induced rates of myocarditis and myopericarditis. Furthermore, the Wuhan SARS-CoV-2 virus was more virulent than later variants that predominated, so this may have also reduced the risks of myocarditis and myopericarditis as the COVID-19 pandemic progressed.

Based on PCR testing alone, by April 26, 2023 over 104 million Americans had been infected with SARS-CoV-2.[178] Studies of serological testing for SARS-CoV-2 anti-nucleocapsid antibodies in Canada up to the same time indicate that at least 75 percent of Canadians had been infected with SARS-CoV-2,[179] and this is probably true for Americans as well. If the risks of myocarditis and myopericarditis from SARS-CoV-2 viral infections were as high as suggested in these earlier studies, then a much higher rate of these diseases would have been evident in North America and worldwide, which apparently has not transpired. One might suggest that this was circumvented due to the wide-spread adoption of COVID-19 vaccines. However, as will be evident in the next subsection, the COVID-19 vaccines have been linked to increased rates of myocarditis. For at least healthy men under thirty years of age, there is a greater risk of myocarditis and myopericarditis from these vaccines than from a SARS-CoV-2 infection.

13.8.3. Myocarditis and Myopericarditis from COVID-19 Vaccines

In the Phase 3 clinical studies with COVID-19 vaccines, the risks of myocarditis and pericarditis following inoculation were not readily apparent. Tracking for COVID-19 vaccine-induced adverse events in VAERS after the dissemination of these vaccines soon flagged this as a problem (see Table 13.1).[180] A very comprehensive study by Barda et al. (2021) was undertaken early on in Israel, which compared pathology from COVID-19 vaccine injury to that produced with COVID-19 from SARS-CoV-2 infection.[181] However, this study, which covered the first five months of the start of the vaccination program in Israel, reflected only up to a second dose of the Pfizer/BioNTech vaccine, and provided comparisons with the risks of COVID-19 injury associated with the Wuhan and earlier variants of COVID-19 that were more severe than from the Omicron variant. The most problematic aspect of this study, despite its comprehensive approach, is that it did not provide a breakdown of the risks by age group or sex. In this study, it was suggested that there was an overall risk of about one in forty-five thousand getting symptomatic myocarditis from the Pfizer/BioNTech vaccine for those over eighteen years of age, but this was still about 3.24-times higher than in the unvaccinated when all ages groups were aggregated.

Montag and Kampf (2022), following analysis of German hospitalized cases of myocarditis or pericarditis, noted that "in 2019 and 2020, there were no or only very few cases (<4) of myocarditis or pericarditis described as adverse events after any type of vaccination."[182] Of these, none of them required intensive-care treatment. In 2020, there were thirty-two hospitalized COVID-19 patients that had myocarditis or myopericarditis and fifteen of them needed intensive-care treatment. However, in 2021, the number of hospitalized myocarditis or pericarditis cases among juveniles (ten- to seventeen years old) more than doubled from 270 (2019) and 196 (2020) to 506 (2021). In total, only eleven cases (2.2 percent) were associated with SARS-CoV-2 infection, whereas 160 cases (31.6 percent) were associated with a COVID-19 vaccine or vaccination in general, and thirty-two of these cases required intensive-care treatment. Similar results were also described for young adults of eighteen to twenty-nine years of age.[183]

Block et al. (2022), using ICD-10-CM billing codes from US doctors filed between January 1, 2021 and January 31, 2022, estimated that the rate of post-vaccination myocarditis was 22.0 per 100,000 males aged twelve to seventeen years, but claimed that "the risk was 1.8–5.6-times as high after SARS-CoV-2 infection than after vaccination," which was estimated as 50.1–64.9 cases per hundred thousand after infection.[184] However, these data were based only on electronic health records and did not include SARS-CoV-2 test results and mRNA COVID-19 vaccinations that were performed in homes, schools, community sites, or pharmacies, and the electronic health records covered only

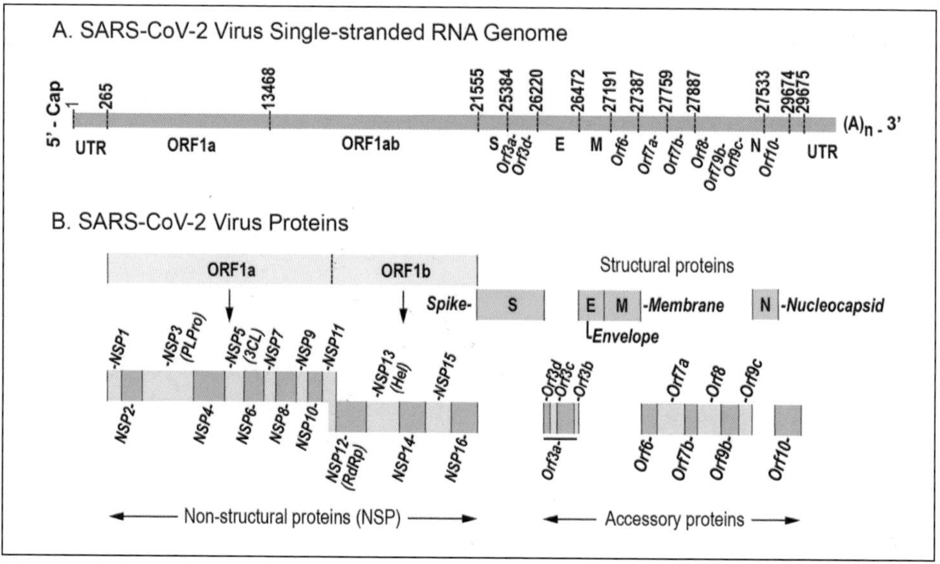

Figure 5.1. Location of protein-encoding genes in SARS-CoV-2 genome (A) and the proteins that they encode (B). Of particular relevance are the Spike (S), Membrane (M), Envelope (E) and Nucleocapsid (N) proteins, which are found in the final virus particle along with a single strand of viral RNA. Adapted from Figure 2 of Tali et al. (2021)[1] and Figure 1 of Yadav et al. (2021).[2] UTR corresponds the untranslated regions of the viral genome, which do not encode viral proteins. At the 3 prime end of the RNA is a poly-adenine tail (An), which may be thirty to sixty nucleotides long. When produced, the ORF1a and ORF1b proteins are further processed by partial proteolysis to generate sixteen non-structural proteins (NSP), which play various roles in the replication of the virus inside of host cells.

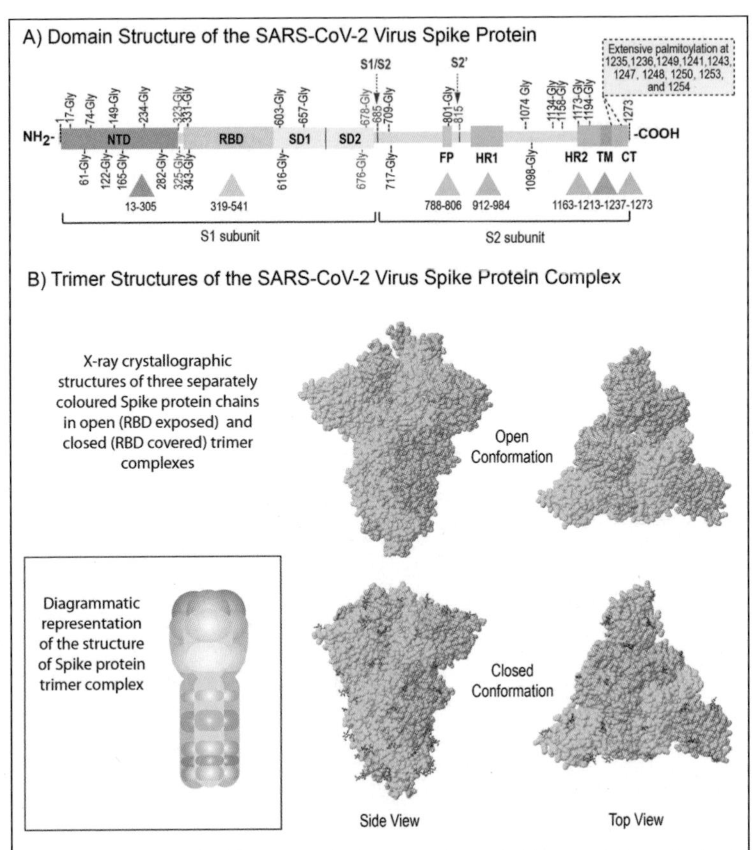

Figure 5.2. Domain structure of the SARS-CoV-2 spike protein (A) and its trimer complex structures (B). Adapted from Huang et al. (2020)[3] and Zhao et al. (2021).[4] Like other coronaviruses, SARS-CoV-2 binds to host cells via its spike protein, which has an affinity for ACE2. The RBD (receptor binding domain) region is critical for binding to ACE2. A protease cleavage site (S1/S2), not found in other betacoronaviruses (like SARS-CoV and MERS-CoV), and targeted by common human proteases including furin and TMPRSS2, increases the infectivity of SARS-CoV-2. The N-terminus domain (NTD) is the first part of the protein that is made during protein synthesis by the ribosomes, and the C-terminus domain (CT) is the last part that is made. Just before the CT is the transmembrane domain (TM), which is a hydrophobic patch of about seventeen amino acid residues in length, which anchors the spike protein into the lipid membrane that envelopes the virus. The C-terminus also features covalently-bound fatty acid side chains (i.e., it is heavily palmitoylated), which further strongly affixes the spike protein complex to lipid membranes.[5] The locations of glycan groups that are also attached to the spike protein are also shown.[6] The spike protein is extensively glycosylated (Gly) at about twenty-six sites: twenty-two glycans are N-linked to asparagine amino acid residues (black) and four glycans are O-linked to threonine amino acid residues (purple). The Fusion Peptide (FP) mediates the fusion of the virus particle with the plasma membrane of the host cell. HR1 and HR2 correspond to heptad repeat domains, which also participate in membrane fusion. The front end of proteins is called the N-terminus, because it usually features a free amino (NH_2) group, and the back end of proteins is known as the C-terminus, because it usually has a carboxyl (COOH) group. The N-terminus features thirteen amino acids that serve as a signal peptide for membrane insertion. Amino acid numbering is based on the UniProt P0DTC2 entry for SARS-CoV-2. The X-ray crystallographic structures from the Research Collaboratory for Structural Bioinformatics (RCSB) Protein Data Base (PDB) of the SARS-CoV-2 spike trimer in open (RBD up) and closed (RBD down) conformations are from PDB files 7DDN and 7DF3, respectively.

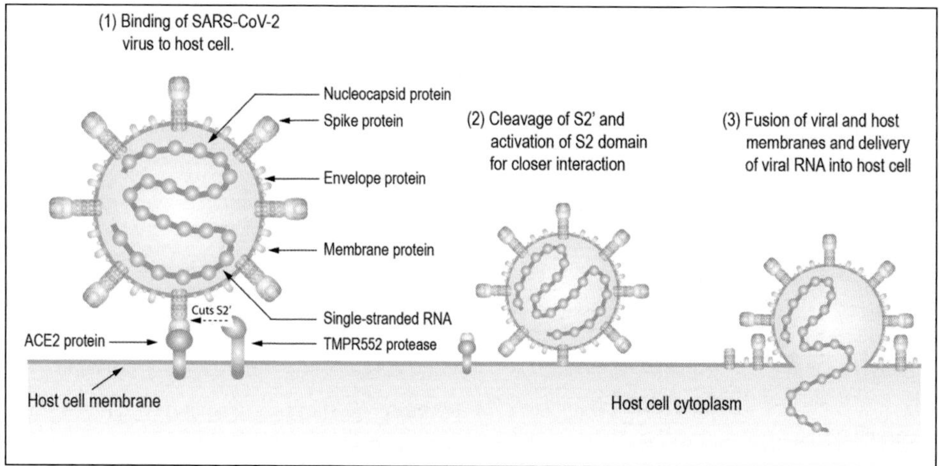

Figure 5.3. Binding and internalization of the SARS-CoV-2 to host cells. The TMPRSS2 cleaves the spike protein into S1 and S2 subunits and facilitates the fusion of membranes of the virus and host cell to permit the entry of the viral genome into the host cell. Based in part on Figure 1 from Lamers and Haagmans (2022).[7]

Variant	311	321	331	341	351	361
Wuhan	GIYQTSNFRV	QPTESIVRFP	NITNLCPFGE	VFNATRFASV	YAW**N**RKRISN	CVADYSVLYN
Alpha/B.1.1.7	----------	----------	----------	----------	----------	----------
Beta/B.1.351	----------	----------	----------	----------	----------	----------
Gamma/P.1	----------	----------	----------	----------	----------	----------
Delta/B.1.617.2	----------	----------	----------	----------	----------	----------
Lambda/C.37	----------	----------	----------	----------	----------	----------
Omicron/BA.1.1.529	----------	----------	--------D-	----------	----------	----------
Omicron/XBB.1.5	----------	----------	--------H-	-----T----	----------	-------I--
Eris/EG.5.1	----------	----------	--------H-	-----T----	----------	-------I--
	371	381	391	401	411	421
Wuhan	SASFSTFKCY	GVSPTKLNDL	CFTNVYADSF	VIRGDEVRQI	APGQTG**K**IAD	YNYKLPDDFT
Alpha/B.1.1.7	----------	----------	----------	----------	----------	----------
Beta/B.1.351	----------	----------	----------	----------	------N---	----------
Gamma/P.1	----------	----------	----------	----------	------T---	----------
Delta/B.1.617.2	----------	----------	----------	----------	----------	----------
Lambda/C.37	----------	----------	----------	----------	----------	----------
Omicron/BA.1.1.529	L-P-F-----	----------	----------	----------	------N---	----------
Omicron/XBB.1.5	F-P-F-----	----------	----------	----N--S--	------N---	----------
Eris/EG.5.1	F-P-FA----	----------	----------	----N--S--	------N---	----------
	431	441	451	461	471	481
Wuhan	GCVIAWNS**N**N	LDS**K**VGGN**Y**N	Y**L**YR**LF**RK**S**N	LKPFERDIS**T**	EI**YQA**GSTPC	NGV**E**G**FN**CY**F**
Alpha/B.1.1.7	----------	----------	----------	----------	----------	----------
Beta/B.1.351	----------	----------	----------	----------	----------	---K------
Gamma/P.1	----------	----------	----------	----------	----------	---K------
Delta/B.1.617.2	----------	----------	-R--------	----------	-------K--	---Q------
Lambda/C.37	----------	----------	-Q--------	----------	----------	---------S
Omicron/BA.1.1.529	---------K	-----S----	----------	----------	------NK--	---A------
Omicron/XBB.1.5	---------K	----PS----	---------K	----------	------NK--	---A-S---S
Eris/EG.5.1	---------K	----PS----	-----L---K	----------	------NK--	---A-P---S
	491	501	511	521	531	541
Wuhan	PL**Q**SYGF**QP**T	**N**GVGYQPYRV	VVLSFELLHA	PATVCGPKKS	TNLVKNKCVN	FNFNGLTGTG
Alpha/B.1.1.7	----------	Y---------	----------	----------	----------	----------
Beta/B.1.351	----------	Y---------	----------	----------	----------	----------
Gamma/P.1	----------	Y---------	----------	----------	----------	----------
Delta/B.1.617.2	----------	----------	----------	----------	----------	----------
Lambda/C.37	----------	----------	----------	----------	----------	----------
Omicron/BA.1.1.529	--K--S-R--	Y---H-----	----------	----------	----------	------K---
Omicron/XBB.1.5	--R--S-R--	Y---H----	----------	----------	----------	------K---
Eris/EG.5.1	--R--S-R--	Y---H-----	----------	----------	----------	------K---
	551	561	571	581	591	601
Wuhan	VLTESNKKFL	PFQQFGRDIA	DTTDAVRDPQ	TLEILDITPC	SFGGVSVITP	GTNTSNQVAV
Alpha/B.1.1.7	----------	---------D	----------	----------	----------	----------
Beta/B.1.351	----------	----------	----------	----------	----------	----------
Gamma/P.1	----------	----------	----------	----------	----------	----------
Delta/B.1.617.2	----------	----------	----------	----------	----------	----------
Lambda/C.37	----------	----------	----------	----------	----------	----------
Omicron/BA.1.1.529	----------	----------	----------	----------	----------	----------
Omicron/XBB.1.5	----------	----------	----------	----------	----------	----------
Eris/EG.5.1	----------	----------	----------	----------	----------	----------
	611	621	631	641	651	661
Wuhan	LYQDVNCTEV	PVAIHADQLT	PTWRVYSTGS	NVFQTRAGCL	IGAEHVNNSY	ECDIPIGAGI
Alpha/B.1.1.7	---G------	----------	----------	----------	----------	----------
Beta/B.1.351	---G------	----------	----------	----------	----------	----------
Gamma/P.1	---G------	----------	----------	----------	----Y-----	----------
Delta/B.1.617.2	---G------	----------	----------	----------	----------	----------
Lambda/C.37	---G------	----------	----------	----------	----------	----------
Omicron/BA.1.1.529	---G------	----------	----------	----------	----Y-----	----------
Omicron/XBB.1.5	----------	----------	----------	----------	----Y-----	----------
Eris/EG.5.1	----------	----------	----------	----------	----Y-----	----------

Figure 5.4. Location of mutations in the receptor binding domain region of the SARS-CoV-2 spike protein encoded by variants of concern. The original Wuhan sequence (UniProt ID P0DTC2) is provided with the single letter amino acid codes for each of twenty possible amino acids from residues 311 to 591, which encompasses the receptor binding domain that interacts with the ACE2 protein on host cells. Those amino acids that are known to be important for direct binding to ACE2 are bolded and underlined. Identical amino acids in the VOC are shown with dashes, and substituted amino acid residues are indicated. It is evident that many of the mutations are shared between the VOC, and they often occur at amino acid positions that are known to be critical for binding to ACE2.

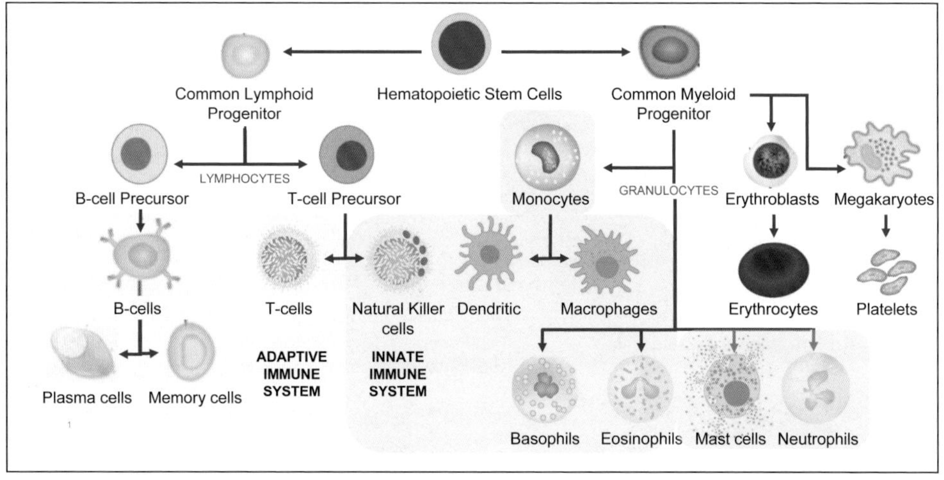

Figure 7.1. Cells of the hematopoietic system.

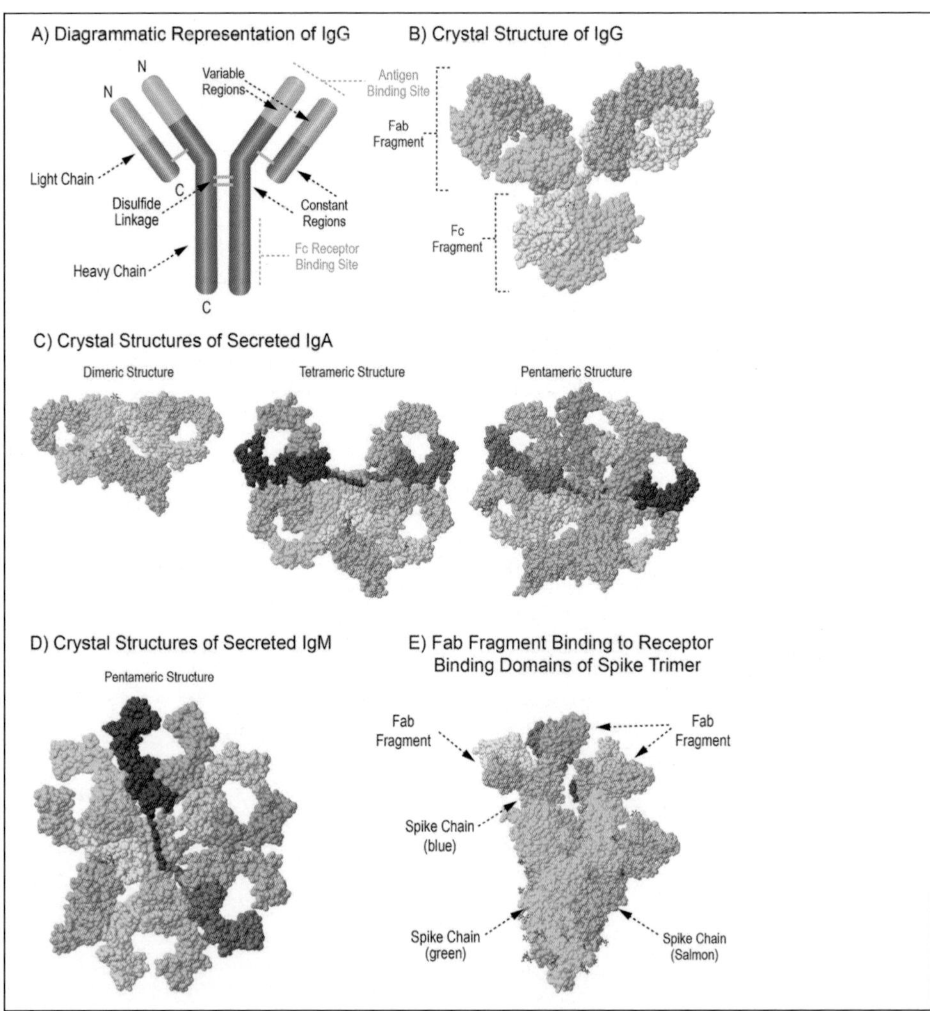

Figure 7.2. Structures of Immunoglobulins. For visualization purposes, the light and heavy chains of the immunoglobulins are shown in different colors as space-filling representations of atoms on each of these macromolecules.

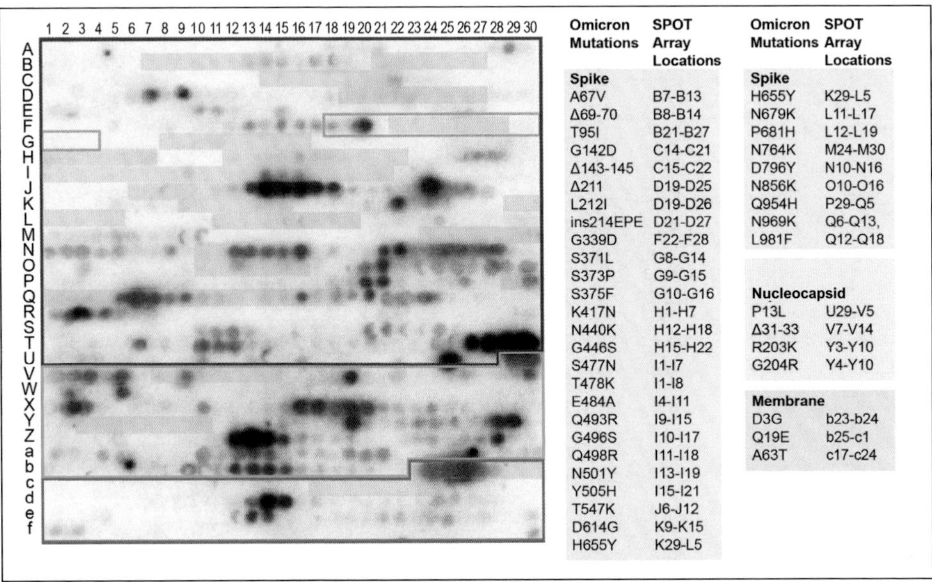

Figure 8.1. Kinexus CDH/CDR SARS-CoV-2 SPOT array overlay of nine images of separate serum sample results from different participants who recovered from COVID-19. Short overlapping peptides that cover the entire structures of the spike (upper outlined section), nucleocapsid (middle outlined section), and membrane (lower outlined section) proteins of the Wuhan strain were produced on arrays that were probed with serum samples that contained antibodies from confirmed COVID-19 cases. Peptides from the RBD of the spike protein are dash outlined.

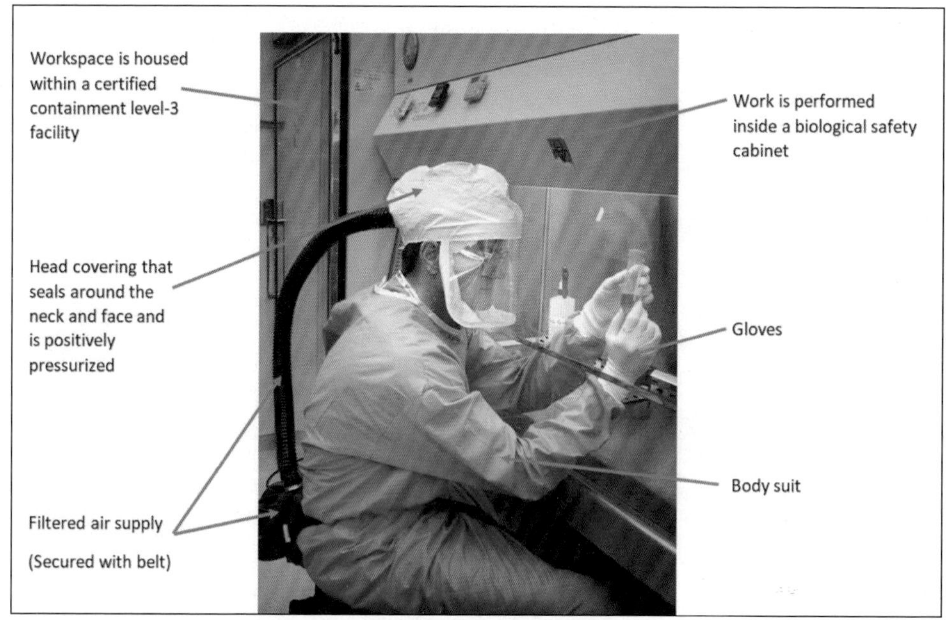

Figure 9.1. Personal protective equipment required to safely work with BSL3 pathogens such as SARS-CoV-2. Image sourced from Wikipedia.[8]

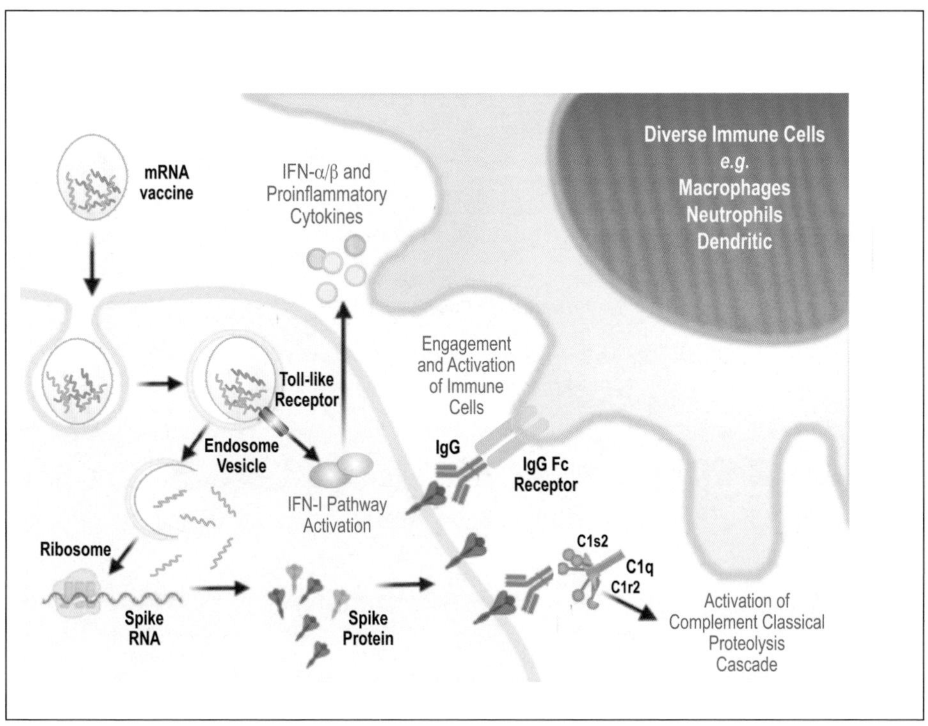

Figure 11.1. Early mechanisms of RNA vaccine action. Toll-like receptors (TLR) sense non-natural lipids present in the lipid nanoparticles and induce the release of cytokines that recruit immune cells to the site of the transfected host cell. Existing anti-spike antibodies may react with the produced spike protein that is expressed on the surface of the lipid nanoparticle-transfected host cell. Innate immune cells that express a receptor (IgG Fc receptor) that recognize the common portion (Fc) of the IgG class antibodies allows the immune cells to attach to the transfected host cell. Not illustrated in this figure is the subsequent attack and generation of small pieces of the host cell within exosomes. These exosomes are coated by spike protein (along with other host cell proteins) and are engulfed and digested by the innate immune cells. Exosomes are a known result of transfection with gene therapy products and are normally assessed for potential excretion into the environment under gene therapy regulations. Fragments of the spike protein that are generated in the innate immune cells are presented with major histocompatibility antigens (MHCs) by these cells to T-cells and B-cells in lymph nodes and other locations where these adaptive immune cells reside. In addition, antibody-bound spike proteins on host cells recruit the activation of proteins of the complement system, leading to formation of holes and destruction of the host cell.

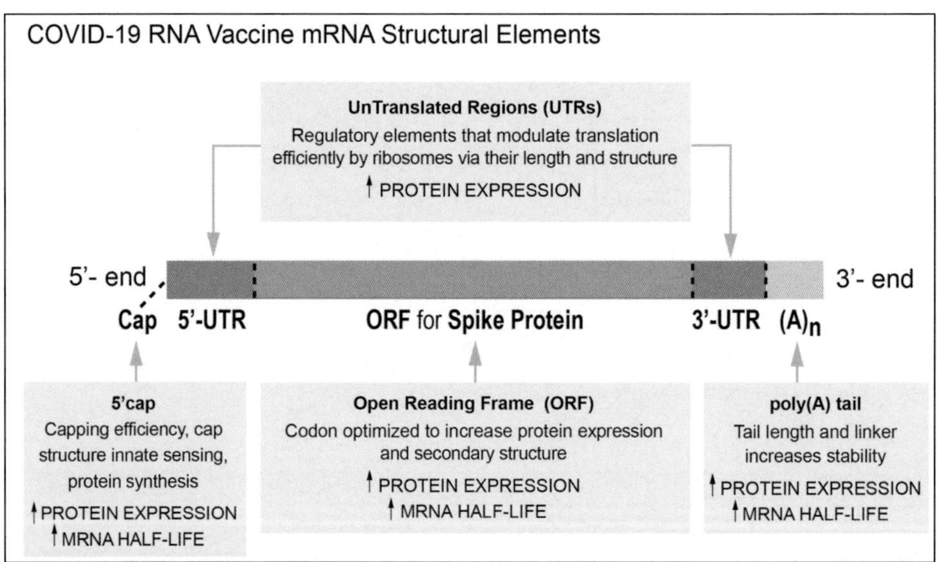

Figure 11.2. mRNA structural elements that control the structure and stability of mRNA and the protein product.[9] In the cases of the Pfizer/BioNTech and Moderna COVID-19 mRNA vaccines, codon optimization involves use of codon triplicates that favor use of guanidine and cytidine nucleotide bases (but still specify the correct amino acids), replacement of uridine bases with 1-N-methyl-pseudouridine (m1Ψ), and the mutation of Lysine-986 and Valine-987 to Proline-986 and Proline-987, which stabilizes the conformation of the spike protein in a pre-fusion state and has been shown to improve the induction of neutralizing antibodies.

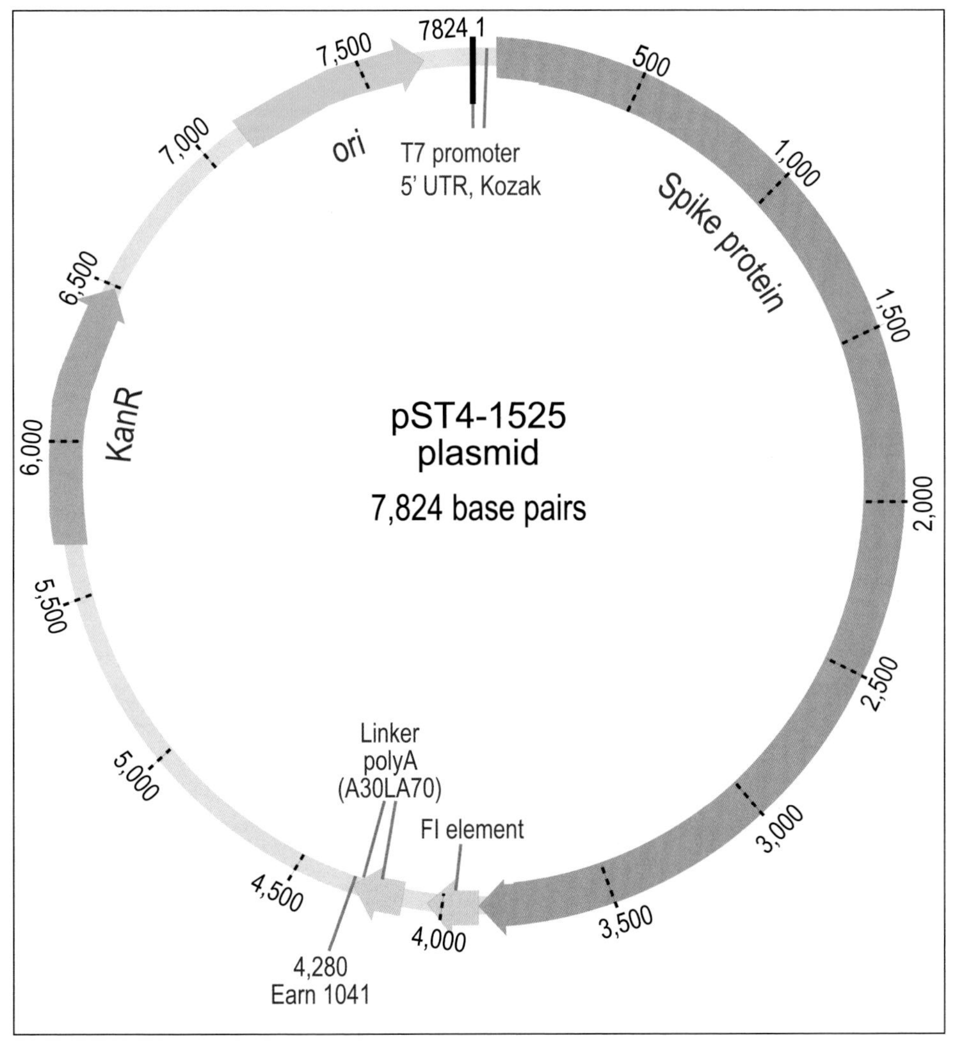

Figure 11.3. pST4-1525 plasmid map. Adapted from Josephson et al. (2020)[10]

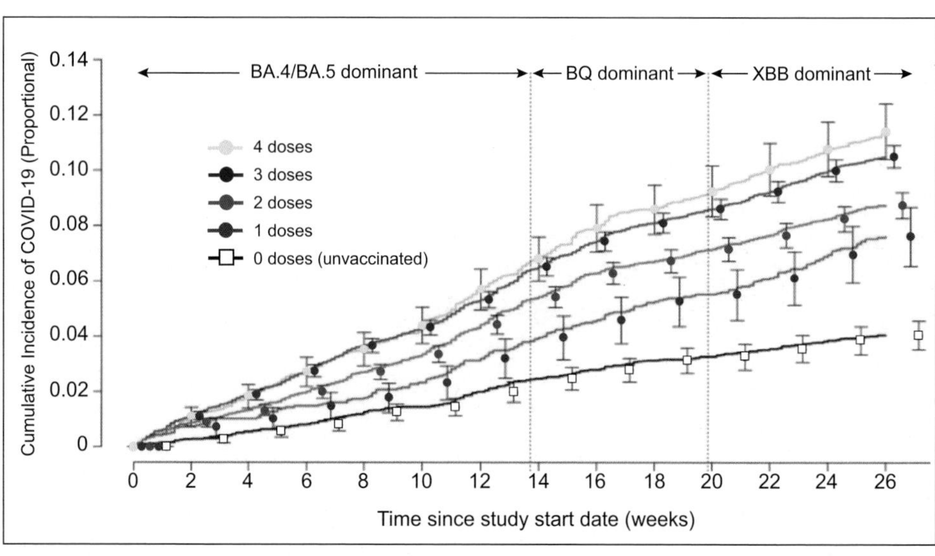

Figure 12.1. Cumulative incidence of COVID-19 disease for Cleveland Clinic study participants stratified by the number of COVID-19 vaccine doses previously received. Day Zero was September 12, 2022, the date the bivalent Wuhan/Omicron BA.4/5 vaccine was first offered to employees. Point estimates and 95 percent confidence intervals are jittered along the x-axis to improve visibility. Adapted from Figure 2 of Shrestha et al. (2023).[11]

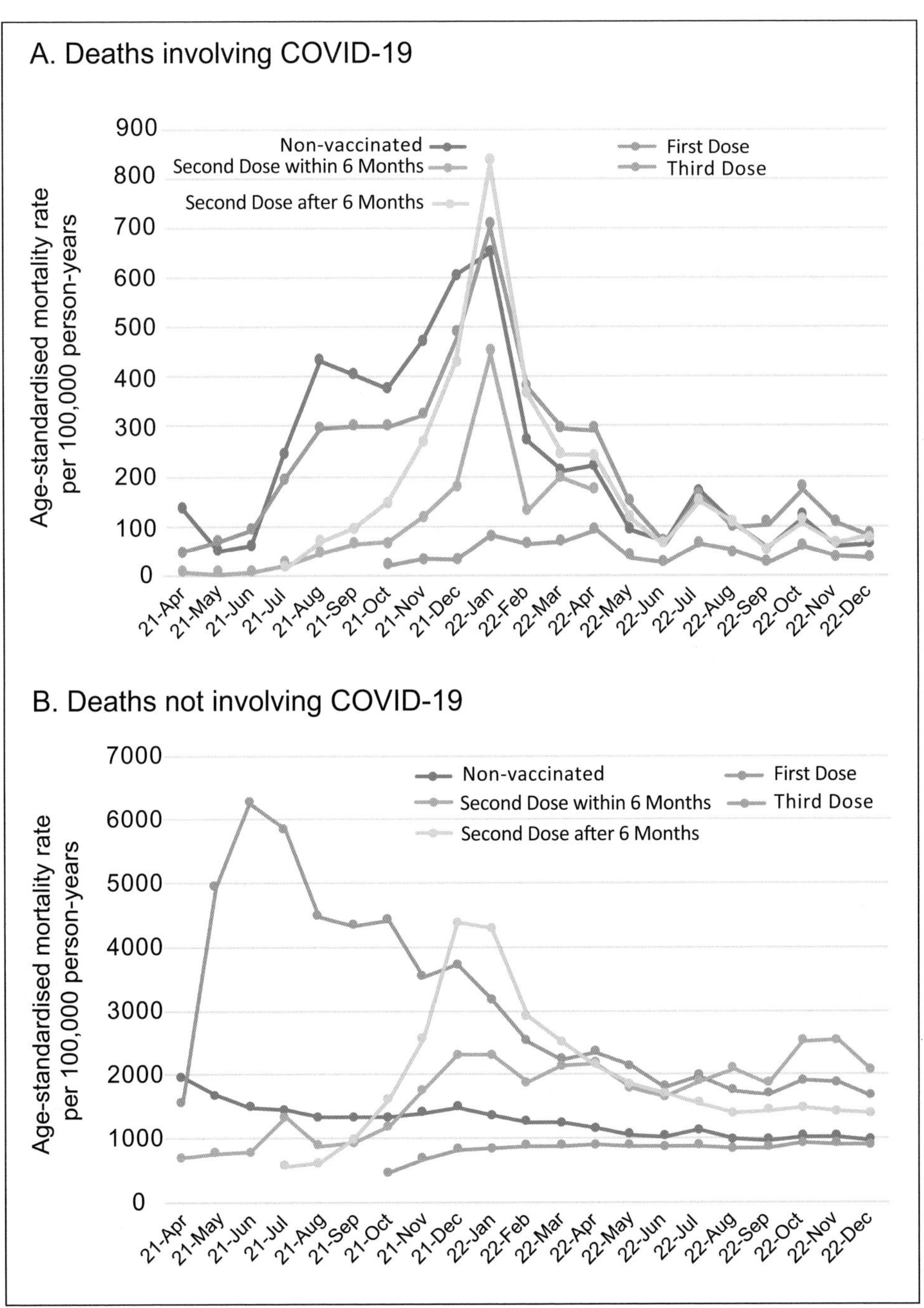

Figure 13.1. England monthly all-cause and COVID-19 mortality rates from April 1, 2021 to December 31, 2022 as a function of COVID-19 vaccine status.[12]

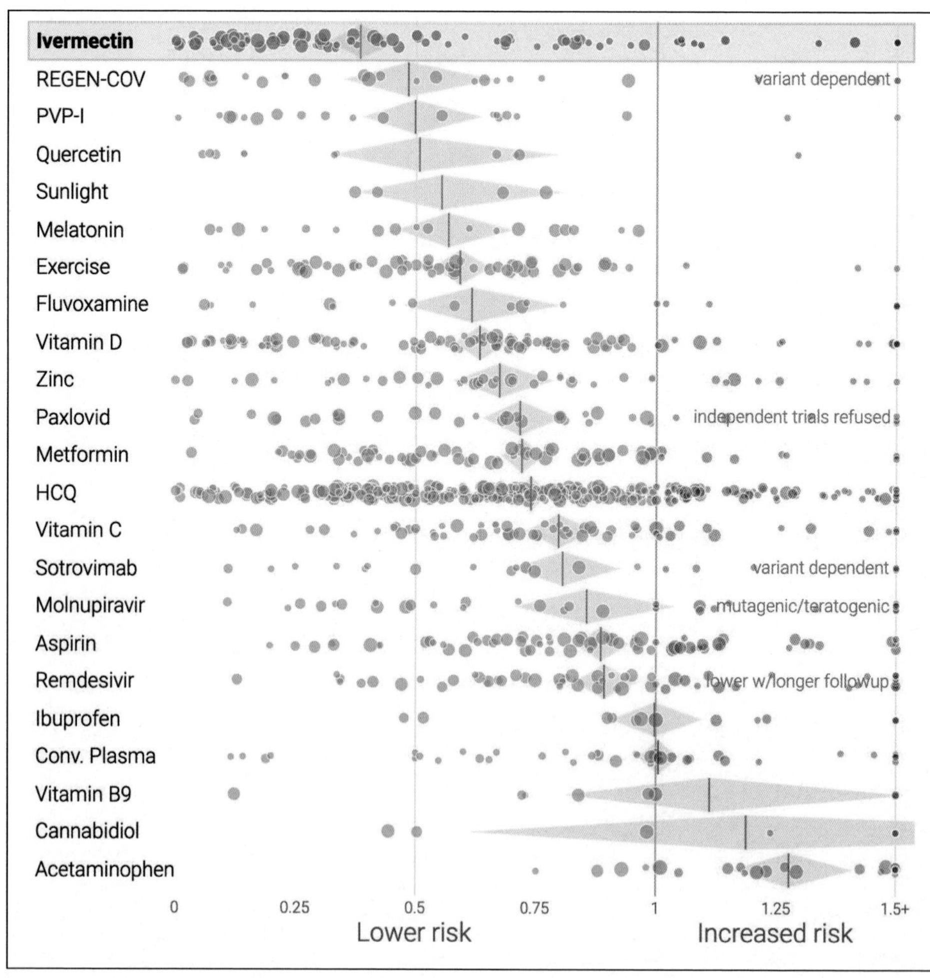

Figure 14.1. Efficacy in COVID-19 studies (pooled effects). Scatter plot showing the most serious outcome in all studies in the context of multiple COVID-19 treatments. Diamonds show the results of random effects meta-analysis for each treatment.[13]

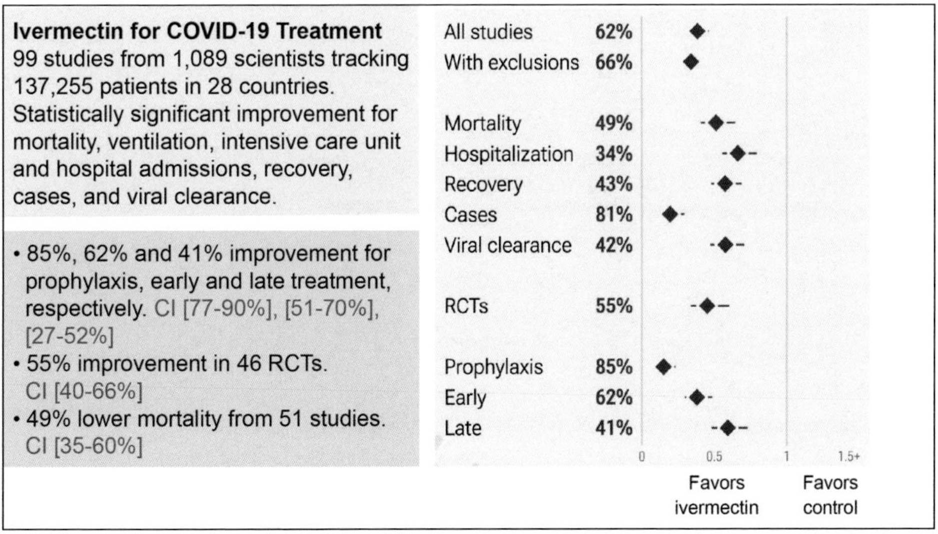

Ivermectin for COVID-19 Treatment
99 studies from 1,089 scientists tracking 137,255 patients in 28 countries.
Statistically significant improvement for mortality, ventilation, intensive care unit and hospital admissions, recovery, cases, and viral clearance.

- 85%, 62% and 41% improvement for prophylaxis, early and late treatment, respectively. CI [77-90%], [51-70%], [27-52%]
- 55% improvement in 46 RCTs. CI [40-66%]
- 49% lower mortality from 51 studies. CI [35-60%]

All studies	62%
With exclusions	66%
Mortality	49%
Hospitalization	34%
Recovery	43%
Cases	81%
Viral clearance	42%
RCTs	55%
Prophylaxis	85%
Early	62%
Late	41%

0 0.5 1 1.5+

Favors ivermectin Favors control

Figure 14.2. Meta-analyses of IVM effectiveness for COVID-19. From https://c19ivm.org/; reproduced under Creative Commons license. Retrieved December 7, 2023.

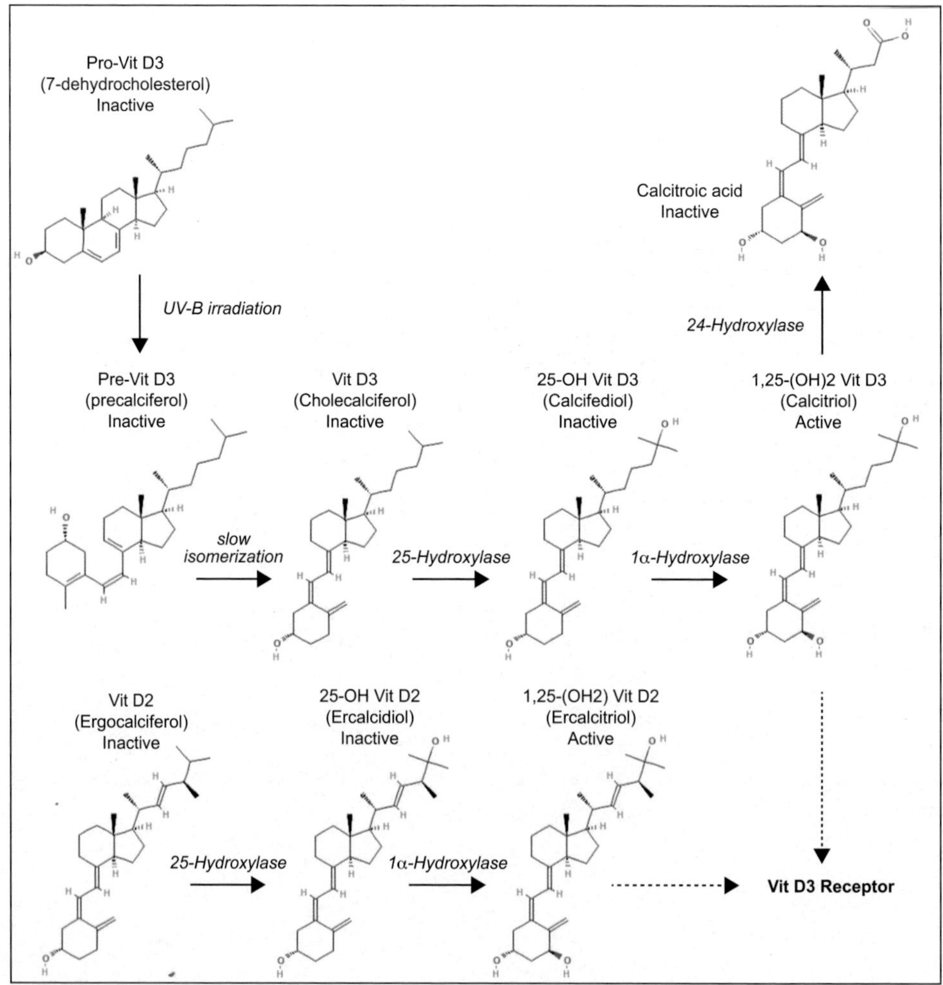

Figure 14.3. Vitamin D2 and Vitamin D3 metabolism. Chemical structures were sourced from PubChem.[14]

28 percent of vaccinees, when 82 percent of the population five years and older was estimated to be vaccinated. Nevertheless, the actual number of people that were likely infected with SARS-CoV-2 by this time was likely at least ten-times higher than based on PCR test results. These diagnostic records were also not confirmed by chart review and were subject to misclassification.

In a meta-analysis of twenty-two published studies following administration of 405 million doses of COVID-19 vaccines, Li et al. (2022) concluded that "there was no statistically significant difference in the overall incidence of myocarditis or pericarditis between those with COVID-19 vaccination and those without. It was also found that the risk of myocarditis was higher with mRNA-based vaccines as compared to non-mRNA vaccines as well as the second vaccination dose posing a higher risk for myocarditis than the first-time doses."[185] The authors also noted that in seven studies of adolescents aged twelve- to nineteen years old, 111 of 1,008,753 (i.e., one in 9,088 or eleven in a hundred thousand) vaccinated youth developed symptomatic myocarditis or myopericarditis, with females in this age group being about 13.9-fold less likely to be afflicted with these diseases. These increased risks of symptomatic myocarditis or myopericarditis with the Pfizer/BioNTech BNT162b2, Moderna mRNA-1273, and AstraZeneca ChAdOx1 COVID-19 vaccines were further confirmed in the recent Global Vaccine Data Network study of 99 million vaccinated individuals in eight countries.[186]

It is now generally recognized that the incidence of symptomatic myocarditis in males who are twelve to twenty-nine years of age with the second shot of the BNT162b2 vaccine ranges from one in five thousand to one in fifteen thousand, depending on the study (Table 13.3). For Moderna's mRNA-1273, with this demographic, the risk of myocarditis is even higher, at around one in 4,400.[187] Similar risks are observed with symptomatic myopericarditis in male adolescents and young adults. When the risks of either symptomatic myocarditis or myopericarditis are considered together, the chances of acquiring one of these diseases becomes even greater, as high as one in 704 with BNT162b2 and one in 264 for sixteen to twenty-four-year-old males following a second dose in one Nordic study.[188] By contrast, in these same studies, there were no recorded female cases with symptomatic myocarditis or myopericarditis (i.e., no measurable risk). However, in most studies with twelve- to thirty-nine-year-olds, the risks of these diseases in young females can be calculated from Table 13.3 to be about 6.2-fold lower on average than in their male counterparts. The reasons for the predominance in myocarditis and myopericarditis in men is not known, but may relate to sex hormone differences in the immune response and myocarditis, and possibly the under diagnosis of cardiac disease in women.

The incidence of myocarditis and myopericarditis following a third dose of BNT162b2 continued to be high in males under thirty years of age according to a study conducted in British Columbia by Naveed et al. (2020) and was further increased for older men in the thirty- to forty-nine-year-old age bracket.[189] For example, with the booster dose of BNT162b2 in men between forty and forty-nine years of age, the incidence of symptomatic myocarditis was one in 3,922. For males under sixty-nine, there was also a trend toward increased myopericarditis with the third dose of BNT162b2, and in the twelve- to seventeen-year-old males, the risk of myopericarditis increased to one in 4,024 compared to one in 6,281 with the second dose. With Moderna's mRNA-1273, there were no data provided in the Naveed et al. study for twelve to seventeen-year-olds, although after the second dose the risk for either myocarditis or myopericarditis was high at around one in 1900 for males that were eighteen to twenty-nine years of age. However, further increases in the rates of myocarditis and myopericarditis were not evident with the mRNA-1273 booster and were lower than seen following the second dose. This may have been in part because fewer people took a third shot of this mRNA vaccine after the stronger adverse effects experienced with earlier inoculations discouraged them. However, in the larger Global Vaccine Data Network study, the risk of symptomatic myocarditis was found to be further increased with a third dose of mRNA-1273 as well as BNT162b2 and ChAdOx1.[190] In an examination of the Permanente Northwest Health Plan with male and female members aged eighteen to thirty-nine years in the United States, Sharff et al. (2022) recorded four males and two females with symptomatic myopericarditis.[191] In the case of the males in the study, the incidence of symptomatic myopericarditis with the BNT162b2 booster worked out to one in 6,800.

Table 13.3. Rates of COVID-19 vaccine-induced myocarditis and myopericarditis in people under forty years after a second dose of the same COVID-19 vaccine.

Vaccine	Disease	Incidence per 100,000	Incidence/ Vaccinated Study Participants	Demographic	Country	Study Period	Reference
Pfizer/ BioNTech -BNT162b2	Myocarditis	6.73	9/133,633	Males, 12–17 years	Canada, BC	December 15, 2020 to March 10, 2022	Naveed et al. (2022)[192]
		1.53	2/130,628	Females, 12–17 years			
Moderna -mRNA-1273	Myocarditis	22,97	25/108,820	Males, 18–29 years	Canada, BC	December 15, 2020 to March 10, 2022	Naveed et al. (2022)[193]
		2	2/99,895	Females, 18–29 years			
Pfizer/ BioNTech -BNT162b2	Myopericarditis	9	12/133,633	Males, 12–17 years	Canada, BC	December 15, 2020 to March 10, 2022	Naveed et al. (2022)[194]
		3.1	4/130,628	Females, 12–17 years			

Vaccine	Disease	Incidence per 100,000	Incidence/ Vaccinated Study Participants	Demographic	Country	Study Period	Reference
Moderna -mRNA-1273	Myopericarditis	32.2	35/108,820	Males, 18–29 years	Canada, BC	December 15, 2020 to March 10, 2022	Naveed et al. (2022)[195]
		5	5/99,895	Females, 18–29 years			
Pfizer/ BioNTech -BNT162b2	Myocarditis	5.24	6/114,450*	Males, 20–51 years (median 25)	United States Military	January to April, 2021	Montgomery et al. (2021)[196]
		0	0/28,350*	Females, 20–51 years (median 25)			
Moderna -mRNA-1273	Myocarditis	4.35	14/321,550*	Males, 20–51 years (median 25)	United States Military	January to April, 2021	Montgomery et al. (2021)[197]
		0	0/79,650*	Females, 20–51 years (median 25)			
Pfizer/ BioNTech -BNT162b2	Myocarditis and myopericarditis	19.31	44/?	Mixed, 12–39 years	United States	December 2020 to October 9, 2021	Klein (2021)[198]
Moderna -mRNA-1273	Myocarditis and myopericarditis	37.51	22/?	Mixed, 18–39 years	United States	December 2020 to October 9, 2021	Klein (2021)[199]
Pfizer/ BioNTech -BNT162b2	Myocarditis and myopericarditis	11.65	56/480,407	Males, 18–25 years	United States	December 18, 2020, to December 25, 2021	Wong et al. (2022)[200]
		3.49	20/572,330	Females, 18–25 years			
Moderna -mRNA-1273	Myocarditis and myopericarditis	14.20	34/239,420	Males, 18–25 years	United States	December 18, 2020, to December 25, 2021	Wong et al. (2022)[201]
		2.84	8/282,057	Females, 18–25 years			
Pfizer/ BioNTech -BNT162b2	Myocarditis and myopericarditis	1.70	60/3,535,806	Males, 13–39 years	England	December 1 2020, to December 15, 2021	Patone et al. (2022)[202]
		0.22	9/4,131,123	Females, 13–39 years			
Moderna -mRNA-1273	Myocarditis and myopericarditis	102.60	36/35,074	Males, 13–39 years	England	December 1 2020, to December 15, 2021	Patone et al. (2022)[203]
		0	0/328,311	Females, 13–39 years			
AstraZeneca -ChAdOx1	Myocarditis and pericarditis	2.21	21/949,865	Males, 13–39 years	England	December 1 2020, to December 15, 2021	Patone et al. (2022)[204]
		0	0/1,437,517	Females, 13–39 years			
Pfizer/ BioNTech -BNT162b2	Myocarditis and myopericarditis	9.42	48/509,590	Mixed, 12–39 years	Denmark	October 1, 2020 to October 5, 2021	Husby et al. (2021)[205]
Moderna -mRNA-1273	Myocarditis and myopericarditis	28.21	21/74,441	Mixed, 12–39 years	Denmark	October 1, 2020 to October 5, 2021	Husby et al. (2021)[206]
Pfizer/ BioNTech -BNT162b2	Myopericarditis	9.74	13/133,477	Males, 12–17 years	Denmark	May 15 to September 15, 2021	Nygaard et al. (2022)[207]
		1.56	2/127,857	Females, 12–17 years			

Vaccine	Disease	Incidence per 100,000	Incidence/ Vaccinated Study Participants	Demographic	Country	Study Period	Reference
Pfizer/ BioNTech -BNT162b2	Myocarditis and myopericarditis	142	59/?	Males, 16–24 years	Denmark, Finland, Norway, Sweden	December 27, 2020 to October 5, 2021	Karlstad et al. (2022)[208]
		0	0/?	Females, 16–24 years			
Moderna -mRNA-1273	Myocarditis and myopericarditis	379	22/?	Males, 16–24 years	Denmark, Finland, Norway, Sweden	December 27, 2020 to October 5, 2021	Karlstad et al. (2022)[209]
		0	0/?	Females, 16–24 years			
Pfizer/ BioNTech -BNT162b2	Myocarditis	8.68	8/92,200	Males, 16–29 years	Israel	June 2 to November 30, 2021	Witberg et al. (2022)[210]
		1.08	1/90,405	Females, 16–29 years			
Pfizer/ BioNTech -BNT162b2	Myocarditis and myopericarditis	13.23	58/438,511	Males, 16–24 years	Israel	December 20, 2020 to May, 2021	Mevorach et al. (2021)[211]
		1.85	8/431,666	Females, 16–24 years			
Pfizer/ BioNTech -BNT162b2	Myocarditis	20.94	38/181,392	Males, 12–17 years	Hong Kong	March 10 to October 18, 2021	Li et al. (2022)[212]
		2.82	5/177,405	Females, 12–17 years			
Pfizer/ BioNTech -BNT162b2	Myocarditis and myopericarditis	4.3	19/442,025	Mixed, 16–18 years	South Korea	July 19 to October 2021	June Choe et al. (2022)[213]

*Exact numbers of military personnel vaccinated with the Moderna and Pfizer/BioNTech vaccines were not provided. However, it was reported that the US Army initially procured 5.9 million doses from Moderna and 2.1 million doses from Pfizer.[214] This ratio was applied to the total numbers of males (436,000) and females (108,000) that were vaccinated to calculate the myocarditis rates.

A small study by Levi et al. (2023) with 324 healthcare workers (59 percent female, median age of fifty-two years) in Israel with a fourth dose of BNT162b2 was undertaken to evaluate whether there was an increased risk of myocarditis with further vaccine boosting.[215] The authors reported that two of the participants had acute vaccine-related myocardial injury, a female who had mild symptoms and the other a male who was asymptomatic. Despite high cardiac troponin levels in their blood, myocarditis was ruled out in both cases. About 41 percent of the participants had some sort of vaccine-adverse reaction, most commonly injection-site local pain, muscle aches and pains, and fatigue. A particularly interesting observation in this study was the elevated levels of troponin in 6.5 percent of the subjects just prior to receiving their fourth vaccine dose, which might be evidence of prior heart damage.

As discussed in the previous subsection, the risk of myocarditis from a SARS-CoV-2 infection by age is much higher in elderly people who are known to also have more severe COVID-19 than younger people. Consequently, the risk to benefit ratio with COVID-19 vaccination versus SARS-CoV-2 infection when it comes to myocarditis and myopericarditis is very different when based on age, sex, and pre-existing morbidities. Yet, almost categorically in these studies, the authors still advocated that everyone should be vaccinated against COVID-19 due to higher risks associated with a SARS-CoV-2 infection, even with the emergence of more benign variants of SARS-CoV-2, such as the Omicron variants that have predominated since December 2021.

As seen with SARS-CoV-2-induced myocarditis, it should be appreciated that risks of undiagnosed asymptomatic myocarditis or myopericarditis would be expected to be much higher in adolescent and younger males, especially since they would normally have a long life before them. The prevalence of asymptomatic myocarditis or myopericarditis was never assessed in any of the clinical studies with COVID-19 vaccines and not quantified in any of the aforementioned studies. However, it was carefully investigated by Mansanguan et al. (2022) in a study of 301 teenagers of thirteen to eighteen years of age in Thailand following their receipt of a second dose of the Pfizer/BioNtech BNT162b2 vaccine.[216] Cardiovascular effects were found in 29.24 percent of the teenagers, ranging from tachycardia, palpitation, and myopericarditis. Of the 201 males, four had evidence of asymptomatic myocarditis, one had myopericarditis, and two had pericarditis for a rate of one in twenty-nine. This involved active monitoring of heart abnormalities, including presence of heart proteins such as troponin in the blood, cardiac MRI, electrocardiogram measurements, and physical examinations. Such a 3.4 percent risk of myocarditis or myopericarditis in adolescent teens following a second COVID-19 mRNA vaccination is about seventy-five-times the risk associated with a SARS-CoV-2 infection in the same age group (i.e., 0.045 percent).[217]

In light of the relatively high frequency of risk for myocarditis and myopericarditis among younger males following COVID-19 vaccination, the question arises whether or not this is serious and potentially lethal. Kracalik et al. (2022) analyzed 519 US individuals (88 percent male) aged twelve to nineteen years (median was seventeen years) three months after the onset of COVID-19 vaccine-induced myocarditis.[218] They noted that while most patients showed marked improvements in cardiac diagnostic markers (e.g., troponin) and testing (echocardiograms, electrocardiograms, exercise stress), 54 percent still showed abnormalities by cardiac MRI.

Barmada et al. (2023) found that 80 percent of those with vaccine-induced symptomatic myocarditis in their US study still had lasting effects on their hearts as revealed by MRI scans over six months after initial diagnosis.[219] Warren et al. (2024) observed with cardiac magnetic resonance (CMR) late gadolinium enhancement (LGE) imaging of sixty-seven patients with COVID-19 vaccine-induced myocarditis between 398 to 603 days after their vaccination that 30 percent still had detectable persistent damage that was detectable with this method.[220]

Patone et al. (2022) reported in their analysis of 2,861 hospitalized English patients that got symptomatic myocarditis following COVID-19 vaccination, 345 (12 percent) died within twenty-eight days of hospital admission with myocarditis or with myocarditis as the cause of death recorded in the death certificate.[221] Cho et al. (2023) in their study of 480 Koreans who experienced COVID-19 vaccine-induced symptomatic myocarditis observed twenty-one had died (4.4 percent) after a year.[222] Within a week of their COVID-19 mRNA vaccination, eight of these individuals, six males and two females all under forty-five years of age, died from sudden cardiac death. These rates of death are consistent with the rates of death observed with symptomatic viral myocarditis.[223]

In a meta-analysis of fourteen publications that described the autopsy results of twenty-eight people who died mostly within a week following their COVID-19 vaccination, Hulscher et al. (2023) noted that twenty-six of them involved exclusively the cardiovascular system.[224] The authors established that all of these twenty-eight deaths were causally linked to COVID-19 vaccination by independent adjudication and stated:

> The temporal relationship, internal and external consistency seen among cases in this review with known COVID-19 vaccine-induced myocarditis, its pathobiological mechanisms and related excess death, complemented with autopsy confirmation, independent adjudication, and application of the Bradford Hill criteria to the overall epidemiology of vaccine myocarditis, suggests there is a high likelihood of a causal link between COVID-19 vaccines and death from suspected myocarditis in cases where sudden, unexpected death has occurred in a vaccinated person.[225]

From internal studies, the US Department of Veteran Affairs were aware of the problem of myocarditis and myopericarditis with the Pfizer/BioNTech COVID-19 vaccine as early as May 13, 2021, and based on surveys conducted by the US CDC, "54 percent of post-vaccination myocarditis patients had an abnormal finding like welling or scarring on follow up cardiac MRIs."[226] Apparently, the CDC decided not to send out a draft May 25, 2021 alert through their Health Alert Network to warn physicians about the risks of myocarditis and myopericarditis to avoid causing a panic.[227]

While myocarditis and myopericarditis are now well-recognized potential adverse events associated with COVID-19 vaccines, other cardiac complications of these vaccines are also reported. In a recent study conducted between September 17 and November 16, 2023, of 804 adult Saudi Arabian participants,

27.11 percent reported being diagnosed with cardiac complications post mRNA vaccination.[228]

13.8.4. Mechanism of COVID-19 Vaccine-Induced Pathology from Autopsy

The mechanism by which COVID-19 genetic vaccines may induce myocarditis has been revealed from careful autopsy studies. This first became apparent in the scientific literature from immunohistochemistry studies performed by German pathologist Dr. Michael Mörz on a deceased male, seventy-six-year-old Parkinson's patient who died within three weeks of receiving his third inoculation with the BNT162b2 mRNA.[229] Using specific antibodies to detect either the spike or nucleocapsid proteins in tissue slices, only the spike protein was detected within the foci of inflammation in the brain and the heart, particularly in the endothelial cells of small blood vessels. No nucleocapsid protein could be detected at these sites, which ruled out an actual SARS-CoV-2 infection to account for the spike protein detection. From inspection of the foci of spike protein detected in the brain and heart slices, it was evident that the spike protein has been locally produced, almost certainly from the spread of the lipid nanoparticles in the COVID-19 vaccines.

Even more extensive analyses of seventy-five people in the Reutlingen area that had died following COVID-19 vaccinations were performed by German pathologist Professor Arne Burkhardt and his international team of nine other pathologists, coroners, biologists, and chemists. These deceased individuals (forty men and thirty-five women with a median age at death of 65.7 years) had died one day to ten months after their last COVID-19 vaccination, most commonly with the BNT162b2 vaccine. The cause of death for sixty-eight of them was previously ruled as "natural" or "uncertain" by pathologists or coroners at the time of death (only seven were possibly linked to COVID-19 vaccination), and nineteen of these cases were examples of unexpected Sudden Adult Death Syndrome. Dr. Burkhardt's team subsequently determined that 77 percent of these deaths (twenty-one beyond reasonable doubt and thirty-seven probable) were caused by their COVID-19 vaccination. The CCCA Scientific and Medical Advisory Committee was privileged to review many of Professor Burkhardt's findings with him, and a video copy of his presentation is posted on the CCCA website.[230] In the immunohistochemistry images of the various tissues retrieved from the deceased individuals that Dr. Burkardt's team analyzed, it was apparent that the spike protein was widely and highly expressed in many of the tissue samples, whereas the nucleocapsid protein was absent, ruling out active SARS-CoV-2 infections. Furthermore, in these images it was clear that there was infiltration of immune cells and clear tissue pathology. This included, as observed by Dr. Matthew Mörz with the deceased Parkinson's patient, spike protein expression, immune cell presence, and cellular damage in the heart muscle. These findings are in line with the expected inflammatory responses that would arise from the expression of spike protein on the surface of cells. Significantly, the detection of spike protein was evident in the deceased who died even ten months after their last vaccination, and the spike protein production was concentrated in the tissue images at the sites of destruction. This means that the detected spike protein was not simply produced at the site of injection in the muscle and released from the muscle cells into the circulation, but rather the lipid nanoparticles or adenoviruses in the vaccines traveled throughout the body and produced the spike protein locally.

With respect to the type of immune cells that could be responsible for the inflammatory attack on spike-producing cells in the heart with myocarditis and myopericarditis, the work of Barmada et al. (2023) provides some insight.[231] These investigators ruled out the production of cross-reactive antibodies that recognized normal cardiac proteins or expansion of the T- and B-lymphocytes. They also noted that there was not an overproduction of spike-recognizing antibodies especially in these patients compared to other COVID-19 vaccinated people. However, there were many immune changes, including more production of interleukins (e.g., IL-1β, IL-1RA, and IL-15) and chemokines (e.g., CCL4, CXCL1, and CXCL10), and activation of cytotoxic T-lymphocytes and natural killer (NK) cells, and inflammatory monocytes. These responses are consistent with the spike protein–induced changes illustrated in Figure 13.1 (in the insert), which result in damage and potentially death to spike protein-producing cells by immune cell attack and the activation of the complement-cascade. Other causes may include the dsRNA contamination, which act as an intrinsic adjuvant and may induce uncontrolled immune-inflammatory reactions. Vaccine lipid nanoparticles preferentially transfect macrophages and dendritic cells residing in peripheral tissue such as myocardium and may induce autoimmunity.[232] Initiatives to reduce dsRNA contamination in the vaccines have been noted by Moderna, who have designed a T7 RNA polymerase that produces very little dsRNA.[233]

In view of the potential mechanisms of how myocarditis and myopericarditis can come about from COVID-19 genetic vaccines, there is no compelling reason to believe that these adverse effects at the cellular and tissue level are not also produced at high levels in many females and the elderly. The symptoms of vaccine-induced myocarditis and myopericarditis may be more manifested in young males, due to their tendency to be much more physically active, which could exacerbate the condition.

It should be noted that a study by Paratz et al. (2023) investigated an Australian out-of-hospital cardiac arrest (OHCA) registry to determine whether rates of OHCA in young people, particularly OHCA attributable to unascertained causes or myocarditis, increased after COVID-19 vaccination.[234] Some 4.49 million people were eligible for COVID-19 vaccination over the study period of April 2019 to the end of March 2022, and 2,242 people were identified with OHCA, of which thirty-eight died (mostly after BNT162b2 or ChAdOx1 vaccination). The authors concluded that:

> Our statewide analysis of OHCA in young people did not demonstrate increased rates of overall OHCA, myocarditis causing OHCA, or unascertained OHCA during the COVID-19 pandemic or after the introduction of nationally mandated COVID-19 vaccination. Causes of death in young people experiencing fatal OHCA within 30 days of their COVID-19 vaccination were consistent with prepandemic causative profiles.[235]

13.8.5. Increased Sudden Cardiac Arrest in Athletes

Prior to the COVID-19 pandemic, the incidences of sudden cardiac arrest (SCA) and sudden cardiac death (SCD) were relatively low in students and professional athletes under thirty years of age. Peterson et al. (2023) collected data in this regard from the US National Center for Catastrophic Sports Injury Research, the University of Washington Medicine Center for Sports Cardiology, searches of student-athlete deaths on the National Collegiate Athletic Association's Resolutions List, the National Federation of State High School Associations, and the Parent Heart Watch.[236] From July 2014 through to June 2018, the authors identified 331 cases, of which 173 were fatal. The majority of these cases occurred in males (83.7 percent), high school athletes (61.6 percent), and during exercise (74 percent), with cardiomyopathies accounting for nearly half (47 percent) of the cases with college and professional athletes. Ice-hockey (one in 23,550) followed by basketball (one in 39,811), and then football (one in 82,587) had the highest incidence rates of SCD for males. From their data, it can be calculated that there was an average of forty-three SCD per year in the United States.

An earlier study by Bille et al. (2006) on SCD in sports in the scientific literature for athletes under thirty-five years of age noted that between 1966 to 2004, there were 1101 reported cases in total.[237] Of these, about 50 percent had congenital anatomical heart disease and cardiomyopathies. The expected rate of SCD in young athletes averaged to about twenty-nine per year.

And yet in recent times, there has been a surge in the number of news and social media reports of collapses and sudden deaths of athletes worldwide since the availability of COVID-19 vaccines. The most comprehensive list of athletes that have lost consciousness or died since January 2021 is available on the social media website goodsciencing.com.[238] Most of these reports arise out of US news sources. While the authors of the website are anonymous, they provide direct

URL links to news sources for most of the 2,024 athletes identified by name up to September 30, 2023, who have collapsed or died (69.4 percent), and who were confirmed or highly suspected to have been vaccinated against COVID-19. This list includes those over forty years of age, but none apparently with reported congenital heart abnormalities. For the entries where the age of the person was provided (1,894), 1,293 (68 percent) were under forty years of age and of these 625 (48 percent) had died. Some of the deaths were also identified as from comorbidities such as cancer. From the 1,417 deaths over the 2.75-years period, this corresponds to a rate of 515 deaths per year on average since the introduction of the COVID-19 vaccine.

Binkhorst and Goldstein (2023) analyzed the incidence of SCA and SCD in US athletes under forty years of age from January 2021 to December 2022, using highly filtered data from the goodsciencing.com website.[239] They recognized that COVID-19 vaccination status of those that experienced SCA or SDA was unverified, and so they tried to apply the strict criteria indicated in the study by Peterson et al. (2021).[240] They noted that the deaths primarily occurred at rest (32.5 percent) (some died in their sleep) or under unknown circumstances (38.6 percent). Binkhorst and Goldstein concluded that the "SCD rate among young US athletes in 2021–2022 was comparable to pre-pandemic estimates." And, that there was at that time, "no evidence to substantiate a link between (mRNA) COVID-19 vaccination and SCD in (young) athletes." Most of the goodsciencing.com website data were omitted from this analysis, because there was insufficient information about COVID-19 vaccination status of the affected people in most of the news reports. However, it is significant that during the time period of the COVID-19 vaccinations, there was a strong correlation between the rates of COVID-19 vaccination and the frequency of news reports of SDA and SCD. As vaccine uptake declined in 2023, so did the number of news reports on the goodsciencing.com website for the same period. It is also important to recognize that there was a strong push for COVID-19 vaccination of athletes in universities and professional sports, so it is highly likely that the vast majority of the cases captured in the goodsciencing.com website were vaccinated individuals. What is needed is the participation of the sporting organizations that supported the Peterson et al. (2023) study to provide equivalent data for their athletes after the release of COVID-19 vaccines.

13.9. Neurological Disorders Linked to COVID-19 Vaccines

A wide range of neurological disorders that affect the central or peripheral nervous systems (CNS, PNS) have also been linked to COVID-19 vaccination. This has been reviewed extensively in the recent scientific literature.[241, 242] In particular, headache, intracerebral hemorrhage, venous sinus thrombosis (VST), Guillain–Barré syndrome (GBS), and facial palsy (e.g., Bell's Palsy) are the most commonly described adverse events. Sudden hearing loss has also been attributed to COVID-19 mRNA vaccination, although this seems to be relatively rare.[243] As pointed out by Finsterer (2023),[244] other neurological conditions that appear to be induced by COVID-19 vaccines in the CNS include cerebrovascular disorders (in addition to VST and intracerebral bleeding, ischemic stroke, subarachnoid bleeding, reversible, cerebral vasoconstriction syndrome, vasculitis, pituitary apoplexy, Susac syndrome), inflammatory diseases (encephalitis, meningitis, demyelinating disorders, transverse myelitis), epilepsy, and a number of other rarely reported CNS conditions. PNS disorders related to SARS-CoV-2 vaccines include neuropathy of cranial nerves, mono-/polyradiculitis (e.g., Guillain–Barré syndrome), Parsonage–Turner syndrome (plexitis),[245] small fiber neuropathy, myasthenia, myositis/dermatomyositis, rhabdomyolysis, and a number of other conditions. CNS diseases can also indirectly arise from adverse effects of COVID-19 vaccines in extra-neural tissues such as myocarditis or vaccine-induced immune thrombotic thromocytopenia (VITT). VITT is a condition characterized by acute blood clots and then a deficiency of platelets, which can lead to easy or excessive bruising and internal bleeding.

Headache has been reported in about 30 to 51 percent of COVID-19 vaccinees with neurological disorders.[246, 247] It was also among the most common side-effects of COVID-19 vaccines in Phase 3 clinical studies.

In the Italian NEURO-COVAX study conducted by Salsone et al. (2023), the investigators aimed to evaluate the neurological complications after the first and/or second dose of different COVID-19 vaccines and identify factors potentially associated with these adverse effects.[248] Adults aged eighteen years and older in Novegro (Milan, Lombardy) who received two vaccine doses of Pfizer/BioNTech's BNT162b2 (15,368 participants), Moderna's mRNA-1273 (2,077 participants), and AstraZeneca's ChAdOx1nCov-19 vaccine (1,651 participants) described any neurological complications from their vaccination between July 7 and 16, 2021. Approximately 31.2 percent of the participants developed post-vaccination neurological complications, particularly with ChAdOx1nCov-19, and about 40 percent of these symptomatic individuals had comorbidities in their clinical histories. ChAdOx1nCov-19 was associated with increased risks of headaches, tremors, muscle spasms, and insomnia. For Moderna's mRNA-1273 vaccine, there were increased risks of paresthesia (burning or prickling sensation on skin), vertigo (dizziness associated with sensation of motion or spinning), diplopia (double vision), and sleepiness. However, in the period that ranged from March to August 2021, none of the participants were hospitalized and/or died of severe complications related to COVID-19 vaccinations.[249]

Of recent concern is the apparent increased risk of seizures/convulsions after BNT162b2 to two- to four-year-olds and mRNA-1273 to two- to five-year olds from an analysis by Hu et al. (2023) of COVID-19 vaccine administered to 4,102,106 US children aged six months to seventeen years old.[250] In this report, in which the corresponding author is from the FDA, twenty-one pre-specified outcomes were tracked from administrative claims data provided by Optum, Carelon Research, and CVS Health, as well as pharmacy claims and data from participating local and state Immunization Information Systems. There were sixty-five observed COVID-19-vaccine-related seizures/convulsions cases among 752,415 doses (8.64 in a hundred thousand risk) given to aged two- to four-/five-year-olds across a seven-day risk window following vaccination. Seizures/convulsions were also observed in six-month- to one-year-olds with an incidence of 5.32 in a hundred thousand doses, and in five-/six- to seventeen-year-olds with an incidence of 3.14 in a hundred thousand doses. In the same analysis, myocarditis/myopericarditis in ages twelve to seventeen years old was the other outcome that met the statistical threshold for a warning signal with 107 cases out of 3,083,412 doses with BNT192b2 for a 3.47 in a hundred thousand risk. The risk of Bell's Palsy for those aged five/six to seventeen years old was 1.97 in a hundred thousand based on 115 cases in 5,837,942 doses.

In another study of COVID-19 vaccination of US children two to five years old, with data collected between June 2022 and May 2023 and retrieved from Optum, Carelon Research, and CVS Health databases, there was a 2.5-times greater incidence of febrile seizures within a day after a Moderna mRNA-1273 shot than in the same children eight to sixty-three days afterwards.[251] Out of 288,754 children vaccinated with BNT192b2, twenty-two experienced febrile seizures and thirty-two experienced seizures/convulsions within seven days of their vaccination (approximately a one in 5,347 risk). With 192,540 vaccinations with mRNA-1273, there were twenty-one cases of febrile seizures and twenty-eight cases of seizures/convulsions within seven days of inoculation of the children (approximately a one in 3,929 risk). When compared to the expected incidence of 5 percent febrile seizures in young children, these adverse events were not considered as statistically significant.

In the next subsections, the discussion focuses on GBS and Bell's Palsy, as these are neuropathies that have been more commonly associated with COVID-19 vaccine adverse effects in previous studies. However, it is important to appreciate that the full spectrum of neurological side-effects of these vaccines is broad, ranging in severity from initially asymptomatic to mild to severe, with outcomes that range from full recovery to death. A wide range of hypotheses have been proposed to account for these side-effects, including effects of the spike protein directly on cellular targets such as Angiotensin 2 and Neuropilin, to the inflammatory responses that the vaccines evoke from their components (e.g., pegylated lipids in the lipid nanoparticles) as they spread through the circulation or spike protein on the expression of cells that take up the lipid nanoparticles or adenoviruses used for delivery of spike mRNA.

13.9.1. Guillain-Barré Syndrome

Guillain-Barré syndrome (GBS) is a neurological disorder in which one's immune system attacks the myelin coating of long axons, primarily of peripheral nerves. Incidence is approximately one to two in a hundred thousand people, and lower in children.[252, 253] While GBS can occur at any age, the incidence rate markedly increases after fifty years of age, by about 20 percent for each additional decade.[254]

GBS typically causes weakness and tingling in the arms and legs that can spread throughout the body. The typical presentation is bilateral. GBS can lead to paralysis and death by respiratory failure. The cause of GBS is unknown,[255] but is typically triggered by an infection with a wide range of bacteria and viruses or even by surgery.[256] A more controversial risk factor is that of vaccination, which may trigger an autoimmune response by a process known as molecular mimicry.[257] In 1976, those that were inoculated with the Swine Flu vaccine had an increased risk of about one to two per hundred thousand doses for developing GBS.[258]

Diagnosis with GBS is usually based on the signs and symptoms with tests such as nerve conduction studies and examination of the cerebrospinal fluid. There are several GBS subtypes known to exist.[259]

Treatment for GBS includes supportive care, intravenous immunoglobulin, and plasmapheresis, with the latter replacing the patient's blood through transfusion to remove anti-myelin antibodies. Recovery from GBS may take years; some 30 percent of patients may retain some longer-term weakness.[260, 261]

From a meta-analysis of eighteen studies published in 2020 investigating GBS incidence in 136,746 hospitalized and non-hospitalized COVID-19 patients, Palaiodimou et al. (2021) estimated an incidence of fifteen GBS cases per hundred thousand COVID-19 cases.[262] Considering that a relatively low percentage of the population was expected to have been infected with SARS-CoV-2 in 2020, this indicates that the overall incidence of GBS would unlikely change appreciably during the first year of the COVID-19 pandemic. Keddie et al. (2021) observed a slight decrease in GBS cases in UK hospitals during the early stages of the COVID-19 pandemic between March and May of 2020.[263]

Ogunjimi et al. (2023), in their meta-analysis of seventy-one publications regarding GBS with COVID-19 vaccination established a rate of 0.8 cases per hundred thousand doses, with a higher prevalence in males (59.4 percent) and in people between forty and sixty years of age.[264] They found the onset of GBS typically occurred within two weeks of vaccination. The highest rates of

GBS were associated with the AstraZeneca vaccine (56 percent of cases), which was 1.4- to ten-fold higher than expected depending on the studies analyzed. About 20 percent of the GBS cases were associated with the Pfizer/BioNTech COVID-19 vaccine and 5 percent with the Moderna product.

An outstanding question is whether prior infection with SARS-CoV-2 and subsequent COVID-19 vaccination may increase the rate of incidence of GBS. Zheng et al. (2023) tried to answer this question, but obtained inconclusive results, and this is worthy of further investigation.[265]

13.9.2. Bell's Palsy

Bell's palsy (BP) is a condition in which damage to the facial nerve (cranial nerve [CN] 7) causes weakness in the muscles on one side of the face, leading that side of the face to droop. It can occur at any age.

Symptoms include lopsided smiles and an impact on eye closure on the affected side of the face. It can result from various forms of inflammation that may affect CN7. It is listed as one of the outcomes of pregnancy and from various infections causing inflammation. The face droop feature of BP is often temporary, but may be longer lasting, sometimes for life.[266]

The incidence of Bell's palsy prior to COVID-19 was fifteen to fifty per hundred thousand people.[267] Tamaki et al. (2021), from an analysis of data from forty-one health organizations collected in 2020, identified 284 BP patients from 348,088 COVID-19 patients for an incidence rate of 81.6 BP cases per hundred thousand COVID-19 cases.[268] About 46.1 percent of these BP patients had a previous history of Bell's palsy. Considering that most people in 2020 were not COVID-19 vaccinated, the rate of BP in the general population was not appreciably different with SARS-CoV-2.

In another meta-analysis, Rafati et al. (2023) picked seventeen published studies to calculate the rate of BP in COVID-19 vaccine recipients and following SARS-CoV-2 infection.[269] By pooling data from four randomized Phase 3 studies with COVID-19 vaccines, it can be calculated that there was a 221 percent increase in BP incidence with vaccination compared to placebo controls, with a rate of 19.3 cases of BP per hundred thousand participants in the COVID-19 vaccinated, and 6.0 cases of BP per hundred thousand unvaccinated participants. The authors claimed that no significant increase was evident when the data from observation studies were also considered, which included a study by Klein et al. (2021) that provided an incident rate that was 20.1 BP cases per hundred thousand unvaccinated participants, but only 4.58 BP cases per hundred thousand vaccinated participants.[270] Apart from having an opposite trend from most of the other studies cited, this data accounted for 88 percent of the people tracked in all the studies combined. However, by excluding the data from Klein et al. (2021) and aggregating the remaining data from the twelve studies presented, it can be calculated that there was a 13 percent decrease in BP incidence with vaccination compared to the unvaccinated, with a rate of 9.0 BP cases per hundred thousand participants in the COVID-19 vaccinated, and 10.3 BP cases per hundred thousand unvaccinated participants. An important caveat for consideration in this type of comparison is the time sampling period for quantifying COVID-19 vaccine-induced cases of BP, which are usually within a few weeks of receipt of the vaccine, whereas in the unvaccinated population, this is based on the duration of the study, which may be over a year. This is why the findings from controlled random clinical studies are much more insightful. The authors did not detect any differences between the rates of BP between the Pfizer/BioNTech and AstraZeneca vaccines.

In the meta-analysis of eighty-six articles on neurological disorders associated with COVID-19 vaccination by Alonso Castillo and Martinez Castrillo (2022), they calculated that 4,936 of 13,809 (35.7 percent) of these patients experienced BP, and it was more prevalent in women (60 percent) than men.[271]

Collectively, these studies indicate that incidence levels for Bell's palsy likely were not appreciably increased by SARS-CoV-2 infection and may not be by the COVID-19 vaccines. However, the diverse findings across the quoted studies justify further investigations as to the relationships between BP, COVID-19, and its vaccines.

13.10. Excess Deaths and All-Cause Mortality Statistics

Since the introduction of the COVID-19 genetic vaccines, there has been at least an eight-fold surge in news reports of collapses and unexpected deaths in otherwise young healthy people, pilots, musicians, and athletes.[272, 273] Sudden Adult Death Syndrome of "unknown" cause became among the top category of deaths in Alberta in 2021 since the rollout of the COVID-19 vaccines.[274] It is hard to ignore the rise of these unusual deaths with the timing of the launch of the COVID-19 genetic vaccines. The question is whether there has in fact been an increase in the total numbers of deaths since the advent of COVID-19 and with the introduction of the COVID-19 vaccines. This is best revealed by examining the available data on excess all-cause mortality.

With respect to deaths with COVID-19, the average age of a person that died of COVID-19 in Canada was about eighty-four years compared to about eighty-two years for all-cause mortality. There was no major increase in all-cause mortality in the first year of the COVID-19 pandemic, when the virus was more virulent, and there were no specific medications for its treatment or vaccination for its prevention. Bearing in mind an increase in the size of the total population in Canada, the total number of deaths from all causes in 2019 in Canada was 285,270, and it was 307,205 in 2020.[275] Infectious diseases accounted for only 8.6 percent of these deaths in 2019 and 12.6 percent of deaths in 2020 in Canada. By comparison, in 2020, cancer, and heart and stroke-related disease accounted for 27.0 percent and 23.2 percent of all deaths, respectively. The total number of deaths with COVID-19 in 2020, which was 16,151 (of which about half was due to a co-morbidity), accounted for 5.25 percent of the total number of deaths. Accidents and suicides killed more people in Canada in 2020 than COVID-19.

There were fewer deaths from other infectious diseases such as influenza and RSV during the first two and a half years of the COVID-19 pandemic, and about half of the deaths ascribed to COVID-19 were people that died with COVID-19, but actually they may have been due to their co-morbidities. Rancourt et al. (2023) have concluded that there was no increase in all-cause mortality in the United States in 2020, especially when compared to 2017.[276] Although there was virtually no increase in overall excess all-cause mortality in 2020, the first year of the COVID-19 pandemic in Canada and elsewhere, it increased significantly in 2021 and 2022, since the introduction of the COVID-19 vaccines.[277, 278, 279] In a study of all-cause mortality in thirty-one European countries, this was positively correlated with increased COVID-19 vaccination.[280] A 1 percent increase in COVID-19 vaccine uptake in 2021 between the countries was associated with a statistically significant monthly increase in mortality in the first nine months of 2022 by 0.105 percent.

The United Kingdom is one of the few jurisdictions where all-cause and COVID-19 linked mortality has been correlated with COVID-19 vaccination status, age, and sex, and this data is available for public scrutiny.[281] Graphic representation of some of the findings provided by the UK Office for National Statistics for England are shown in Figure 13.1. The data indicate that with the emergence of Omicron variants, there has been no real benefit of single or double COVID-19 vaccination for preventing COVID-19 deaths compared to not being vaccinated against SARS-CoV-2. There is evidence that triple vaccination might have reduced COVID-19 deaths prior to September 2022, but not significantly afterwards. This might be due to a temporary protection afforded by the booster vaccination in vulnerable groups and that many who were particularly susceptible to dying from COVID-19 may have already succumbed by the time a third vaccine dose was available. However, with all-cause mortality, especially with the first dose of the COVID-19 vaccines early in the vaccination program, and the second dose subsequently after September 2021, the inoculations are associated with higher rates of death. After May 2022, there is little support that even a third shot of COVID-19 vaccines provided any significant benefit in reducing all-cause mortality. Interpretation of the data in Figure 13.1 (in the insert) is complicated, since the virulence of SARS-CoV-2 was steadily reduced with the evolution of new variants, and the extent of natural immunity in the UK population also increased.[282] However, it is evident by comparison of the top and bottom panels of Figure 13.1 (in the insert) that COVID-19 associated deaths only accounted for a small portion of the excess deaths in England.

While such a temporal link in these increased deaths with COVID-19 vaccination exists, it does not necessarily have to be causal. However, in considering the proposed mechanisms of action of the COVID-19 genetic vaccines, their inadequate testing prior to wide-spread dissemination, and the unacceptably high risks for these vaccines for adverse reactions, it is not surprising that they do correlate.

More recent publications have also documented excess deaths in 2022 following the introduction of COVID-19 vaccines at the end of 2020 in the United Kingdom[283, 284] and other countries, including the United States,[285] Germany,[286] and Japan.[287] Alegria and Nunes (2024) investigated the UK trends in death rates and disabilities for malignant cancers for individuals aged fifteen to forty-four by computing excess death rates and excess disability claims.[288] They reported:

> We show a large increase in morbidity (disabilities) and mortality due to malignant neoplasms that started in 2021 and accelerated substantially in 2022. The increase in disability claims mirrors the increase in excess deaths in 2022, and both are highly statistically significant (extreme events). The results indicate that from late 2021 a novel phenomenon leading to increased malignant neoplasm deaths and disabilities appears to be present in individuals aged 15 to 44 in the UK.[289]

Alegria and Nunes (2024) showed similar trends in the United States starting in 2020 with increased excess mortality of +3.4 percent in 2020, +9.2 percent in 2021, and +16.4 percent in 2022.[290] They observed that excess deaths from cancers occurred for most age groups, with the strongest effect in ages fifteen to twenty-four years and individuals sixty-five years and older. The increase in 2020 was suggested by the authors to be due to COVID-19-related or other negative effects from lockdowns, stress, reduced exercise, worse food habits, and reduced medical care. However, they implicated adverse effects from COVID-19 vaccines in 2021 and 2022.

In Japan with an estimated 115,799 excess deaths following a third COVID-19 shot in 2022 to two-thirds of the population, Gibo et al. (2024) noted:

> No significant excess mortality was observed during the first year of the pandemic (2020). However, some excess cancer mortalities were observed in 2021 after mass vaccination with the first and second vaccine doses, and significant excess mortalities were observed for all cancers and some specific types of

> cancer (including ovarian cancer, leukemia, prostate cancer, lip/oral/pharyngeal cancer, pancreatic cancer, and breast cancer) after mass vaccination with the third dose in 2022.[291]

Of the excess deaths in 2022 in Japan, only about 39,060 could be ascribed to SARS-CoV-2 infections. The six specific types of cancer that showed the greatest increases in incidence were estrogen receptor-alpha (ER-alpha) sensitive cancers. Coincidently, in another study involving the screening of a possible nine thousand human proteins, ER-alpha as among the strongest binders to the spike protein of SARS-CoV-2, and this binding stimulates the transcriptional activity of ER-alpha.[292] Another mechanism that has been proposed to account for increased rates of cancers associated with three or more doses of COVID-19 vaccines has been the disruption of the immune system toward tolerance with IgG class switching to IgG4, as discussed in chapter 12.7. Rubio-Casillas et al. (2024) have suggested that the 100 percent replacement of uridine with N1-methyl-pseudouridine in the COVID-19 vaccine mRNA reduces cytokine production and anti-tumor immune suppression that may contribute to cancer growth and metastasis.[293] Addition of 100 percent of N1-methyl-pseudouridine (m1Ψ) to an mRNA vaccine in a melanoma model inhibited interferon type-1 anti-tumor immunity leading to cancer growth and metastasis, while non-modified RNA had an opposite effect.[294]

Interestingly, a recent study by Fürst et al. (2024) noted what appeared at first blush to be evidence based on all-cause mortality (ACM) data from 2.2 million individual records in the Czech Republic that ACM was consistently lower in vaccinated groups for COVID-19 than in the unvaccinated.[295] However, the investigators found that this pattern was also observed in periods outside of "pandemic waves" of sickness and death, where "the ACMs in groups more than 4 weeks from Doses 1, 2, or 3 were consistently several times higher than in those less than 4 weeks from the respective dose." They ultimately attributed this to what is known as the "Healthy Vaccinee Effect" (HVE), which they further corroborated by mathematical modeling. HVE has likely been a general phenomenon in retroactive studies of COVID-19 vaccine efficacy. HVE can occur when one cohort contains fewer or greater numbers of people with a comorbidity than another cohort with which it is being compared. Reassessment of ACM data in a previous Italian study of the effectiveness of COVID-19 vaccines also identified biases such as HVE, and when Alessandria et al. (2024) recalculated the ACM, they found that two doses of COVID-19 vaccination reduced life expectancy in the Pescara population by 3.6 months, and with three or four doses, it further reduced it by 1.31 months.[296]

13.11. The Changing Response of Public Health Abroad to COVID-19 Vaccination

While most Canadian public health authorities still zealously embrace COVID-19 vaccines, public health authorities in Quebec[297] and many other countries are much less enthusiastic. As a consequence, the COVID-19 adenovirus vaccines and Medicago, while initially approved by Health Canada, have all since been discontinued in 2023.

In view of the mounting and disturbing data about the limited efficacy and serious safety issues associated with the COVID-19 genetic vaccines, health regulatory agencies around the world have begun to discourage or ban the use of these vaccines, especially in younger people. Denmark was the first nation in Europe to invoke this step by halting vaccination invitations on May 14, 2022.[298] By autumn 2022, Denmark recommended vaccination only to those over fifty years old and some vulnerable populations.[299]

Many European countries as well as Australia and some US states such as Florida have stopped recommending vaccinations for COVID-19 to anyone under forty, fifty, or sixty years of age and especially children. Even in 2021, France and Scandinavian countries did not recommend the Moderna vaccine for people under thirty years of age.[300, 301] The United Kingdom Joint Committee on Vaccination and Immunisation (JCVI) no longer recommends vaccination of healthy individuals under fifty years of age in the United Kingdom except for those in clinical risk groups or those attending to such individuals.[302] The Federal Office of Public Health in Switzerland also no longer recommends COVID-19 vaccination for healthy people in all age groups, and will not pay for COVID-19 vaccination for anyone, unless medically indicated by a physician for a patient with a clear risk-benefit analysis.[303] The Australian government has advised that as of February 2023 a booster dose is not recommended for children and adolescents up to eighteen years who do not have any risk factors for severe COVID-19, and only for those eighteen to sixty-four years of age who have undergone a risk-benefit analysis with their health-care provider.[304] The German Federation of Hospitals (DKG) has called for the mandatory vaccination obligation of health-care personnel to be revoked after the German Ministry of Health admitted that one in five thousand COVID-19 vaccination shots led to serious side-effects.[305]

In April 2023, the European Medicine Agency and the European Parliament finally recognized that at least 11,448 deaths in the European Union occurred following COVID-19 vaccination, and that there were 50,648 deaths linked to these vaccines in the EudraVigilance database as of April 10, 2023.[306] It would appear that health regulatory agencies in Europe and elsewhere have come to realize the clear and present dangers of the COVID-19 genetic vaccines.

It seems that the populations of Canada and the United States have also finally come to recognize the efficacy and safety issues of the COVID-19 vaccines, despite the heavy messaging from public health officials in Canada and the United States to the contrary. For example, only about 16 percent of those six months or older in Ontario within the past year had received a COVID-19 vaccination by September 14, 2023.[307] Canada-wide, only about 3.4 percent of Canadians chose to be vaccinated between March 10 and September 10, 2023.[308] In the United States, only about 5.4 percent of children and 14.8 percent of adults eighteen years and older received the updated XBB1.5 COVID-19 vaccines by November 17, 2023, whereas 35.1 percent of children and 36.3 percent of adults opted to be vaccinated against influenza.[309] By the end of the first quarter of 2024, worldwide sales of Pfizer's and Moderna's COVID-19 vaccines plummeted by 88 percent and 92 percent, respectively, compared to the same period the year before.[310]

The question remains: When will the health regulatory agencies that are tasked to protect Canadians and Americans catch up with their European counterparts?

CHAPTER 14

Therapeutic Treatment of COVID-19

Christopher A. Shaw, Steven Pelech, Philip Oldfield, Anna Kreynes, Wendi Roscoe, & Kanji Nataksu

"The responsible physician knows that 'first do no harm' does not mean: 'do nothing.' Doing nothing, especially for the high-risk patient, is unacceptable. It is lethal folly to withhold a safe medicine that, when viewing the totality of the evidence, shows great promise at negligible cost. Such policies effectively deny to dedicated clinicians the ability to practice medicine."

—Edmund Fordham, Theresa Lawrie, Katherine MacGilchrist, and Andrew Bryant

"You can't judge the ability of a doctor by the amount of praise the undertakers give him."

—Evan Esar

14.1. Introduction to COVID-19 Therapeutic Options

Of all the topics that have kindled debate and acrimony during the COVID-19 pandemic, perhaps none has been as intense as those concerning non-vaccine treatment paradigms for the disease. Very soon after the WHO's declaration of the COVID-19 pandemic in March 2020, public health officers around the world, along with heads of government, Big Pharma, and the media began their expensive campaigns to convince the public that the only way out of the pandemic was though the application of vaccines against the virus. Such statements were so uniformly identical that an independent observer might well conclude that a worldwide master plan to vaccinate the entire world's population was not only afoot but had been in the works for years.

Non-vaccine alternatives were routinely described as ineffective at best and harmful at worst. Two well-studied and incredibly safe, well-known anti-viral compounds, ivermectin and hydroxychloroquine, were declared to be unsafe, spurring a strong negative public reaction to both, with ivermectin routinely labeled as "horse paste," simply because in veterinary practice as in humans, it had been successfully used to treat various parasitic infections. The FDA had to retract in 2024 by court order their earlier statements arguing against the safety of ivermectin and its use in humans.[1] The fact that several research papers denying any benefit to the compounds were soon retracted as being fraudulent were overlooked in the rapid acceptance of mRNA and viral vector vaccines by the regulatory agencies, which were deemed to have Emergency Use Authorization (EUA) in the United States or Interim Order status in Canada. It is worth noting that EUA status for drugs can only be attained normally if there is no alternative treatment. Hence, in brief, the steps were to convince the public that vaccines, and only vaccines, would allow a return to "normal."

The stages used to convince the public that vaccines were essential in the fight against COVID-19 were thus rolled out: Declare a deadly pandemic, convince the public who have already been conditioned to have positive views on vaccines in general that any COVID-19 vaccine, no matter how novel and experimental, would be "safe and effective," and that such vaccines would arrive "soon." To complement the wave of positive COVID-19 vaccine enthusiasm, governments, the health establishment, and the media fueled months of COVID-19 fear almost to the point of hysteria. Mandates and lockdowns served to endlessly reinforce the message. All of those responsible for the hysteria supplemented their message of fear with declarations that only "anti-vaxxers" and other malcontents could possibly refuse such life-saving treatments for themselves, thus presumably putting the elderly and immune compromised at great risk by their obstinacy. Such was the fear in the general population that many lined up to receive the vaccines when they became available, even crossing borders to be first in line. Doing so was widely considered to be not only self-defense for the individual, but also a means of protecting others.

Over three years after the rollout of the vaccines, with much of the population vaccinated with the initial two doses, followed by boosters, much more is known about the disease and the problems with the efficacy and safety of the COVID-19 vaccines. As discussed in the preceding chapters, much, perhaps most, of the official narrative about COVID-19 has been misleading and false, perhaps even deliberately so. In other words, "white lies for the greater good."

This conclusion must then lead to a fundamental question that needs revisiting: Were the other methods/medications against COVID-19 truly ineffective and unsafe or were they deliberately dismissed to serve the purpose of encouraging mass vaccination with still experimental vaccines?

Most of this chapter will deal with some of the treatments that were either dismissed or outright ignored by public health officers, particularly those in the global West.

14.2. Intubation and Ventilation

While for most people breathing is effortless and occurs without conscious thought, it actually involves complex coordination between the brain and respiratory system. Breathing adjusts to minute-to-minute variations in blood chemistry and the body's metabolic needs.[2]

The breathing or the respiratory cycle begins as air enters the upper airways (mouth and nose) and flows through the trachea (windpipe) into an ever-narrowing series of tubes called bronchi and then bronchioles. Each bronchiole ends with a small sac called an alveoli. Capillaries, the blood vessels that surround the tiny alveoli, are the site of gas exchange—where oxygen from breathed air enters the blood and carbon dioxide produced in the body enters the lung airspace. This air is exhaled, completing the cycle.

Several scenarios will limit the ability of the body to respond to its respiratory needs through voluntary breathing. At these times the body will either not receive adequate levels of oxygen (hypoxia) or is unable to exhale carbon dioxide resulting in its accumulation in the blood (hypercapnia). Either of these scenarios is dangerous and requires urgent supportive medical care, often in the form of mechanical ventilation. Mechanical ventilation involves connecting the patient's respiratory system to a machine called a ventilator. The ventilator is connected to an endotracheal tube that is placed into the patient's trachea. The medical procedure to do this is called intubation where a specially trained health-care provider inserts the endotracheal tube into the trachea via the mouth or nasal passage. The ventilator "breathes for the person," pushing air into the lungs, providing them with oxygen, and sucking out the air, removing the carbon dioxide from the body. The ventilator settings are adjusted to control the volume of air, the rate of "breathing," the amount of oxygen, and the pressure of the air delivered.

One important difference between voluntary breathing and mechanical ventilation is the way the air enters the lungs. When breathing naturally, air is sucked into the lungs due to the negative pressure generated by muscles expanding the chest wall (the area of the body where the lungs are contained), thus expanding the lungs. These muscles include those between the ribs (intercostal muscles) and the diaphragm. In contrast, mechanical ventilation pushes air into the lungs, using positive pressure to expand the lungs. This is a significant difference, because ventilator use may cause direct lung damage by either delivering too much volume of air (volutrauma) or too much pressure (barotrauma), which can damage the lining of the alveoli.[3] Mechanical ventilation has other associated risks including prolonged immobilization, issues with fluid management, nutritional needs, neurological issues, and the potentially significant risk of additional infections, particularly when used long-term.[4, 5] These factors must be considered when deciding if mechanical ventilation is the most appropriate form of clinical management for a patient.

Early in the COVID-19 crisis, international health authorities, including the World Health Organization, defined the serious respiratory illness of COVID-19 as Acute Respiratory Distress Syndrome (ARDS) and published guidelines for its management.[6] ARDS is a life-threatening condition affecting the lungs that occurs in response to a number of other medical conditions.[7, 8] Some of these conditions, such as pneumonia, directly affect the lungs, while others, such as pancreatitis, are issues outside the lungs. Patients suffering from ARDS present with low blood oxygen level (hypoxia) as well as signs of respiratory distress: increased rate of breathing (tachypnea) and a sensation of difficulty breathing (dyspnea). ARDS creates diffuse damage throughout the lungs resulting in both mechanical challenges (stiff lungs) and impaired gas exchange from swelling and leakage of the blood vessels and alveolar damage.[9, 10]

Many of these patients require mechanical ventilation to optimize gas exchange in the injured lungs while the initiating medical condition is treated. It is important for a clinician to recognize a patient who has ARDS, because there is a specific set of recommended parameters for its management that are tailored to the underlying pathophysiology of the disease.[11, 12, 13, 14] Mechanically ventilated ARDS patients are cared for in an intensive care unit and require a multidisciplinary team who attempt to maintain normal physiology and manage any issues that may complicate the clinical course. ARDS management introduces additional challenges, including maintaining positive pressures to optimize air distribution through the lungs.[15, 16] Mechanical ventilation for COVID-19 was recognized as a poor prognostic factor with a higher mortality rate (up to 84.4 percent[17] to 97 percent[18]) than expected in comparison to traditional ARDS patients.[19]

Viral pneumonia is a recognized trigger for ARDS. Indeed, clinicians have reported that COVID-19 patients fit into the criteria for the diagnosis of ARDS.[20, 21, 22, 23, 24, 25] However, it soon became clear to front line clinicians that some acutely ill COVID-19 patients did not have the clinical features of ARDS. As early as March 2020, New York emergency room physician Dr. Kyle-Sidell made a YouTube appeal to clinicians to apply their clinical assessment in their approach to managing COVID-19 patients rather than following guidelines for ARDS parameters,[26] which he believed were not only ineffective but potentially harmful for some patients. Physicians reported that mechanically ventilated

COVID-19 patients were developing higher than expected rates of damage to the lungs.[27, 28, 29, 30, 31, 32, 33] Many of these patients did not exhibit the signs of respiratory distress typically associated with ARDS, earning them the nickname the "Happy Hypoxic." COVID-19 patients required a different clinical approach to the management of their hypoxia.

Mechanical ventilation is supportive, not curative. The differential diagnosis for COVID-19 associated hypoxia needed to be expanded, allowing earlier application of appropriate treatments, and potentially preventing unnecessary exposure to the risks of mechanical ventilation. A variety of alternate reasons for COVID-19-related hypoxia have been presented. Some of these are primary lung conditions such as bacterial infections[34] or organizing pneumonia.[35] Others involved disorders of the blood system impairing blood flow to the lungs due to microthrombosis,[36, 37, 38] or the ability of red blood cells to become oxygenated.[39, 40, 41, 42, 43, 44, 45, 46] Without appropriate treatment of these underlying conditions, mechanical ventilation may be futile and even harmful.

Mechanical ventilation may be life-saving, providing a person with the ventilator assistance needed to optimize the exchange of gases. As with other medical procedures, there are a number of potential complications, many of which in themselves may worsen a patient's prognosis. Ventilatory guidelines for the management of COVID-19 respiratory disease were established early in the COVID-19 crisis, but was the ARDS protocol the appropriate treatment? With a deeper understanding of the progress of the illness, the differential diagnosis included other reasons for hypoxia of the COVID-19 patient, many of whom may have been spared unnecessary exposure to the risks of mechanical ventilation with treatment. This illustrates the importance of an open dialogue among frontline clinicians that is vital to determine best practices particularly in the event of a declared emerging novel disease.

The two terms, intubation and ventilation, are often used interchangeably, and, although related, are different things.

Basically, intubation is the standard procedure used by medical personnel to create a stable airway in patients who may not be able to breathe successfully on their own. It is usually performed on patients whose airway is compromised by injury and/or who are unconscious. It involves the placement of an endotracheal tube into the patient's mouth with one end positioned in the trachea. This procedure allows the patient to receive oxygen if required from any oxygen source, including a ventilator.

Ventilation is the act of moving air in and out of the lungs. When ventilation is inadequate, various methods can be used to overcome the problem, including supplying oxygen-enriched air via face mask or nasal prongs in the hospital or by mouth-to-mouth resuscitation, in emergency situations.

Sometimes mechanically-assisted ventilation is required, for which the patient is intubated to allow air to be forced into and out of the lungs by a ventilator machine. Typically, ventilators are used on patients who cannot breathe spontaneously during surgery or due to a diminished level of consciousness.

The Cleveland Clinic lists the following conditions for which mechanical ventilation may be useful: Acute respiratory distress syndrome, pneumonia, obstructive pulmonary disease, stroke, traumatic brain injury, coma, and anaphylaxis.[47] Included in this list is the intense use of mechanical ventilators during the early stages of the COVID-19 pandemic, a use that may have contributed to a significant number of deaths attributed to COVID-19.[48] The survival rate of COVID-19 patients that required mechanical ventilation after twenty-eight days was estimated to be only 39 percent in the greater New York City area in the first COVID-19 wave in 2020, but this was not different than typically seen with other infectious respiratory diseases that required ICU care.[49]

Patients can be kept on mechanical ventilation for various periods ranging from a few hours (as during surgery) to years. Of note, patients with amyotrophic lateral sclerosis (ALS), also known as Lou Gehrig's disease, often need to be ventilated as the disease progresses.

One consequence of this use of ventilators is that patients may suffer secondary respiratory infections, such as bacterial pneumonia. This is termed ventilator-associated pneumonia (VAP). It can also cause lung damage, lead to a collapsed lung (pneumothorax), and alter heart function. It is noteworthy that most COVID-19 deaths were ultimately due to pneumonia,[50, 51] as were those of the Spanish flu pandemic of 1918.[52]

New York City experienced an unusually high rate of COVID-19 deaths early in the spring of 2020. According to Dr. Joseph Merola, "76.4% of COVID-19 patients (aged 18 to 65) in New York City who were placed on ventilators died. Among patients over age 65 who were vented, the mortality rate was 97.2% . . . But venting COVID patients wasn't recommended because it increased survival. It was to protect health care workers by isolating the virus inside the vent machine."[53] The bacterial infections associated with VAP likely contributed to the high mortality early on during the COVID-19 pandemic. From a study of mechanically ventilated patients, of which 190 had COVID-19, Gao et al. (2023) reported "secondary pneumonia is present in up to 40% and pneumonia or diffuse alveolar damage is present in over 90% of autopsy specimens obtained from patients with acute SARS-CoV-2 infection."[54] The authors further speculated that "a relatively low mortality rate directly attributable to primary SARS-CoV-2 infection is offset by a greater risk of death attributable to unresolving VAP."

14.3. Off-Label Medications

As the COVID-19 pandemic unfolded, the professional colleges regulating doctors, nurses, and pharmacists instructed their members not to use treatments that lacked a college-approved imprimatur. If a patient tested positive for COVID-19 and had symptoms, what was the clinician to do? The message from the professional colleges can be paraphrased as, tell the patient to "go home and isolate, take acetaminophen (Tylenol) for headaches and if/when your lips turn blue, go to the Emergency Department of your local hospital."

This directive to health-care professionals was issued despite reports from around the world that COVID-19 could be treated effectively, especially if it was treated early, using existing, well-known generic drugs that had low to moderate risks if used at the correct dosages and times. It has been hypothesized that using these treatments could have saved most people who died from COVID-19 (perhaps 80 percent of the 7.04 million stated in the WHO's Coronavirus (COVID-19) Dashboard);[55] these treatments would have provided time for new therapies, such as novel antivirals and mRNA "vaccines," to be subjected to the normal widely established safety evaluations. Significantly, using existing drugs would have removed the imperative for fast-tracking the new therapies, which was not in the fiscal interests of the manufacturers of these novel products. One outcome of this discordance was society-wide dismissal of many drugs (e.g., ivermectin), as will be further detailed.

What generic, cheap drugs were effective as early treatment for COVID-19? See drugs in the Forest plot in Figure 14.1 (located in the insert).

Paxlovid, Molnupiravir, Remdesivir, and acetaminophen have been approved by most Canadian professional colleges for symptomatic treatment of COVID-19. Ironically, acetaminophen is one of the few drug treatments to show worsening of COVID-19 symptoms. An explanation for this may be its anti-febrile effect to reduce fever, since elevated body temperatures have an antiviral action as part of the immune response.

Many diverse protocols have been developed by many different doctors using many different drugs; most of the drugs used are from Figure 14.1 (in the insert). Representative doctors, countries, approximate numbers treated, and success (as mortality rate) are shown in Table 14.1.

Table 14.1. Representative doctors and success for treatment of COVID-19 patients. The numbers are based on personal communications that were provided to the Canadian Citizens Care Alliance.

Doctor(s)	Country	Number Patients	Mortality %
Dr. Ira Bernstein	Canada	>1,000	0
Dr. Flavio Cadegiani	Brazil	>3,450	0
Dr. Shankara Chetty	South Africa	>14,000	0
Drs. Bryan Tyson & George Fareed	USA	>20,000	0
Dr. Edward Leyton	Canada	>800	0
Dr. Abdulrahman Mohana	Saudi Arabia	2,733	0
Dr. Carlos Nigro	Brazil	5,000	0.5
Dr. Didier Raoult	France	8,315	0.1
Dr. Vladimir Zelenko	USA	2,200	0.1

Several Canadian doctors have lost their positions/licenses or are under investigation by their professional college for treating COVID-19 patients with off-label drugs. Such medications are those that have already been approved for one purpose, but may have utility for treatment of other illnesses based on new evidence in the scientific literature. As result of these threats of professional discipline, Canadian doctors and nurse practitioners have been reluctant to reveal their data. Unfortunately, many others have simply declined treating patients with COVID-19 as well as those with mRNA vaccine injuries.

Most doctors used combinations of re-purposed drugs shown in Figure 14.1 (in the insert). Ivermectin was used widely in virtually all nations, despite being censored (see subsequent section for full description). Ivermectin was most commonly used for early COVID-19 treatment followed closely by hydroxychloroquine, while vitamin D was the prime example of prophylaxis via immune support. Space limitations in this book do not allow a full description of all therapies used.

14.4. Ivermectin

Ivermectin (IVM) is a cheap medication used for over thirty years and has been given to billions of people as a generic drug, primarily for the treatment of parasitic infections like worms, lice, and mites in humans and livestock. It has also been shown to have antiviral activity against several RNA and DNA viruses, including alphaviruses chikungunya, Avian influenza A, BK polyomavirus, cow herpesvirus 1, dengue virus, Hendra, human immunodeficiency virus type 1, mouse pseudorabies virus, pig circovirus 2, Semliki Forest and Sindbis virus, Venezuelan equine encephalitis, West Nile virus, yellow fever flavivirus, and Zika virus.[56, 57] Early on in 2020, it was reported that ivermectin also inhibited the replication of the SARS-CoV-2 virus in isolated cultured cells.[58]

In view of the wide range of applications of IVM, it appears to have multiple mechanisms of action. For SARS-CoV-2, its proposed activities include: preventing entry of the virus into the cell, anti-inflammatory actions, and additional actions to prevent viral replication and prevention of the complications of the infection. In particular, the anti-inflammatory actions of IVM (notably its ability to dampen the activity of two major inflammatory cytokines, i.e., Tumor necrosis factor-alpha and Interleukin-6 [IL-6]) are critical to reducing the destructive cytokine storm; the severity of which is a critical phase in determining disease severity and recovery.[59]

14.4.1. Ivermectin Efficacy for COVID-19 Treatment

Since the initial reports of IVM's inhibitory effects on SARS-CoV-2 replication, there have been over a hundred studies that support its use for the prevention and treatment of COVID-19. While there have been many individual reports that have been compelling for the effectiveness of IVM,[60] there have been several meta-analyses described by the most experienced and non-conflicted authors that document the effectiveness and safety of IVM for COVID-19 treatment.[61, 62, 63] For example, the second author in the Bryant et al. (2021) review, Dr. Theresa Lawrie, has several Cochrane Collaboration reviews to her credit. These authors concluded that "moderate-certainty evidence finds that large reductions in COVID-19 deaths are possible using ivermectin. Using ivermectin early in the clinical course may reduce numbers progressing to severe disease. The apparent safety and low cost suggest that ivermectin is likely to have a significant impact on the SARS-CoV-2 pandemic globally."[64] A smaller number of meta-analyses type studies of IVM have indicated that it is ineffective, including a Cochrane review by Popp et al. (2022),[65] which relied on only eleven of the published studies on IVM use for treatment of COVID-19. These kinds of meta-analyses have been critically reviewed by Fordham et al. (2021), who identified at least eleven major issues with the Popp et al. Cochrane review.[66] In virtually every study in which IVM did not perform well, conflicts of interest and deficiencies in experimental design protocols could be identified. Examples of the latter are: administration of IVM on an empty stomach to ensure that it stays in the gastrointestinal tract and is not absorbed; under-dosing IVM in obese people that are at higher risk of severe disease; conducting studies in environments in which IVM is freely available to the public resulting in both treated groups and controls taking IVM; and ignoring the status of natural immunity to COVID-19 in participants.

The ACTIV-6 (Accelerating COVID-19 Therapeutic Interventions and Vaccines) trial lower dose IVM arm was published after peer-review.[67] Even only a cursory review of this paper reveals several shortcomings of methodology and statistical analysis that may invalidate the authors' interpretations. Some of these problems included:

A. The treatment drug, IVM, was under-dosed.
   a. The doses were approximated on weight ranges to accommodate for dose per tablet. People at the upper end of the weight range would be under-dosed for the variants circulating at the time.
   b. Maximum dose was capped, leaving patients over eighty-eight kilograms (44 percent of participants) in receipt of inadequate dosing. This was even more problematic for obese patients, because IVM is lipophilic (fat attractive) and distributes into fat tissue, leaving less drug available for therapeutic effect.
   c. Authors instructed patients to take IVM on an empty stomach—"Ivermectin should be taken on an empty stomach with water" (Protocol Section 16.3.3). Taking IVM on an empty stomach is suitable for treatment of intestinal parasites but not systemic diseases, because IVM is lipophilic and administration with a fatty meal facilitates absorption.
   d. IVM following a high-fat meal has resulted in an approximately 2.5-fold higher bioavailability relative to administration in the fasted state.[68]
   e. The lead author of the ACTIV-6 trial acknowledged that there was supporting evidence in the clinical literature for the use of higher doses of IVM as she stated in a video that, "when we looked at the data, frankly we thought it justified a study with a higher dose."[69] Later, a second IVM arm was introduced in the study of 0.6 mg/kg/day for six days.

B. The IVM treatment was delayed or not provided.
   Early treatment (ET) (five days or less following symptom onset) is recognized as a key component for the successful management of COVID-19. Table 1 of the *JAMA* article showed that treatment was not started until a median time of six days following symptom onset.[70] Some patients did not receive their treatment for as long as two weeks after symptom onset, thereby negating the potential benefit of *early* treatment that could have prevented progression to the more severe inflammatory phase of the illness, which required a more aggressive treatment regime.

In her grand rounds presentation, Dr. Naggie acknowledged that the one patient who died in the treatment arm had not received their medication.[71] Of additional concern was that "participants had already consented to participate but had not received [the] study drug, and these participants continued in their assigned study group."[72] Allocating patients to a treatment group when they in fact did not receive treatment skews the results in favor of the placebo group that was without IVM.

C. IVM was used as a monotherapy.
COVID-19 is a multifaceted disease with recognized treatment protocols using multi-drug regimens based on addressing the known underlying pathophysiologic disease mechanisms. However, in ACTIV-6, IVM was used as a monotherapy.

D. Participants in the treatment arm were sicker than those in the placebo arm.
The Supplemental Online Content eTable 1 indicates that a higher proportion of patients assigned to the treatment group experienced severe shortness of breath (dyspnea) compared to the patients assigned to the placebo group.[73]

E. Preprint results show benefit for the IVM treatment arm.
Despite these methodological concerns, a benefit for the treatment arm was evident in the study's preprint. Bayesian statistical analysis was used, and Table 2A in the preprint shows a treatment benefit of 97 percent and 98 percent probabilities on days seven and fourteen, respectively.[74]

F. Conflict of Interest.
The study was funded by the US National Institutes of Health (NIH), which is involved in public-private partnerships with numerous pharmaceutical companies. The lead authors received funding from pharmaceutical companies, including those that make patented antiviral treatments for COVID-19. Interestingly, authors of most of the fewer trials and meta-analyses that concluded that IVM was ineffective had connections to large pharmaceutical companies. Moreover, critical aspects of many such trials rendered them "designed to fail," as described the leader of a small generic company that withdrew from one of the "failed" trials.[75]

The TOGETHER trial, published in the *New England Journal of Medicine* in March 2022, was a large, randomized control trial whose IVM arm has been used by vested interests as conclusive evidence against the use of IVM in COVID-19.[76] Of the many shortcomings identified, the IVM dosage regimen was very problematic; 0.4 mg/kg/day for three days on an empty stomach is clearly inadequate for the reasons described previously. Moreover, the trial was conducted in an area of Brazil where IVM was freely available to control subjects via over-the-counter sales. Even with these design flaws that would deter the detection of positive impacts of IVM treatment, the data nestled in the supplemental section still supported the validity of IVM use in COVID-19. A full critique of this IVM study has been written by Halgas (2022).[77]

The TOGETHER trial's lead authors also received funding from pharmaceutical companies, including those that would financially gain from a preferential marketing and sale of patented antiviral treatments for COVID-19. Regretfully, the public pronouncement of the failure of the TOGETHER trial was made several months before the altered and flawed methodology of the study was finally revealed at the time of publication.[78]

The PRINCIPLE (Platform Randomised Trial of Treatments in the Community for Pandemic and Epidemic Illnesses) study conducted in the United Kingdom is another clinical trial where the investigators claimed that there was no demonstrated meaningful improvement by IVN for COVID-19 in terms of recovery, hospital admissions, or longer-term outcomes.[79] This trial suffered from many of the shortcomings listed previously, including: treatment limited to three days; no more than 0.36 mg/kg/day even for people over eighty-four kilograms in weight; given without food; and commencement of the treatment could begin up to fourteen days after presentation of COVID-19 symptoms as long as they were ongoing (the median was five days after onset of symptoms). About 71 percent of those that received ivermectin had comorbidities. The participants were also given standard treatments, including corticosteroids, and in some cases, monoclonal antibodies and antiviral drugs, which would have confounded the interpretation of the benefits from IVN alone. Nevertheless, as reported by Hayward et al. (2024), "In the SARS-CoV-2 positive primary analysis population, there were 34/2157 (1.6%) COVID-19 related hospitalisations/deaths in the ivermectin group (33 hospitalisations, of whom 2 died, 1 death without hospitalisation), and 144/3256 (4.4%) in the usual care group (143 hospitalisations, of whom 11 died, 1 death without hospitalisation)."[80] These relative risk reductions of 63 percent in hospitalizations and 73 percent in deaths in the IVN group, as well as a 2.06-day shorter recovery period (median of fourteen days in the IVN group and sixteen days in the usual care group) were deemed as not meeting the prescribed cut-offs for a meaningful effect by the authors.

Many examples of IVM mass distribution campaigns—in Mexico City, several states in India, and several Argentinian provinces—have demonstrated rapid population wide decreases in morbidity and mortality, indicating the safety and effectiveness of IVM in all phases of COVID-19.[81] In another recent study conducted with 159,561 subjects in Itajaí, Brazil, 113,845 (71.3 percent) were regular IVM users and 45,716 (23.3 percent) were non-users.[82] Of these, 4,311 IVM users were infected, among which 4,197 were from the city of Itajaí (3.7 percent infection rate), and 3,034 non-IVM users (from Itajaí) were infected (6.6 percent infection rate), with a 44 percent reduction in the COVID-19 incidence rate. Non-use of IVM was associated with a 12.5-fold increase in mortality rate and a seven-fold increased risk of dying from COVID-19 compared to those with IVM treatment.

In early January 2023, MedinCell Pharmaceutical released the data from their SAIVE study (NCT 05305560) that was conducted from March to November 2022.[83] This was a Phase 2, multicenter, randomized, double-blind, placebo-controlled, parallel-group clinical study that evaluated the safety and efficacy of IVM tablets taken orally for twenty-eight days (200 μg/kg on day one then 100 μg/kg daily until day twenty-eight). The study targeted unvaccinated adults who had been exposed to the virus within five days of screening after documented close contact with a person who had a PCR-confirmed SARS-CoV-2 infection. Participants in the IVM group showed no signs of drug safety concerns and experienced a significant 72 percent reduction in laboratory-confirmed infections (thirty/two hundred) versus placebo (105/199), which is a high statistical significance of $p<0.0001$. This only added to the mounting evidence of IVM's significantly favorable level of protection against SARS-CoV-2 infection, especially during the highly transmissible Omicron-variant phase of the pandemic. At least forty countries have officially or unofficially approved IVM usage for treatment of COVID-19.[84]

With respect to the effectiveness of IVM for COVID-19 treatment, the Front Line COVID-19 Critical Care (FLCCC) Alliance website has provided extensive documentation for its utility.[85] Figure 14.2 (found in the insert) is reproduced from the FLCCC website and provides a summary of a meta-analysis of ninety-nine published studies. IVM clearly ranks well above Paxlovid, Molnupiravir, and Remdesivir with respect to effectiveness against COVID-19 from analyses of over ninety-nine studies by the C19early.org group as shown in Figure 14.2. Moreover, its cost is just pennies a day compared with thousands of dollars for the three newer drugs, which are all still protected by patents and approved under Emergency Use Authorization in the United States, with two approved under Interim Order in Canada.

While there remains a lack of consensus on the utility of IVM for COVID-19 treatment among health regulatory agencies, there are nonetheless numerous advocates promoting its use for this indication as demonstrated in the cited literature. Thousands of doctors worldwide have prescribed it for their patients. Multiple organizations, including North American physicians highly experienced in treating COVID-19, i.e., the FLCCC (led by Drs. Paul Marik and Pierre Kory), the British Ivermectin Recommendation Development (BIRD),[86] and the World Council of Health[87] are strong advocates for the use of IVM to treat COVID-19.

14.4.2. Ivermectin Safety for COVID-19 Treatment

IVM has been used internationally for decades, affording the accumulation of a large amount of data related to its potential for toxicity in human use. While there has been controversy with respect to the efficacy of IVM for COVID-19 treatment, there is no dispute about the safety of IVM. Occasionally, IVM side-effects have been noted to include skin rash, nausea, vomiting, diarrhea, hepatotoxicity, and neurologic adverse events (including seizures and confusion). These particular symptoms are more associated with the parasitic die-off when used to treat parasite infections. They would not occur with the treatment of COVID-19, in the absence of a parasite. With over four billion IVM treatments administered, as of June 19, 2023, only twenty-five deaths have been recorded since 1992 according to the WHO.[88] All drugs, including those prescribed for the stated indications for which they are approved, can have side-effects. IVM is clearly one of the best tolerated drugs known. There were no adverse effects in Merck's Phase 1 clinical trial when healthy subjects were administered with IVM at a dosage appropriate for a horse.[89]

In March 2021, Dr. Jacques Descotes published an extensive analysis addressing the toxicity potential of this drug.[90, 91] In his overall summary, Dr. Descotes commented: "Safety analysis of >350 articles show[s] that ivermectin has an excellent safety profile." He noted that "no severe adverse event has been reported in dozens of completed or ongoing studies involving thousands of participants worldwide to evaluate the efficacy of ivermectin against COVID-19."

Further key findings from the Descotes report included:

- Mild to moderate adverse effects of IVM usage have been infrequent and temporary;
- More severe neurological complications are possible with IVM, but are rare and affect susceptible individuals, especially those with severe parasitic disease;
- Serious adverse events relate mainly to the body's efforts to rid itself of an overwhelming parasite load as a result of IVM's therapeutic effects—rather than any potential drug toxicity;
- IVM safety has been confirmed with its long history of therapeutic use, spanning over thirty years.

Dr. Descotes added this statement of particular interest:

> The often-reiterated claim, even today, that ivermectin can be lethal in treated patients only rests on a one-page correspondence to *The Lancet* published in 1997. This claim is deemed to be unfounded as

> it has never been further substantiated until today and instead, subsequent publications repeatedly showed this claim was either incorrect or methodologically inaccurate. ... No severe adverse reactions have seemingly so far been described in relation to off-label studies or clinical trials of ivermectin as a potential prophylactic or curative treatment of COVID-19.[92]

There are many additional resources pointing to extensive IVM safety data:

- IVM has been an approved medication internationally for human use for decades. It continues to be listed on the WHO list of essential medications.[93]
- Safety data of standard doses of IVM is widely established; safety of doses up to ten times the highest FDA approved dose of 200 ⊠g/kg have been well tolerated.[94]
- Adverse events, if they occur, are typically non-severe.[95, 96]
- The ACTIV-6 and TOGETHER trial data found no concerns with safety in their IVM treatment groups.[97, 98]

As documented in Figure 14.1 (found in the insert), IVM is much safer to use than is acetaminophen/Tylenol, which professional health colleges have recommended for management of pain in COVID-19 patients who have been advised to isolate at home. This over-the-counter medication was associated with approximately 186,000 adverse events on the vigiaccess.org website over the same period (October 23, 2022 cumulative since 1992) in which IVM was associated with approximately seven thousand events. Moreover, there is some evidence that acetaminophen prolongs rather than shortens COVID-19; this would be expected on the basis of knowledge that the virus is sensitive to raised temperatures, and acetaminophen lowers elevated temperatures, which would in turn reduce the effectiveness of the immune system to fight infectious diseases.

The use of IVM in some populations remains cautionary. This includes pregnancy, breastfeeding, pediatric patients less than fifteen kilograms, and geriatric patients.[99]

Concerns had been expressed that the demand for IVM for COVID-19 could have resulted in a shortage of the drug available in Canada to treat parasitic infections. Any difficulty that patients may have had in Canada in obtaining IVM for any purpose is the fault of its main supplier, Merck Canada, Inc., and the health-care professional colleges, who worked to actively discourage its use for COVID-19 treatment. While IVM marketed by Merck as Stromectol was out of stock in many Canadian pharmacies, it was readily available in the United States. Moreover, generic IVM was fully available in most other countries, such as in India in the state of Uttar Pradesh, where it was cheaply provided by the authorities in kits for prevention and treatment of COVID-19.[100] From consultation with many Canadian compounding pharmacies, the Canadian Citizens Care Alliance learned that such pharmacies possessed ample supplies of IVM. The pharmacists' main concern was the threats to their licenses issued by the provincial colleges of pharmacy if they filled prescriptions of IVM for COVID-19 treatment. Likewise, doctors that prescribed IVM for their patients were also at risk of disciplinary action from their provincial colleges of physicians and surgeons. The Canadian Citizens Care Alliance's position is that medical and pharmacy colleges should not be barring their members from considering the off-label use of IVM in a multifaceted COVID-19 prevention and early treatment protocol. Of note, the inability of Canadians to obtain IVM legally led to a robust black-market trade in the drug.

Global use of IVM has exploded, with more than half of the states in the United States now recognizing IVM for early treatment of COVID-19,[101] as well as an array of regions around the world, including countries in South America, Japan, India, and the European countries of Germany, Portugal, Ukraine, and Slovakia. As of August 2023, at least 44 percent of fifty sampled countries and 28 percent of the world population have used IVM for COVID-19 prevention and treatment.[102]

14.5. Hydroxychloroquine (HCQ)

In 2020, many people were introduced to HCQ when then US President Donald Trump declared that he was using it for his case of COVID-19. The political situation of the day facilitated the polarization and politicization of HCQ. Former President Trump's praise of HCQ was enough to rally his supporters behind it, while his opponents (read: US Democrats) lined up in opposition. Neither side was particularly well informed about the drug, its prior usages such as prevention and treatment of malaria, and its safety profile.

In various jurisdictions, HCQ became part of the standard of care for patients with COVID-19. For example, Entrenas Castillo et al. (2020) in Spain employed HCQ as "standard care, (per hospital protocol), of a combination of hydroxychloroquine (400 mg every 12 h on the first day, and 200 mg every 12 h for the following 5 days), azithromycin (500 mg orally for 5 days)."[103]

In the same year, other published reports noted the ineffectiveness of HCQ for COVID-19 treatment. The most controversial of these was Mehra et al. (2020), in which the authors stated that they were "unable to confirm a benefit of hydroxychloroquine or chloroquine, . . . on in-hospital outcomes for COVID-19. . . . was associated with decreased in-hospital survival and an increased frequency of ventricular arrhythmias when used for treatment of COVID-19."[104] This led to severe criticism via an open letter published in the journal *Lancet* and signed by over a hundred international doctors and scientists.[105] Subsequently, three of the four authors published their withdrawal of the publication, stating that the owner of the data (Surgisphere) would not provide adequate access to the original details sufficient to address these criticisms.[106]

As of June 2023, HCQ was listed by the FLCCC in their protocol for early treatment of COVID-19.[107] It has not been approved by any of the Canadian professional colleges for COVID-19 treatment.

14.6. Dexamethasone

The anti-inflammatory steroids were the least controversial of all the drugs used in the treatment of COVID-19. In part this was due to their previous application in SARS and MERS, where rapid deterioration or death was partly attributed to the "cytokine storm" discussed in chapter 6.[108] Thus, the immune regulation properties of corticosteroids in treating SARS and MERS helped to pave the way for introduction of these drugs for COVID-19. This does not mean that the corticosteroids were universally accepted. In fact, influential bodies such as the CDC and WHO initially expressed reservations. This was understandable, as it is well known that corticosteroids have substantial adverse effects.

This reservation led to a two-pronged attack on the question of corticosteroid use. There were parties that organized formal clinical trials with proper registration through the ClinicalTrials.gov website. A snapshot in July 2023 revealed ninety-three trials using the search words "COVID-19" and "corticosteroids." There were also many doctors dealing with COVID-19 on a daily basis accepting their professional responsibilities by developing treatment protocols based on their education and experience.

An example of the latter is Dr. Shankara Chetty, a South African family practitioner, who has written an excellent rationale for treating the inflammatory phase of COVID-19 as one would treat well-known hypersensitivity reactions. This was published in the Aug-Sep 2020 edition of *Modern Medicine*.[109] By this time, he had accumulated experience with over two hundred COVID-19 patients that he had treated successfully with a variety of common prescription and non-prescription drugs. With a full range of severity of COVID-19 in this cohort, none died or required oxygen or hospitalization. His treatment protocol included prednisone 50 mg on the first day of treatment with subsequent daily decreases of 5 mg.

Another individual who advanced the treatment charge was Dr. Peter McCullough, who led a substantial number of doctors in writing an approach to COVID-19 titled, "Pathophysiological Basis and Rationale for Early Outpatient Treatment of SARS-CoV-2 (COVID-19) Infection." which was published online on August 7, 2020.[110]

Although Dr. McCullough had impressive academic credentials and appointments, he experienced considerable adverse criticism after presenting his opinions on the prevention and treatment of COVID-19. In the present discussion, the McCullough protocol included the use of dexamethasone "for outpatients starting on day 5 or the onset of respiratory symptoms is prednisone 1 mg/kg given daily for 5 days with or without a subsequent taper."

In one of the clinical investigations of dexamethasone, the RECOVERY trial found that it "reduced deaths by one-third in patients receiving invasive mechanical ventilation" and "by one-fifth in patients receiving oxygen without invasive mechanical ventilation."[111] Although the results of formal clinical trials did not match those of Dr. Chetty, corticosteroids were still seen as useful treatments for COVID-19. Dexamethasone, 6 mg PO/IV daily, was listed by the Ontario Science Table on December 22, 2021 for moderately and critically ill patients. Inhaled budesonide was added for mildly ill COVID-19 subjects by the same group. Alberta Heath Services guidelines stated, "In hospitalized adult patients who meet criteria for severe disease (defined by the IDSA as SpO2 <94% on room air), and requiring supplemental oxygen, mechanical ventilation or extracorporeal membrane oxygenation, clinicians should prescribe dexamethasone 6 mg IV/PO daily for 10 days (or equivalent glucocorticoid dose), or until off oxygen or discharged, whichever is earlier."[112] This contrasts with Dr. Chetty who used these steroids to keep his patients out of the hospital and off oxygen. In British Columbia, the recommendations for hospitalized patients as of October 2023 was "Dexamethasone 6 mg IV/SC/PO q24h for up to 10 days is strongly recommended (RECOVERY trial), ... Hydrocortisone 50 mg IV q6h is recommended as an alternative (REMAP-CAP trial). If dexamethasone and hydrocortisone are not available, methylprednisolone 32 mg IV q24h or prednisone 40 mg PO daily are recommended."[113] It is interesting to note that as of June 2023, Dr. Chetty had treated over fourteen thousand patients without any deaths or hospitalizations, while some provinces have followed the RECOVERY Trial protocol in which "482 of 2,104 patients (22.9%)" died.

The respected FLCCC MATH+ protocols refer to the use of anti-inflammatory corticosteroids (Methylprednisolone), high-dose intravenous Vitamin C (Ascorbic acid), Vitamin B1 (Thiamine), and an anticoagulant (Heparin), plus co-interventions such as antivirals and supplements to treat COVID-19. The "core principle of MATH+ is the use of anti-inflammatory agents to dampen the 'cytokine storms,' together with anticoagulation to limit the microvascular and macrovascular clotting and supplemental oxygen to help overcome the hypoxia." These protocols employed methylprednisolone or prednisone in the pulmonary phase.[114]

In summary, anti-inflammatory corticosteroids have been recommended and used widely for the treatment of COVID-19. While virtually all drugs in the class are useful, the selection of specific drugs depends on many factors, including personal experience, availability, cost, desired route of administration, and duration.

14.7. Remdesivir

When COVID-19 arrived in 2020, the biotech company Gilead was primed and ready—ready in the sense that it already had Remdesivir available for application to the novel viral disease. While Remdesivir had not been successful in the battle against Ebola, there were hopes that it would be the effective antiviral needed for the SARS CoV-2 virus. Remdesivir is an antiviral drug sold under the brand name Veklury by Gilead, who claimed it to be "the first antiviral drug approved to treat COVID-19." While it has been supported by clinical trials, it has several disadvantages, including its high cost of approximately US $3,000 per course of treatment, requirement for intravenous dosing, and significant adverse effects, especially liver and kidney damage.

As early as March 2020, Remdesivir was reported to have good antiviral activity *in vitro* with 50 percent inhibition of growth of SARS-CoV-2 at 1.13 μmoles/liter concentration.[115] By May 2020, a clinical trial of Remdesivir for COVID-19 was reported on hospitalized patients in ten countries.[116] There were 541 participants assigned to Remdesivir, and 521 participants treated with a placebo. The median time from symptom onset to treatment initiation was nine days. With respect to the primary outcome, the Remdesivir group had a shorter time to recovery than patients in the placebo group (median, ten days, as compared with fifteen days, statistically significant $p<0.001$). The FDA issued Emergency Use Authorization (May 1, 2020) for COVID-19 in hospitalized adults and children. The authors acknowledged the limitations of Remdesivir as it did not prevent deaths; all-cause mortality was 11.4 percent with Remdesivir and 15.2 percent with placebo. This is not surprising, because treatment was initiated at nine days, which would be either late in or after the viral replication phase of COVID-19. Several subsequent trials have revealed mixed results for Remdesivir in COVID-19.[117] At best, prevention of death was modest and at worst was negative, as seen with the DisCoVeRy trial.[118] In February 2022, the Association of Medical Microbiology and Infectious Disease Canada (AMMI) Clinical Research Network and the Canadian Critical Care Trials Group assumed the position that "Remdesivir, when compared with standard of care, has a modest but significant effect on outcomes important to patients and health systems, such as the need for mechanical ventilation."[119] On November 22, 2020, the WHO issued a conditional recommendation against the use of Remdesivir in hospitalized patients based on the evidence at that time.[120] On August 5, 2022, the WHO recommended Remdesivir for those at highest risk for severe complications and less than seven days after symptoms started.[121] The Ontario Science Table recommended Remdesivir for the moderately ill on low flow oxygen; it stated further that it "does not appear to be associated with significant adverse effects."[122]

At the end of 2021, some Canadian doctors were using Remdesivir for COVID-19 but seemingly without conviction that it was based on sound evidence. Accordingly, Dr. Zain Chagla, Infectious Diseases, St. Joseph's Hospital, said on X (formerly Twitter) at 9:55 p.m. on December 30, 2021: "We've been giving some high risk mild remdesivir while admitted. Maybe works, maybe makes us feel better?" On the same platform Dr. Isaac Bogoch, an infectious disease physician, on December 31, 2021 stated, "I've been giving it."

In summary, Remdesivir was recommended by various international and Canadian "authorities" for the treatment of COVID-19 in certain circumstances even in the face of poor and sometime negative evidence. The accumulating evidence as shown in the Forest plot in Figure 14.1 (in the insert) revealed that this expensive antiviral drug was far down the list of COVID-19 treatments. It is intriguing how supportive health authorities were for Remdesivir, but quickly dismissed IVM and hydroxychloroquine for COVID-19 treatment, despite much stronger evidence for their effectiveness in scientific, peer-reviewed publications.

14.8. Paxlovid

The Pfizer drug Paxlovid is a combination of nirmatrelvir and ritonavir. Nirmatrelvir works by inhibiting the NSP5/3CL protease of the SARS-CoV-2 virus, which is essential for SARS-CoV-2 replication. Nirmatrelvir is cleared from the body by an enzyme classified as cytochrome P450 3A4. Ritonavir is an inhibitor of this enzyme. Thus, the combination of nirmatrelvir and ritonavir results in better inhibition of the viral protease than nirmatrelvir alone.

In the United States, the FDA issued an Emergency Use Authorization for Paxlovid on December 22, 2021 for the treatment of COVID-19. On January 17, 2022, Health Canada authorized Paxlovid "to treat adults with mild to moderate COVID-19 who are at high risk of progressing to serious disease, including hospitalization or death." By this date, Canada had received the first shipment of 30,400 treatment courses for Paxlovid and had announced plans for the distribution of the drug to provinces and territories.[123] The Government of Canada had secured one million courses of Paxlovid treatments.

In human clinical trials, Paxlovid did not demonstrate an improvement of the disease symptoms of COVID-19 in patients with a standard risk of illness due to SARS-CoV-2 infection. In the EPIC-HR (Evaluation of Protease Inhibition for COVID-19 in High-Risk Patients) study, symptomatic improvement was measured, but it was not reported. Similarly, the interim analysis of the EPIC-HR study revealed that "the novel primary endpoint of self-reported sustained alleviation of all symptoms for four consecutive days as compared to placebo, was not met."[124]

In the EPIC-HR study, Paxlovid was reported to dramatically lower the combined outcome of COVID-19 related hospitalizations (five of 697) or death (zero of 697) compared to placebo (forty-four of 682 hospitalized with nine subsequent deaths) when expressed as a relative risk reduction of 88.9 percent up to twenty-eight days if administered within five days of the onset of symptoms of COVID-19. However, these results are far less impressive when expressed as an absolute risk reduction of less than 6 percent. A Cochrane Review in September 2022 concluded only low-certainty evidence that nirmatrelvir/ritonavir reduced the risk of all-cause mortality and hospital admission or death in unvaccinated patients.[125] Since then, another major clinical study with 1,296 participants tracked for COVID-19 treatment with Paxlovid between August 25, 2021 and July 25, 2022 also concluded that there was marginal benefit with a reduction of the median time for alleviation of all COVID-19 symptoms to twelve days from thirteen days in the placebo controls.[126]

Paxlovid is administered at a dose of 300 mg (two 150 mg tablets) of nirmatrelvir with one 100 mg tablet of ritonavir, given twice daily for five days. There is a significant number of rebound cases of COVID-19 following five-days of initial Paxlovid treatment. In one study conducted during the Omicron period with 11,270 COVID-19 patients, the seven-day and thirty-day COVID-19 rebound rates after Paxlovid treatment were 3.53 percent and 5.40 percent for COVID-19 infection, 2.31 percent and 5.87 percent for COVID-19 symptoms, and 0.44 percent and 0.77 percent for hospitalizations.[127]

Prevention of transmission of SARS-CoV-2 was not included in the EPIC-HR study, and there was no measurable difference in the viral load between the placebo and Paxlovid treatment group at the end of the study, as shown in Figure 3A of the study publication, although the Pfizer press-release indicated a ten-fold reduction in viral load.[128] Thus, suggestions regarding an impact on transmission of clinical significance were not well supported.

In Canada, Paxlovid was recommended only for high-risk patients. In contrast, the EPIC-HR study, which justified Paxlovid use, comprised mostly participants who were not at high risk of developing severe illness.[129] In a February 23, 2022 document, the Ontario Science Table raised this concern, stating "young age and lack of details on concomitant medication use limit study generalizability."[130] Furthermore, the study included only non-vaccinated patients, not the vaccinated, who then comprised the majority of the Canadian population.[131]

The WHO VigiAccess database showed over twenty thousand reported adverse events for Paxlovid by October 28, 2022. This was based on less than one year of reporting, in sharp contrast with IVM, which had fewer than seven thousand reported events after over thirty-five years of use. At the time of introduction, long-term safety data on Paxlovid were not available, as clinical trials had been too short to allow for this information. Another area of concern was adverse effects due to drug interaction, especially with other drugs cleared from the body by cytochrome P450 3A4, as mentioned previously. The Paxlovid monograph produced by Health Canada[132] listed an impressive number of potential drug interactions and other areas of concern for adverse effects.

When the safety concerns are taken into account in conjunction with potential benefit to a select portion of the population, it is not hard to suggest that the utility of Paxlovid for COVID-19 was at most of marginal benefit.

14.9. Molnupiravir

The reluctance of Merck to conduct a clinical trial of IVM, the drug it brought to the world marketplace, was initially surprising because of the profit from increased sales that the company stood to gain. Granted, this profit would have been modest as this drug was already off-patent. Nevertheless, the enhanced reputation and goodwill accruing to Merck would have been substantial.

The rationale for this behavior becomes apparent with a bit of "following the money" investigation. At the beginning of the pandemic, in cooperation with Ridgeback Biotherapeutics, Merck was developing a novel antiviral agent, Molnupiravir (Lagevrio), which was eventually marketed for the treatment of COVID-19. This was facilitated by a grant from the US government of $356 million for the development of Molnupiravir. Subsequently, Merck received a contract to supply this novel antiviral to the US government with a value of US $1.2 billion.

Molnupiravir is an inhibitor of the SARS-CoV-2 RNA-dependent RNA polymerase NSP7/NSP8/NSP12 complex, by binding to NSP12, which renders it potentially useful for the treatment of COVID-19. It works by creating errors in the replication of RNA in viruses, known as lethal mutagenesis. Experiments in cultured cells exposed to different RNA viruses revealed that Molnupiravir was effective against several of these viruses and held promise for activity against viral illness in humans, such as COVID-19.[133] However, as a mutagenic ribonucleoside antiviral agent, there is a hypothetical risk that Molnupiravir might be metabolized by the human host cell and incorporated into the host DNA, leading to genetic mutation.[134]

Clinical trials such as the MOVe-OUT trial were conducted on COVID-19 high-risk, unvaccinated, non-hospitalized adult subjects. The authors reported that Molnupiravir reduced the rate of hospitalization or death by 31 percent compared to placebo.[135] However, this study was undertaken before the emergence of Omicron. The PANORAMIC trial was conducted during a period when the Omicron variants predominated.[136] Subjects in this clinical trial were non-hospitalized adults with COVID-19, at high risk of progressing to severe disease, and most had been administered three or more doses of a COVID-19 vaccine. The outcome was disappointing in that Molnupiravir did not reduce hospitalization or death rates. Nevertheless, Molnupiravir did show some benefit for secondary clinical endpoints as it appeared to speed recovery by an average of four days.

Like Paxlovid, there have been a significant number of rebound cases of COVID-19 following five days of initial Molnupiravir treatment. In a study conducted during the Omicron period with 2,374 COVID-19 patients, the seven-day and thirty-day COVID-19 rebound rates after Molnupiravir treatment were 5.86 percent and 8.59 percent for COVID-19 infection, 3.75 percent and 8.21 percent for COVID-19 symptoms, and 0.84 percent and 1.39 percent for hospitalizations.[137]

Molnupiravir was approved for EUA in the United States on December 23, 2021. However, the approval process in Canada had a different outcome, after its initial filing for approval on August 13, 2021. Public Services and Procurement Canada and the Public Health Agency of Canada secured access to five hundred thousand courses of Molnupiravir on January 17, 2022, prior to any Health Canada approval.[138] The oral tablets were manufactured in Canada but were sold elsewhere.[139] On April 26, 2023, Merck canceled its request for Interim Order approval of Molnupiravir in Canada.[140] It also withdrew its marketing authorization application in the EU on June 27, 2023.[141]

14.10. Monoclonal Antibodies

One of the early strategies to treat COVID-19 was to develop monoclonal antibodies (mAb) that would specifically block the ability of the SARS-CoV-2 virus spike protein to bind to the host target protein ACE2. Several monoclonal antibodies were successfully produced and marketed for COVID-19 treatment. However, with the mutations that occurred in the SARS-CoV-2 variants of concern, which increased the affinity for the spike protein for ACE2, this often reduced the binding ability of many of these therapeutic antibodies for the spike protein and loss of their neutralizing activities. Coupled with the high expense of these commercial antibodies, this has largely resulted in failure and abandonment of this form of COVID-19 treatment. FDA approved broadly neutralizing monoclonal antibodies that were effective against the early SARS-CoV-2 variants, but these agents turned out to be mostly ineffective against Omicron BA.1 with the exception of sotrovimab (Xevudy), and even this monoclonal antibody was poorly effective against Omicron BA.2.[142]

14.11. Cannabinoids

To treat COVID-19 vaccine injuries and neurological complications of SARS-CoV-2, there is a demand for easily accessible natural compounds that can alleviate both the short-term effects and chronic consequences of spike protein exposure. For this purpose, compounds are needed that can disrupt the binding of the spike protein to its host cell receptors, interfere with its systemic distribution, suppress inflammation, reduce the disturbances of metabolism regulation caused by spike protein, and attenuate the potential development of chronic neurodegenerative disease.

The *Cannabis sativa* plant has over five hundred bioactive compounds, including terpenes, cannabinoids, and flavonoids, many of which have well documented anti-inflammatory, antioxidant, and neuroprotective properties. The cannabinoids most widely studied in the medical literature, including cannabidiol (CBD), tetrahydrocannabinol (Δ9-THC) and cannabigerol (CBG), are found in cannabis plants in their acidic forms, as cannabidiolic acid (CBDA), tetrahydrocannabinolic acid (THCA-A), and cannabigerolic acid (CBGA), respectively, each of which have their own unique medicinal properties. Minor cannabinoids such as tetrahydrocannabivarin (THCV) and cannabichromene (CBC), and many more, are also emerging as important medicinal compounds, with their own unique biochemical properties. In addition to cannabinoids, cannabis flavonoids, cannflavin A and cannflavin B, have potent anti-inflammatory properties.[143, 144] Terpenes, such as those associated with flavors in cannabis, like limonene (citrus), α-pinene (pine), and β-caryophyllene (pepper), are present in other plants and have been recognized for their anti-inflammatory, neuro-protective, and anti-oxidant properties.[145]

Cannabinoids impart many of their neuroprotective and anti-inflammatory properties through the cannabinoid receptors CB1 and CB2, which are found abundantly in the neurons of the CNS, and immune cells, respectively.[146, 147] Additionally, some cannabinoids can activate additional receptors (i.e., peroxisome proliferator–activated receptors (PPAR) - alpha and gamma), which have anti-inflammatory and neuroprotective functions and play an important role in metabolism and maintaining health.[148] Because of the biochemical diversity of compounds in *Cannabis sativa* and multiple molecular targets, the plant can provide a multi-targeted approach to treatment of inflammation and a wide range of chronic ailments that have been increasing since the introduction of the COVID-19 pandemic vaccination programs.

14.11.1. Cannabis Compounds Bind SARS-CoV-2 Spike Protein

While the spike glycoprotein remains in circulation, its ability to bind a variety of receptors and a few other proteins becomes a source of persistent stress, inflammation, and metabolic de-regulation. For instance, binding of the spike protein to ACE2 leads to inflammation, mitochondrial fragmentation, and disruption of blood vessels,[149, 150] in addition to downregulation of ACE2,[151] which leads to hypertension (i.e., high blood pressure).[152] Full-length spike protein can bind to the protein fibrin and its precursor fibrinogen found in blood plasma, and initiate abnormal blood clots that are more resistant to degradation, thus evoking a coagulatory cascade that can impede blood circulation as well as trigger fibrin-induced inflammatory responses and production of reactive oxygen species that can mutate DNA and damage proteins.[153]

Several compounds from cannabis can bind spike protein and prevent its interaction with its receptor ACE2. The acidic cannabinoids, CBDA, CBGA, and THCA-A, can bind to S1 subunit of the SARS-CoV-2 spike protein.[154] CBDA and CBGA are able to block entry of pseudoviruses engineered to present the SARS-CoV-2 spike protein into cells grown in cultures,[155] as does β-caryophyllene (BCP),[156] which is a terpene present in cannabis and other plants. Importantly, these compounds have no psychoactive effects and negligible toxicity, making them good candidates for treatment of chronic conditions linked to spike protein exposure.

14.11.2. Cannabis Compounds Suppress Exosome Trafficking and Promote Autophagy

Exosomes are extracellular vesicles that export RNA, proteins, and signaling molecules from cells. While exosomes play an important part in cell-to-cell communication, they can also contribute to disease progression by exporting pathogenic RNA and proteins from diseased cells to healthy cells in other parts of the body. In vaccinated individuals, circulating exosomes carrying spike protein are evident fourteen days after vaccination and persist for months, contributing to systemic distribution and prolonged exposure of various body organs and tissues to spike protein.[157] When spike protein is produced in cells in culture, it leads to increased exosome release and altered exosomal cargo that can lead to deregulation of microglia cells (resident macrophage immune cells that are found in the brain and spinal cord), which contribute to central nervous system inflammation and damage.[158] CBD and Δ9-THC were shown to suppress the release of exosomes carrying pathogenic proteins from HIV-infected cells, (a process linked to neurocognitive decline known as HIV-associated dementia),[159] and CBD was shown to inhibit exosome trafficking from several cancer cell lines.[160] These findings indicate that these cannabinoids could play a role to reduce the release of exosomes that may contribute to pathogenesis.

CBD can enhance autophagy,[161, 162, 163] which is a vital degradative and recycling process required for turnover of damaged and harmful cell components, misfolded proteins, and pathogens. Impaired autophagy is a driver of neurodegenerative disease progression, as it leads to accumulation of misfolded protein aggregates, such as amyloid-β plaques in Alzheimer's, α-synuclein in Parkinson's, mutant superoxide dismutase in amyotrophic lateral sclerosis (ALS), and huntingtin protein in Huntington's diseases.[164] Spike glycoprotein can de-regulate autophagy. Inflammatory responses triggered by spike protein were shown to drive autophagy, leading to excess cell death through programmed cell suicide known as apoptosis,[165] but in some cases spike protein can impair autophagy, leading to accumulation of toxins in cells.[166] As in SARS-CoV-2-infected cells, autophagy can play an important role in degrading spike protein in vaccine-transformed cells and therefore prevent export of this pathogenic protein via exosomes. Therapeutic effects of cannabinoids (Δ9-THC and CBD), through activation of autophagy, have been documented in several cancer models,[167, 168, 169, 170] and their autophagy-driven neuroprotective action has been demonstrated in animal models of Alzheimer's [171, 172] and Parkinsons' diseases.[173, 174] Furthermore, cannabinoids' ability to enhance autophagy can promote neuronal health and longevity.[175, 176] Increase in autophagic flux, driven by cannabinoid receptor (CB2) activation, has been shown to reduce inflammation after neuronal injury[177] and autoimmune encephalomyelitis,[178] by driving degradation of pro-inflammatory cytokines. In addition to CB2, autophagy can be activated by CB1,[179] PPAR-gamma,[180] and PPAR-alpha receptors,[181] indicating other cannabis compounds may have a positive impact on autophagy.

14.11.3. Cannabis Compounds with Anti-inflammatory Properties

Spike glycoprotein can trigger the inflammatory cascades associated with severe COVID-19 by driving release of pro-inflammatory cytokines and chemokines,[182, 183] as well as the production of highly reactive oxygen species (ROS), including superoxide anion (O_2-), hydrogen peroxide (H_2O_2), and the hydroxyl radical (HO•).[184, 185] ROS cause mutations in DNA and damage to proteins and lipids. Cytokine release leads to activation of pro-inflammatory enzymes, such as those that are important for production of prostaglandins and nitric oxide, respectively, leading to oxidative stress, pain, and inflammation.[186, 187] Spike protein can activate several pro-inflammatory signaling pathways,[188, 189, 190] which further increases cytokine and chemokine production and release, as well as the recruitment of leukocytes to the site of inflammation.

Cannabis compounds have a wide range of anti-inflammatory and immune modulatory properties that subdue acute and chronic inflammation. Cannabinoids can suppress production of ROS and pro-inflammatory cytokines, such as tumor necrosis factor-alpha (TNF-α), interferon-gamma (IFN-gamma) and interleukins (IL) IL-1β, IL-6, and IL-8.[191] In a recent study, crude cannabis extract, high in CBD, CBG, THCV, and several terpenes, was shown to suppress production of pro-inflammatory cytokines, in lung epithelial cell lines, treated with TNF-α, to simulate inflammatory conditions observed during SARS-CoV2 infection.[192] In another study Δ9-THC and CBD-rich cannabis preparations were able to quell inflammation in lung fibroblast cells, by downregulating expression of inflammatory mediators (e.g., TNF-α and IL-6) associated with SARS-CoV-2-induced inflammation and autoimmunity.[193] In human cell lines that model the intestinal epithelium (e.g., Caco-2 cells) and express ACE2, cannabidiol prevented spike protein-induced cytotoxicity, and significantly reduced production of pro-inflammatory cytokines, including TNF-α, IL-1β, IL-6, and IL-18. Additionally, cannabidiol suppressed spike protein-driven increase in toll-like receptor 4 (TLR4) and ACE2 expression.[194] CBG, CBD, and Δ9-THC suppress immune-cell infiltration in a variety of tissues, by reducing production of chemokines and adhesion molecules that facilitate their migration.[195, 196] Δ9-THC can promote the apoptosis of immune T cells, which can ameliorate autoimmune and neurodegenerative conditions.[197] The terpene BCP, which has a wide range of antioxidant and anti-inflammatory properties, has been demonstrated to have protective actions in a wide range of ailments, including autoimmune and neurodegenerative disease, as well as heart, pulmonary, and vascular inflammation.[198] BCP can attenuate release of inflammatory cytokines associated with COVID-19 and spike protein[199] and was recently used in a formulation to treat long COVID patients, with significant reduction in multiple symptoms in 72–84 percent of tested participants.[200]

14.11.4. Cannabis Compounds Alleviate Symptoms of Neuropsychological Disorders

Spike protein-driven inflammation, hypertension, and disruption of the blood-brain barrier render the nervous system vulnerable to the development of chronic inflammatory conditions that can lead to neurodegenerative disease. The S1 subunit of the spike protein can cross the blood-brain barrier[201] and accumulate in the brain,[202] cause damage to brain endothelium,[203] and trigger microglia activation and oxidative stress,[204, 205] as well as protein misfolding and aggregation.[206] Microglia-driven neuroinflammation and build-up of plaque from misfolded protein aggregates cause neurological damage and disease progression in many neurodegenerative conditions, including multiple sclerosis (MS), amyotropic lateral sclerosis (ALS), Parkinson's, Alzheimer's, and Huntington's diseases.

Several clinical trials showed that cannabis, particularly Δ9-THC and CBD, improved symptoms of spasticity and reduced pain and motor dysfunction in MS patients.[207, 208] SATIVEX (a one-to-one CBD and Δ9-THC formulation) has been approved for treatment of MS symptoms since 2005.[209] Δ9-THC and CBD were shown to have benefits for Alzheimer's disease, alleviating learning impairment in animal models and reducing amyloid and tau plaque accumulation, as well as microglia activation and inflammation.[210, 211, 212] Anti-inflammatory effects of CBD were also reported in animal models for autoimmune encephalomyelitis and MS, along with inhibition of pathogenic T cells, and observable reduction in MS-like symptoms.[213] In Parkinson's disease patients, although CBD did not ameliorate motor dysfunction, it was shown to improve quality of life[214] and alleviate psychotic symptoms.[215] In the case of Alzheimer's disease, a cross-sectional survey showed that CBD is effective for management of behavioral symptoms.[216] These observations indicate that there may be utility of cannabis for treatment of neurological symptoms arising from Long COVID and COVID-19 vaccine injury.

As with all natural compounds, caution must be exercised when employing cannabis to treat patients, because of deleterious side-effects such as immune-suppression and intoxication, as well as interactions with other drugs. Cannabis research has been plagued with prohibitive legal status, biochemical inconsistency between strains and cultivars, and differences in experimental conditions. For these reasons, many studies have been conducted with synthetic agonists and blockers of cannabinoid receptors and molecular targets. While this approach can be effective in understanding the molecular underpinnings of endocannabinoid signaling, it fails to capture the synergistic actions of medicinal compounds found in this plant, which has a history of medical use going back as far as five thousand years.[217]

14.12. Vitamin D3

14.12.1. General Requirements for Vitamin D3

Before the arrival of COVID-19, vitamin D3 (vit D3) was known for its role in bone health and as the "sunshine vitamin" due to its production in skin from exposure to sunlight. This pro-hormone not only regulates calcium and bone balance, but also plays a pivotal role in modulating the immune system. What was not universally known was the vitamin's importance for combating viral diseases, such as COVID-19.

Vitamin D comes in two major forms, vit D2 (ergocalciferol) and vit D3 (cholecalciferol) (vit D3). Vit D2 is derived from ergosterol found in plants and fungi, while vit D3 is produced in the skin upon exposure to UVB radiation and is therefore found in animal products. Vit D3 is inactive when it is made in the skin or even when it is taken as a supplement and absorbed into the bloodstream. Both forms require conversion to calcitriol (1,25-$(OH)_2$Vit D3) to become biologically active.

Prior to discussing the relationship between vit D3 and COVID-19, it may be helpful to review useful background information, much of which was described by Dr. Glenville Jones, a Canadian biochemist.[218] Vit D3 is formed from products of the cholesterol biosynthetic pathway through the actions of enzymes as shown in Figure 14.3, which can be found in the insert.

7-dehydrocholesterol is acted upon by sunlight (UVB) and body heat to create vit D3 (cholecalciferol), which is inactive. It must be activated by metabolism, first to calcifediol (25-hydroxyvitamin D3) by the liver and calcitriol (1,25-dihydroxyvitamin D3) by the kidney. The first activation step is rate-limiting and takes about a week to ten days. This means that it will take almost two weeks to achieve the acute benefit of treatment with substantial doses of this vitamin. Calcitriol can be inactivated by further hydroxylation by a 24-hydroxylase enzyme to calcitroic acid. Apparently, induction of the 24-hydoxylase and excessive sunlight are capable of inactivation and preventing the accumulation of excessive quantities of the active 1,25 (OH)2 vit D3. The half-life of calcitriol is very short, typically six to eight hours.[219]

Natural dietary sources include fatty fish (e.g., salmon, mackerel, and sardines), cod liver oil, and specific mushrooms, like shiitake. Plants are also a source of vitamin D, usually in the form of vitamin D2 (ergocalciferol). In some countries like the United States and Canada, certain products, such as dairy products, are fortified with vitamin D to support bone health.[220] Dietary intake typically supplies less than 20 percent of daily vitamin D. Dietary vitamin D is initially absorbed in the small intestine and bound to chylomicrons where it is transported to the lymphatic vessels, where it is further transported into the circulation bound to vitamin D binding protein (VDBP). Ultimately, individuals' vitamin D status varies widely, influenced by factors such as genetics, geographic location, skin pigmentation, lifestyle choices, and dietary habits.[221]

Most Canadians are vit D3 deficient as described in a review of sixteen studies by Schwalfenberg et al. (2010).[222] They documented that 70–97 percent of Canadians were vit D3 insufficient (less than 72–80 nmol/L) and 14–16 percent were clearly deficient (less than 25–40 nmol/liter). It is widely accepted that north of the thirty-fifth parallel, there is insufficient UVB exposure from October through March to allow the skin to make vit D3. This leads to a vit D3 insufficiency season. Clearly, for Canadians to maintain optimal vit D3 health, it is necessary to consume supplementary vit D3. Since this review was written, it has become apparent that the amount of vit D3 required for optimal immune health is even greater than the standard used in 2013. A requirement of 100 to 150 nmol/liter appears to be the level of calcifidiol needed for optimal functioning of the immune system. To attain these concentrations, most people must take much more that the 800 IU currently recommended by Health Canada. The doses used for optimizing the immune system range from 3000 IU to more than 10,000 IU daily, depending upon the individual.

Vit D3's benefits go well beyond bone health. In their review, Gröber et al. (2013) summarized the roles of vit D3 in a number of functions beyond bone health.[223] Diseases associated with vitamin D deficiency include autoimmune diseases (multiple sclerosis, type 1 diabetes), inflammatory bowel disease (Crohn's disease), systemic lupus erythematosus (SLE), infections (such as infections of the upper respiratory tract), immune deficiency, cardiovascular diseases (hypertension, heart failure, sudden cardiac death), cancer (colon cancer, breast cancer, non-Hodgkin's lymphoma), and neurocognitive disorders (Alzheimer's disease).[224] This is fully consistent with the information that has accrued about the distribution of vit D3 receptors in tissues since they were discovered half a century ago.

Vit D3 acts as an immunomodulator that aids infected lungs by improving both innate and adaptive immune responses and downregulating inflammatory cascades that can be lethal in COVID-19.[225] Importantly, certain immunological cells (leukocytes) like monocytes, macrophages, and dendritic cells are able to convert inactive calcidiol to active calcitriol locally for immunomodulation.[226] Moreover, numerous leukocyte types, particularly T-lymphocytes and macrophages, have high expression of the vitamin D receptor (VDR). Vit D's effects vary depending on the cell type and activation status. For example, it enhances antimicrobial peptide production in monocytes and macrophages, aiding in pathogen defense.[227, 228, 229] In dendritic cells, vit D promotes a less differentiated and more tolerogenic phenotype, supporting immunological tolerance—i.e., tolerance to self-antigens and beneficial microbiota.[230] Vit D also influences T cells by modulating the function of antigen-presenting cell (APCs) including dendritic cells, suppressing self-reactive T cells, and activating regulatory T cells (Tregs).[231] B cell differentiation and function are also influenced by vitamin D, contributing to immune system homeostasis[232, 233, 234] Vit D's ability to stimulate anti-inflammatory cytokines like TGF-β and IL-4 may also suppress hyperactive T cell responses implicated in these diseases thereby supporting the healing process.[235]

In the context of COVID-19, a germane property of vit D3 is its antiviral action. Vitamin D promotes the activity of both the adaptive immune response and the innate immune response. One mechanism by which the innate antiviral effect is enhanced is through up-regulation of cathelicidin and defensin, which are antiviral and anti-microbial peptides.

14.12.2. Vitamin D3 for COVID-19 Treatment

Vit D3 appears to be prophylactic against infectious diseases, although this is qualified by acknowledging the limitations of the studies attempting to address the question. Unlike normal drug trials, there can be no vit D3-free placebo groups for comparison to those supplemented with vit D3. Many of the studies compare groups of subjects based on levels of vit D3 sufficiency. Unfortunately, the circulating levels of vit D3 used to define sufficiency varied among the research groups.

It is crucial to recognize that recommended daily vit D intake guidelines are primarily focused on bone health, not immune function. Vit D's role in immune system support indicates higher doses may be necessary during immune challenges.[236] Current guidelines do not account for the metabolic demands of an active immune response. While vit D toxicity is a concern, studies have shown that doses up to 10,000 IU/day are safe for most individuals, especially during infections.[237] Including vitamin K2 with vit D is becoming more widely accepted due to their proposed synergy in contributing to bone and cardiovascular health, as well as lowering any adverse calcification that might be due to higher levels of vit D, alone.[238] Higher doses of vitamin D have also successfully been used in research studies (see Table 14–1). Individual factors like obesity, diet, and skin type influence the threshold for efficacy and toxicity, and assessing serum 25(OH)D concentrations can provide a more accurate measure of vitamin D status, with levels above 100 nmol/liter being associated with optimal immune and overall health.[239] Various companies, including the Canadian company, ImmunoCeutica Inc. (www.immunoceutica.ca), now offer vit D testing, using a convenient mail-order home test kit. This is important to empower individuals to determine if they are adequately supplementing for their geographical location, skin color, genetic makeup, time of year, and so on. For example, supplemental doses may need to be increased in fall and winter when light levels are lower, particularly in the Northern hemisphere.

A running meta-analysis of vit D3 for COVID-19 prophylaxis has been maintained in the www.c19early.org website by the c19 group and dedicated to COVID-19 early treatment.[240] The overall conclusion, after reviewing multiple studies on vit D3, is that ensuring sufficiency in vit D3 results in a 50 percent or greater reduction in the probability of contracting COVID-19. An example of such a report is that of Abdollahi et al. (2020), who conducted a case-control study with 201 patients and 201 matched controls in Iran and showed that vit D3 sufficiency was associated with a 53.9 percent decrease in cases ($p=0.001$).[241] In a study conducted in England, involving 80,670 participants, the median serum 25-hydroxyvitamin D in non-hospitalized participants with COVID-19 was 50.0 nmol/liter versus 35.0 nmol/liter in those admitted with COVID-19 ($p<0.005$).[242] Hospital admissions were 2.3- to 2.4-times higher among those with serum 25-hydroxyvitamin D less than 50 nmol/liter.

Borshe et al. (2021), in their recent review, addressed the question of whether low vit D3 is caused by COVID-19 infection, or whether vit D3 deficiency predisposes to the disease.[243] They included studies in which patients' pre-infection vit D3 levels were documented, and some in which vit D3 levels up to the day after hospitalization were recorded. Their analysis revealed a significant (p=0.019) negative correlation between vit D3 pre-infection concentrations and mortality. Extrapolation of the regression line to the X-axis showed that the risk of death virtually disappears at 125 nmol/liter (50 ng/milliliter). Using vit D3 in this manner may offer prophylaxis equivalent to that claimed by the mRNA and adenovirus vaccinations without the waning off effect reported with the genetically modified RNA injections. This also indicates that our numerical standard of vit D3 sufficiency should be increased.

Multiple studies indicate that vit D3 improved treatment of COVID-19. Two studies conducted in Spain illustrated the effectiveness of treating infected patients with calcifidiol (aka calcidiol or 25-OH vit D3). In a retrospective study, seventy-nine patients treated with calcidiol had a lower risk of death, as four of the seventy-nine (5.1 pecent) calcidiol-treated subjects died compared with ninety of 458 (19.7 percent) untreated subjects, which indicates that the treatment prevented approximately 80 percent of death in this study.[244]

In an earlier randomized clinical study, Castillo et al. (2020) found that calcidiol treatment in a smaller cohort resulted in no COVID-19 deaths in fifty treated subjects, while there were two deaths in the twenty-six untreated controls from COVID-19.[245] Moreover, only one of the twenty-six calcidiol-treated patients was admitted to ICU compared with thirteen of twenty-six of the control patients. Note that in both successful studies, an activated form of vit D3 was used.

In a recent review by Sartini et al. (2024), they concluded that "vitamin D supplementation (~5,000 IU daily) was associated with 40–60 percent reduced risks of COVID-19 and a 69 percent reduced chance of ICU admission."[246] There have also been reported trials in which no benefit of vit D3 was observed when treating active cases of COVID-19, and this has sometimes been highlighted by people who subscribe to the idea that vaccines are the only way out of the pandemic. Unfortunately, the form of vit D3 used in the failed trials was vit D3 *per se*. This is the inactive form that takes several days to be activated and useful.

In one such unblinded, clinical trial that was conducted in the United Kingdom between May and October 2021, Joliffe et al. (2022) randomized 3,100 participants (median age of sixty years) to a vit D test and either high dose (3,200 IU/day) or low dose (800 IU/day) of vit D3 for six months if their initial blood 25-hydroxyvitamin D concentrations were less than 75 nmol/liter.[247] Another 3,100 controls received no test and no supplementation. They reported that neither dose of vit D had any effect on the incidence of COVID-19 compared to those without vit D3 supplementation. One of the issues with this trial was that participants were aware whether they were receiving vit D supplements or not. About half of the untreated controls also took at least one vit D3 supplement on their own during the testing period. Another issue was that the study was conducted between May and October of 2020, when sunshine levels would have ensured the natural production of vit D3. The study was also conducted during a period in which there were relatively low COVID-19 cases in the United Kingdom, i.e., between their first and second COVID-19 waves.[248]

In a Norwegian study conducted between November 2020 and June 2021, 34,741 participants were randomized to take either five milliliters of cod liver oil (a surrogate for low dose [400 IU/day] vit D supplementation) or five milliliters of placebo oil (corn oil) daily for six months.[249] The authors reported no effect of cod liver oil on any outcome, including PCR-confirmed COVID-19. However, Norwegians have a very high fish diet, including salmon, which is high in vit D. Most participants (75.5 percent) did not use vit D supplements before enrolling in the trial, but 61.5 percent consumed fatty fish, and 59 percent reported greater than thirty hours of exposure to the sun from July to October 2020. Between a hundred and 160 days in Fig. 2 of the publication there appeared to be a slight reduction (12.5 percent) with the cod liver oil supplementation on the probability of being infected by SARS-CoV-2, but the vit D3 levels were only increased on average by 4.4 percent in this group following this supplementation. About 86 percent of the trial participants had 25-hydroxyvitamin D levels greater than or equal to 50 nmol/liter to begin with.

Considering the significance of vit D3, it is disappointing that not one of the political or mainstream medicine leaders who was contacted about vit D3 in 2020 was willing to give serious consideration to its use. Given the recent history of vit D3 for overall health and immune health in particular, public health could have informed citizens about this important nutrient at a time of great need.

14.12.3. Current Status of Vit D3 and COVID-19

There are abundant data showing a strong relationship between vit D3 status of individuals and their susceptibility to COVID-19.[250] While it would have been desirable to have more randomized, double-blinded clinical trials showing that vit D3 supplementation was prophylactic, it can be argued that it would be unethical to wait for this. With such delays, people may have unnecessarily gotten sick and died. Unfortunately, no pharmaceutical company was willing to sponsor clinical studies to test this off-patent nutrient. Promotion of supplementary vit D (equal or greater than 2000 IU/day) should have been promoted for the Canadian population by the health establishment rather than discouraged.

Vit D is a standout immunoceutical with multifaceted immunomodulatory properties. Its influence spans the innate and adaptive immune systems, contributing to immune defense, immune tolerance, and reduced risk of autoimmune diseases and cancers. Understanding its importance in maintaining immune health, and considering individual factors, can guide appropriate vitamin D dosing strategies for optimal immune support. If political and mainstream medical leaders had advocated to Canadians the efficacy of vit D3 sufficiency when the "pandemic" was declared, as opined by various researchers such as Brenner and Schottker,[251] morbidity and mortality could have been reduced by 90 percent. The cost for vit D3 supplementation would have been pennies a day and ordinary citizens may well have paid for it themselves. The cost of testing for vit D3 levels would have been minimal compared to the cost of vaccines and PCR tests. The economic savings of protecting the public from COVID-19 could have been immense.

14.13. Boosting the Immune System with Nutraceuticals

When COVID-19 was declared a pandemic, the authorities had little to offer citizens in terms of prevention and treatment. Concerned that there would be overwhelming numbers of cases, they promoted the slogan "flatten the curve," meaning that cases would be spread out over longer periods, thus preventing the collapse of hospital services. There was little discussion of the medical treatments that could be offered. Nor was there much encouragement by health officials for the population to eat healthier and exercise, even though obesity and diabetes were major risk factors for severe COVID-19. But there was ample discussion of the need for more mechanical ventilation.

This concept, coupled with the creation of fear through incessant broadcasting of COVID-19 cases, hospitalizations, and deaths, led many people to consider complementary and alternative medicine for solutions. One of the sources mined for options was nutritional therapy or nutraceuticals. People looked for nutrients that had the potential to bolster their immune systems. Such nutrients may be referred to as "immunoceuticals," which is a fusion of the words "immunity" and "pharmaceutical," describing a subset of nutraceuticals with proven immunomodulatory mechanisms.

Immunoceuticals are a special class of nutraceutical with the potential to optimize an individual's immune-competence. As described earlier, vit D would be an excellent example. These substances span beyond mere nutrition, demonstrating therapeutic potential when consumed at specific concentrations. These compounds optimize immune function and modify immunological status, making them valuable in defending against diseases like cancer, infections, and autoimmune disorders. Immunoceuticals encompass a wide range of substances including, but not limited to, vitamin D3, fungal β-glucans, plant-derived ergosterols, flavonols, terpenoids, carotenoids, aloe-associated polysaccharides, quercetin, omega-3 fatty acids, melatonin, and micronutrient elements like zinc and selenium. Despite structural differences and distinct modes of action, all immunoceuticals work toward optimizing the function of the immune system. The term "optimize" is used here rather than "enhance," since in some cases it is not desirable to enhance but rather attenuate excessive immunological responses.

Assessing immunocompetence is vital in understanding the effectiveness of immunoceuticals. Various methods, including counts of the various leukocyte subsets, cytokine profiling, and T cell and antibody assays can determine an individual's immune status. These tests help evaluate the need for immunomodulation and the impact of specific immunoceuticals on the function of the immune system.

At the same time, it became apparent that a major factor in COVID-19 pathology was an overactive, hyperinflammatory immune system as demonstrated with "cytokine storms" in advanced COVID-19. Thus, it was essential to optimize the immune response and not simply boost it. The immune system is a sophisticated complex comprising myriad cell types, chemicals, and signaling molecules that have been addressed in chapter 7.

Many aspects of immunology are still under active investigation and much remains to be elucidated. An important development of the last two decades has been a greater appreciation for the role of the microbiome—the total collection of microbes that live on and in our bodies. The story of how the microbiome interacts with the immune system may remain incomplete for many years to come.

As a result of the developing knowledge regarding the microbiome and immune systems, the public was left to fend for themselves to find nutraceuticals to protect themselves against a newly recognized virus. But they had another source of knowledge, which is not widely appreciated or respected by mainstream medicine—traditional or folk remedies. Many of these possessed properties associated with nutrition and also pharmaceuticals, which compelled the search for nutraceuticals that worked against COVID-19.

As described elsewhere in this book, two key properties that are beneficial in combating COVID-19 are antiviral and anti-inflammatory activities. These are important to keep in mind while reading the following section.

14.13.1. Sources of Nutraceutical Information

For Canadians, a leading source of information was the FLCCC, founded in March 2020 by leading US critical care specialists, including Drs. Paul Marik and Pierre Kory. Its purpose was to help prevent and treat COVID-19. This was followed by the Canadian Citizens Care Alliance (CCCA), whose mission was to provide Canadians with balanced, evidence-based information on COVID-19. These are just two of many sources of information used by Canadians who sought knowledge about nutraceuticals and other treatments for the prevention and treatment of COVID-19.

14.13.2. Plethora of Nutraceuticals

The FLCCC website identified a large number of nutraceuticals that were claimed to be effective for COVID-19.[252] The list included the following: vitamins A, B, C, D, and K, vitamins B7 (biotin), B9 (folate) and B12, ashwaganda, berberine, bromelain, Coenzyme Q10, curcumin (turmeric), dandelion, elderberry, ginger, honeysuckle, iron, magnesium, melatonin, N-acetyl cysteine (NAC), Nigella sativa, Omega 3 fatty acids, probiotics, quercetin, reservatrol, selenium, spermidine, L-theanine, and zinc.

The C19early.org website described many re-purposed drugs and nutraceuticals including: *Nigella sativa*, cannabidiol, curcumin, lactoferrin, life style (exercise, sleep, diet, sun), melatonin, minerals (zinc, selenium), quercetin, and vitamins A, B9, C, and D.

14.13.3. Specific Nutraceuticals

Not all of the nutraceuticals mentioned have benefited users to the same extent and space limitations restrict this subsection to an exemplary selection of substances. The following describes some of the nutraceuticals that were used for COVID-19. (Vit D has already been described). Note that all of the substances named in this section are supported by peer-reviewed publications. While this list may seem exhaustive, not every nutrient has been included that has proven to be beneficial against COVID-19.

Curcumin gives the spice known as turmeric its brilliant yellow color and is a bioactive compound credited for the pharmacological properties of turmeric. Curcumin is known for its potent anti-inflammatory and antioxidant properties.[253] Curcumin can suppress NF-κB-regulated inflammatory genes implicated in conditions like osteoarthritis. It can also inhibit NF-κB activation and reduce IL-8 production in human macrophages exposed to cigarette smoke.[254] However, the impact of curcumin on inflammation can vary. Some studies showed no significant change in inflammation markers or cytokine levels.[255] Conversely, other studies show that it can ameliorate intestinal inflammation and improve gut barrier function.[256] Additionally, curcumin can influence gut microbiota and modulate the TLR4 signaling pathway, ultimately enhancing intestinal immune function.[257]

Kaempferol is a flavonol that exhibits significant immunomodulatory and anti-inflammatory properties and is found in a wide variety of fruits and vegetables. It inhibits the NF-kB regulatory pathway involved in immune cell activation, reduces the release of various inflammatory cytokines, and affects enzymes involved in prostaglandin and leukotriene production.[258] It also has immunomodulatory effects on dendritic cells, disrupting key signaling pathways and activating anti-inflammatory transcription factors like PPARγ.[259]

Melatonin is a hormone produced by the pineal gland in the brain, and it plays a role in regulating the circadian basis of the sleep-wake cycle. It is often used as a supplement to promote sleep. Various peer-reviewed publications have reported health benefits in COVID-19, including less thrombosis, sepsis, and death.[260]

Quercetin is a flavonol that entered the pandemic with a strong reputation in the alternative medicine world as a well-known antioxidant that can be beneficial in various ailments through its broad-spectrum anti-inflammatory, antioxidant, antiviral, anticoagulant, and immune-modulatory properties. Its dietary sources include citrus fruits, apples, berries, onions, parsley, sage, tea, and red wine.[261] Any time a health benefit can be garnered from fermented grapes, wine drinkers are happy to embrace it. One of the more important properties of quercetin appears to be its ability to facilitate the transport of zinc into cells, i.e., it is a zinc ionophore and enhances the antiviral effect of zinc.

Quercetin reduces inflammation by inhibiting key regulatory pathways in cells that mediate inflammation and also by enhancing the production of the anti-inflammatory cytokine IL-10, while inhibiting pro-inflammatory proteins like IL-1β and TNF-α. Additionally, quercetin influences the expression of adhesion molecules and reduces inflammation-related tissue damage. Quercetin directly inhibits enzymes like cyclooxygenase (COX) and lipoxygenase (LOX) (which produce prostaglandins and leukotrienes, respectively), down-regulates nitric oxide production, and influences the maturation of dendritic cells, thus affecting antigen uptake and cytokine secretion. Furthermore, quercetin exhibits anti-allergic properties by stabilizing mast cell membranes and inhibiting histamine release, making it useful for treating allergic inflammatory diseases.[262]

Resveratrol gained much attention as the health benefitting component of red wine. Although it is a component of grape skins, it is also found naturally in berries and peanuts, and plants like white hellebore. It protects cells from oxidative stress and shows promise in preventing conditions such as cancer, inflammation, and diabetes. However, it also exhibits immunosuppressive activities, affecting leukocyte function. Resveratrol can down-regulate inappropriate immune responses by inhibiting the activity of T cells and B cells, leading to reduced proliferation, antibody production, and cytokine secretion.[263, 264] In the context of COVID-19, it possesses both anti-inflammatory characteristics and inhibits the replication of SARS CoV-2.[265, 266]

Zinc is the second most abundant metal in the human body and is necessary for numerous functions within cells, including enzyme cofactor action and intracellular structure. Its anti-inflammatory, antiviral, and antioxidant actions are relevant in the treatment of COVID-19. Zinc was a component of the highly successful Zelenko protocol for treatment of COVID-19.[267] While the Zelenko protocol was highly successful, it required azithromycin and hydroxychloroquine in addition to zinc. COVID-19 patients who did not have access to doctors willing to prescribe these medicines could avail themselves of a pseudo-Zelenko approach by using the nutraceutical combination of zinc plus quercetin. More details of the actions of zinc are described by Derwand et al. (2020)[268] and many other publications.

Selenium is an essential mineral important for many body functions, but its role in treating or preventing COVID-19 does not equate to that of zinc. Studies abound relating selenium deficiencies to sub-optimal health in the face of diseases like COVID-19. For example, Moghaddam et al. (2020) conducted a small study in which the selenium status was higher in surviving COVID-19 inpatients (n = 27) compared to those that died (n = 6).[269] Selenium deficiency has been associated with a variety of viral illnesses.[270] Given this background, it is not surprising that selenium has been used in attempts to prevent or treat COVID-19.

N-Acetylcysteine (NAC) has been used for decades in the laboratory as an anti-oxidant, because it provides cells with precursors for the synthesis of glutathione, an essential cellular anti-oxidant. It is generally regarded as safe and regulated in the United States as a dietary supplement. Its reputation as a mucolytic (to breakdown and thin mucus), antioxidant, antiviral, antithrombotic modulator of the immune and inflammatory response was sufficient to entice many people to use NAC with or without medical supervision.[271]

Nigella sativa, sold widely in Canada as black cumin, is a remedy that has been used in traditional medicine for centuries, especially in China and other parts of Asia. Some of its applications have been for the treatment of diarrhea, indigestion, appetite loss (stomachic), rheumatoid arthritis, edema, dysmenorrhea, and amenorrhea. In the context of COVID-19, its historical use for inflammatory diseases of the airways, such as asthma and bronchitis, attracted the attention of those infected with SARS CoV-2.[272]

Vitamin A is of interest in pulmonary infections, in part because of its role in the development of normal lung tissue and tissue repair after infection injury.[273] It is also known to have immune regulatory functions affecting both the innate and adaptive immune responses. Vitamin A deficiency can compromise antibody-forming cells and immunoglobulin development in the upper and lower respiratory tracts. Conversely, vitamin A supplementation can reduce the risks of severe illness with measles and influenza. Therefore, it was not surprising that the public would respond to the COVID-19 pandemic by purchasing over-the-counter dietary vitamin A.

Vitamin C (ascorbic acid) is a water-soluble vitamin that is essential for various bodily functions, including immune system support, collagen synthesis, antioxidant protection, and iron absorption. It is found widely in various fruits and vegetables; it promotes a perception of overall well-being and optimal health. Vitamin C gained public prominence during the 1970s when Nobel Laureate Linus Pauling disseminated his ideas that the vitamin could cure or at least shorten the common cold and even enhance intelligence. Although Pauling's ideas have not been confirmed by subsequent clinical trials, the legacy of vitamin C being valuable for respiratory tract infections remains to this day.[274] This has resulted in citizens supplementing with vitamin C for COVID-19 and other respiratory tract infections.

The use of high dose, intravenous vitamin C has produced inconsistent results with some groups reporting benefits[275] and others being less enthusiastic.[276]

14.13.4. Medicinal Mushrooms

The use of medicinal mushrooms is a practice rooted in Chinese traditional medicine dating back to 200–300 AD and has gained significant recognition in modern times. The global mushroom market is growing and is projected to grow at an annual growth rate of 9.7 percent from 2022 to 2030.[277] Notable medicinal mushroom species include *Lentinula edodes* (shiitake), *Grifola frondosa* (maitaki), *Flammulina velutipes* (enoki), *Pleurotus spp* (oyster), *Ganoderma lucidum* (reishi), and *Trametes versic*olor (turkeytail). While *Ganoderma lucidum* and *Trametes versicolor* may not be palatable due to their bitterness and texture, they have been used medicinally as hot water extracts.[278]

Lentinan, which is derived from shiitake mushrooms, is a 1,3 β-glucan cell wall component that activates various cells of the immune system, including macrophages, dendritic cells, neutrophils, NK cells, and lymphocytes through pattern recognition receptors such as Dectin-1 and toll-like receptors.[279, 280] Through these pathways, lentinan induces the production of inflammatory cytokines, phagocytosis, and reactive oxygen species, which have the ability to destroy pathogens.

Krestin (PSK) is a β-glucan complexed with polysaccharopeptide (PSP) from *Trametes versicolor*, which possess the ability to boost white blood cell counts and cytokine production, with PSP primarily inducing pro-inflammatory cytokines like TNF-α and IL-12.[281] PSP also enhances T cell proliferation and activation, which can contribute to cell-mediated immunity. PSK also helps restore immune system balance following immunological depression caused by tumor burden, or chemotherapy. PSK stimulates cytokine gene expression, including TNF-α, IL-1β, IL-6, and IL-8, which contribute to immune responses against tumors, antibody production, and T lymphocyte activities[282, 283] Both PSP and PSK exhibit extensive *in vitro* anticancer activity against human cancer cell lines, and also show similar activity in human clinical trials.[284]

14.13.5. Probiotics

Probiotics are live organisms that can be taken into the body to alter the microbiome—that collection of bacteria, viruses, and other microbes that live in and on humans, primarily in the gut. The microbiome, also known as the resident flora, is critical to health, especially when it is maintained in balance, because it destroys many substances that are detrimental and creates many others substances that are beneficial. The term probiotics is generally taken to mean a mixture of (usually) bacteria that are intended to change the intestinal microbiome in a beneficial way. Investigations have reported ambivalent results regarding their use in the treatment of COVID-19.

Nevertheless, probiotics have entered the world of mainstream medicine for the treatment of resistant intestinal infections due to *Clostridium difficile*; when a fecal microbiota transplant (donor fecal matter) is placed in the recipient colon, the success rate for this procedure is as high as 90 percent.[285]

It now appears that the term probiotic is inadequate to describe developments in the understanding of the interaction between the immune system and living organisms. Some members of the CCCA have facilitated a way forward by explaining the evolving nomenclature. Drs. Bridle, Karrow, and Mallard define immunoceuticals as "nutraceuticals that demonstrate immunomodulatory mechanisms" and immunobiotics as microbial strains that can regulate the mucosal immune system.[286]

Australian Dr. Robert Clancy and his colleagues have been developing a strain of bacteria, Non-Typable Hemophilus influenza (NTHi), for oral administration that results in increased protective activity of the innate immune system of the bronchi. Their strategy involves the creation of tablets containing significant doses of NTHi, which are delivered to Peyer's patches on the small intestine. This results in activation of T cells that migrate to the bronchial mucosa to induce enhanced activity of the mucosal immune system therein.[287] The latter is not a vaccine but may be superior when applied to large populations, because it is selective in activation and non-selective in effect. Dr. Clancy has suggested that this oral tablet might be taken a few times each winter to protect one against a variety of airborne infections. Because it enhances the mucosal immune system, it should protect against both bacteria and viruses. If NTHi fulfills this potential, it might obviate the rollout of novel mRNA "vaccines" for several viruses, including the RSV (respiratory syncytial virus).

14.13.6. Is There a Unifying Theme?

Nutraceuticals are valuable therapeutics, especially when access to mainstream medicine becomes limited or unavailable. A question that might arise is why is there such a variety of compounds with some beneficial effect in the treatment of COVID-19? This has been addressed in the CCCA article "Stress proteins in COVID-19: Is carbon monoxide formed by heme oxygenase important in drug therapy?"[288] Prior to his retirement, one of the coauthors (Dr. Kanji Nakatsu) of this chapter conducted research in carbon monoxide and heme oxygenase pharmacology at Queen's University. Heme oxygenase is anti-inflammatory by virtue of breaking down heme into carbon monoxide and bilirubin/biliverdin. Many different chemicals have the ability to increase the amount of heme oxygenase in the body (enzyme induction); consequently, they have anti-inflammatory properties.

According to Dr. Nakatsu, curcumin, resveratrol, quercetin, and melatonin are all known to increase heme oxygenase activity. They are among the nutraceuticals with anti-inflammatory properties and are useful in COVID-19 treatment as described by Kunnumakkara et al. (2021).[289]

14.14. Preventative Measures with Gargles and Nasal Sprays

The aforementioned treatments and measures may be effective early on in the treatment of an active SARS-CoV-2 infection, and proper hygiene will be helpful in reducing potential exposures to the virus in the environment. Another strategy is to mitigate the virus at the site of entry into the body, i.e., the nose and mouth.

The FLCCC recommends the use of an antiseptic antimicrobial mouthwash to reduce the viral load:[290] "Gargle twice daily (do not swallow. Choose mouthwashes containing chlorhexidine, povidone-iodine, cetylpyridinium chloride (e.g., Scope™, Act™, Crest™), or the combination of eucalyptus, menthol, and thymol (e.g., Listerine™)."

The FLCCC also recommends the use of a nasal spray such as Betadine.

In Canada, Vancouver-based biotech company SaNOtize developed a patented nitric oxide (NO) releasing solution platform technology (NORS™), which was used to create a nasal spray that has been proven in clinical trials to reduce viral loads of SARS-CoV-2, influenza, RSV, and other viruses by greater than 99 percent in less than two minutes. Nitric oxide, a naturally occurring antimicrobial molecule in the human body, possesses known antiviral properties.

Although Health Canada approved initial testing of the SaNOtize NO nasal spray (NONS) in April 2020, securing institutional participation and lengthy institutional review board delays resulted in delays in commencement of trials until the fall of 2020 in Quebec. This trial involved 103 individuals utilizing the NONS five times daily for fourteen consecutive days, with forty individuals receiving standard care. Regrettably, from a study perspective, no participants in either group tested positive for COVID-19. Nevertheless, from a safety standpoint, over seven thousand self-administered treatments revealed no drug-related adverse effects. NONS demonstrated a commendable safety profile.

Over the next eighteen months, SaNOtize continued to conduct studies to further validate the safety and antiviral efficacy of NONS. In a randomized, double-blind, placebo-controlled Phase 2 clinical trial conducted in the United Kingdom, seventy-nine patients with mild COVID-19 infections received NONS over nine days. The results were promising, with early NONS treatment significantly reducing SARS-CoV-2 viral loads, even in patients with high viral loads. Within seventy-two hours, the viral load dropped by over 99 percent, and 47 percent of NONS users reported feeling better after four days compared to only 8 percent in the placebo group. No serious adverse effects were observed among the thirty-nine participants who received NONS.[291]

Based on these encouraging findings, NONS was approved as a medical device in the European Union, Israel, Bahrain, Thailand, and marketed under the names Enovid™ and VirX™. Despite its low NO concentrations and topical effects in the nasal cavity, regulatory agencies in Canada and the United States classified NONS as a prescription drug due to nitric oxide's previous approval for selective pulmonary vasodilation to treat full-term infants. This classification, coupled with agencies' insistence on using hospitalization or death as clinical endpoints during the vaccine era, posed substantial hurdles for a small pharma-tech company like SaNOtize to obtain approval. Despite approaching the Canadian innovation fund three times during the pandemic, SaNOtize received no financial support.

In 2021, a Phase 3 randomized double-blind placebo-controlled trial with NONS in 306 non-hospitalized patients with mild COVID-19 infection was undertaken in India.[292] The SaNOtize NO nasal spray produced reductions in PCR-tested SARS-CoV-2 levels to below detection in four days as compared to eight days for this endpoint in participants treated with a placebo control. These compelling data led India's Central Drugs Standard Control Organization (CDSCO) to grant emergency use approval for NONS on February 9, 2022 for treating adult COVID-19 patients at risk of disease progression. The product continues to be marketed in India and Southeast Asia as FabiSray™.

Following the UK study, NONS was approved as VirX™ in Thailand. A study conducted at Srinakharinwirot University in Thailand demonstrated this product's effectiveness in preventing COVID-19 infection, with statistically significant results favoring its use.[293] In this observational preventative study with 625 participants, VirX^{TM} demonstrated a relative risk reduction of SARS-CoV-2 infection by 75 percent, and an absolute risk reduction of 19.2 percent.

In summary, a Canadian company developed an antiviral nasal spray that swiftly reduces initial viral loads of all SARS-CoV-2 variants. Retrospectively, the product could have halved quarantine times and protected the majority of individuals in close contact with COVID-19 cases. Additionally, it could have served as a bridge to protect high-risk individuals between vaccine upgrades for new variants with many of the vaccines showing low efficacy as previously documented. Unfortunately, challenges in finding manufacturing, clinical support, and financial backing in Canada led to foreign manufacturing, funding, and clinical trials. Despite approval in fifteen countries worldwide, NONS remains unavailable in Canada and the United States due to practical and financial barriers imposed by current regulatory requirements for a small biopharma company.

14.15. Concluding Remarks

Given this chapter's material, it is difficult to avoid the conclusion that several treatment options existed for COVID-19 prior to the release of the EUA/Interim Order vaccines. Indeed, many of these treatments were well established for treating viral infections, including for COVID-19. These treatments should also have been explored in greater detail and likely would have been had it not been for the obsession on the part of the medical establishment, government, and media that only vaccines would return the world to "normal." Such pronouncements were seemingly the result of some fixed agenda that may have had little to do with health.

An important consideration is the costs of COVID-19 treatments for implementation in the community. Choices should reflect the need for equitable and positive patient outcomes from safe products at a sustainable and efficient cost. The C19early.org website, which performed real-time analysis of over 3,156 studies, has estimated the costs per treatment of many of the aforementioned medications, which are summarized in Table 14.2. As many of the cheaper alternatives were relatively inexpensive medications and vitamins with proven safety records, it is unconscionable that they were dismissed so easily and actively vilified by public health officials.

Table 14.2. Cost per life saved. COVID-19 treatment cost times the median NNT (number needed to treat) from studies reporting mortality results with calculable NNT. The costs are provided in US dollars and are estimated based on widespread distribution by governments. Based on data presented from the C19early.org website.[294]

Treatment	Treatment Cost (US $)	Number of Hospitalization Studies	Hospitalization Studies Number of Patients	% Reduced Hospitalization	Number of Mortality Studies	Mortality Studies Number of Patients	% Reduced Mortality
Melatonin	8	3	366	19	9	2,054	48
Vitamin D	10	23	86,202	20	66	63,148	36
Vitamin C	14	14	18,349	16	38	45,489	20
Zinc	16	14	6,454	19	20	13,290	29
Ivermectin	24	29	44,784	34	51	122,827	49
Hydroxychloroquine	27	16	50,759	41	250	380,893	25
Alkalinization	28	2	134	39	5	954	42
Vitamin A	30	5	6,373	10	6	441	42
Colchicine	31	17	12,405	17	39	29,219	33
Aspirin	41	9	12,578	-2	59	159,603	11
Curcumin	59	12	13,478	27	8	714	63
Famotidine	94	6	587	15	20	86,617	19
Probiotics	99	5	890	13	8	1	61
Quercetin	127	3	301	48	5	790	61
Metformin	163	20	85,983	18	55	196,283	32
Antiandrogens	175	15	8,854	30	33	113,013	38
Nigella Sativa	279	5	1,410	34	4	1,192	73
Nitazoxanide	680	6	1,864	61	6	1,877	42
Budesonide	887	2	1,578	44	11	20,597	26
Favipiravir	1,258	20	6,562	-4	36	23,835	14
Fluvoxamine	1,283	12	6,712	26	9	4,976	43
Paxlovid	46,111	14	48,708	37	18	53,217	45
Molnupiravir	137,653	18	79,431	2	15	83,307	23
Casirivimab/ imdevimab	181,694	12	46,106	42	8	32,929	40
Bamlanivimab/ etesevimab	269,237	11	28,252	39	11	29,105	59
Sotrovimab	352,800	6	14,171	37	10	16,383	49
Remdesivir	549,014	8	5,979	-5	51	154,591	11
Bebtelovimab	737,601	5	12,858	33	4	12,478	60
Tixagevimab/ cilgavimab	14,894,456	7	13,390	56	6	15,721	36
Conv. Plasma	N/A	12	3,290	4	41	23,179	0
Acetaminophen	N/A	4	704	-34	14	144,648	-24

The means by which "regulatory capture" of mainstream medicine and media and the connivance of governments have exacerbated the pandemic and has led to needless deaths is a topic for our next book.

CHAPTER 15

The Past, Present, and Future of COVID-19: Lessons Learned

Christopher A. Shaw

"People will forgive you for being wrong, but will never forgive you for being right."

—Thomas Sowell

"It was their choice and nobody ever was going to force anyone into doing something they don't want to do [speaking about people who are not vaccinated against COVID-19]. *But there are consequences when you don't. You cannot choose to put at risk your co-workers. You cannot choose to put at risk the people sitting beside you on an airplane."*

—Justin Trudeau, CBC Radio, The House, June 25, 2022

According to Epimenides, a Cretan, an "aporia" is an irresolvable internal contradiction or logical disjunction in a text, argument, or theory; for example: ". . . the celebrated aporia whereby a Cretan declares all Cretans to be liars."

It would be challenging to find another statement, distinct from the above by the prime minister of Canada, that better typifies what an aporia sounds like. Indeed, this one statement contains two such aporias. The first aporia: The prime minister, one who prides himself on being "progressive" (whatever that term means anymore), who extols the COVID-19 vaccines as being the "*only way out of the pandemic*" and who spouted the usual "*safe and effective*" mantra, before demanding that everyone take them or face various restrictions and punishments. Justin Trudeau's claim that it was people's "choice" to take or not take the vaccines was hardly a real choice given that it came with severe consequences for those who hoped to follow their own medical and social path. The Nuremburg code was developed as a consequence of the forced experimentation on Jewish and other prisoners in World War II by the Nazis. As the

Nuremburg Code clearly specifies, the concept of "informed consent" does not permit coercion or pressure to be used, no matter if the coercion involves either rewards or punishments.[1]

The second aporia: The vaccines, according to Trudeau and the government of Canada (and until recently virtually all the mainstream media) was that the vaccines are safe and effective, period. But if they are so effective, how would an unvaccinated person possibly become a "risk [to] the [vaccinated] people sitting beside you on an airplane"? The short answer, as has been well-documented in the preceding chapters, is that Trudeau's statement arises from a profound misunderstanding of science and the actual data, the latter which clearly show that those vaccinated can both become infected again and transmit the disease. Yet, here it is, a prime minister of a supposedly educated country spouting utter nonsense, presumably as a political ploy.

Justin Trudeau's comments might simply reflect the tendentious views of a politician running for re-election by using the unvaccinated as convenient scapegoats to score cheap points against his political adversaries without any apparent regard for the overall health of the nation. The same can be said of President Joe Biden in the United States and other heads of government, particularly those "young global leaders" that the World Economic Forum (WEF) has been training for the organization's purposes.

As clearly demonstrated in this book, and in numerous peer-reviewed studies over the last three years, the COVID-19 mRNA vaccines are not effective, hence the apparent need for endless boosters. One hallmark, at least theoretically, for conventional vaccines (i.e., non-mRNA vaccine platforms) is that they are intended to stop disease transmission to the vaccine recipient and to their intended or unintentional contacts. Hence, a two-handed aporia.

As for the vaccines being safe, in chapter 13 it was clearly shown that the opposite is true. They are not safe for many people and only time will tell how many people will be adversely affected. Thus, the "choice" that many made to not accept the COVID-19 vaccines, the choice that got them banished from much of society and which saw unvaccinated Canadians unable to leave their own country, was, in reality, a very valid health and freedom choice based on the most fundamental of all natural rights, i.e., security of the person.

This book has demonstrated that, along with the official aporia, much of what governments and their health agencies stated during the pandemic was simply untrue. Indeed, not only were many of the statements false, but they were often deliberately false, fitting the now widespread distinction between "misinformation" and "disinformation."

The information gaps were apparent in the computer models developed to evaluate the level of harm that the pandemic might cause. Not only were the models simply wrong, but they were so wrong as to leave little doubt that they were designed to elicit fear propaganda, rather than be accurate predictors of COVID-19 pandemic outcomes.

In other words, much of what citizens were told by their governments about COVID-19, in Canada and elsewhere, consisted of outright lies. The powers that be withheld and suppressed data, instead choosing their selected sources to bolster the pre-selected narrative. The fact that this narrative was wildly inaccurate never seems to have crossed the minds of Justin Trudeau, those in his government, or officials in most Western governments until more recently. In Canada, provincial health officers were apparently less concerned with overall health as they brought in endless mandates and restrictions, many of which also had wider negative health, economic, and social consequences.

As discussed in chapter 14.4 and 14.5, some of the reports that ivermectin or hydroxychloroquine were ineffective and harmful were literal frauds that led to very beneficial treatments not being more widely adopted. The simple reason for not using them, based on scientific fraud, provided the COVID-19 genetic vaccine companies (Moderna, Pfizer, Johnson and Johnson, and AstraZeneca) the means to escape the problem of potentially competing treatment options in order to get Interim Order approval in Canada or Emergency Use Authorization (EUA) in the United States for their vaccines. It seems likely that the decision to not use ivermectin or hydroxychloroquine contributed to many avoidable deaths associated with COVID-19.

There are compelling reasons to believe that the SARS-CoV-2 virus most likely originated from the Wuhan Institute of Virology after it was almost certainly manipulated by gain-of-function (GoF) research to make the coronavirus more transmissible, if not more pathogenic. Crucially, the manufacturers of the various experimental mRNA COVID-19 vaccines knew from *in vivo* animal biodistribution studies that the mRNA construct with its lipid nanoparticle coating would be distributed in multiple organ systems, including the central and peripheral nervous system. This could be a grave concern for the future as the short- or long-term consequences of these molecules passing into neural cells are still unknown. Nevertheless, there are strong initiatives now in process to expand the use of mRNA for other infectious diseases in both humans and livestock.

In regard to the pathophysiology of COVID-19 and some of the numerous adverse effects that have arisen from the vaccines,[2] myocarditis and myopericarditis have probably gained the highest public profile.[3] Moreover, the full extent of this damage is not known, because the total extent of cardiac harm may not become appreciated for decades.

Nevertheless, these adverse effects on the heart as well as highly aggressive cancer, "brain fog," and a host of cognitive issues, as cited in previous chapters, pale in comparison to the potential effect of the mRNA injections on human reproduction. Given their accumulation in reproductive organs and the already apparent decrease in birth rates, these lipid nanoparticle-enclosed genetic materials may be capable of further accelerating the forecasted world population decline.[4] In some circles, this is reason for great concern—see "The Great People Shortage is coming—and it's going to cause global economic and social chaos."[5]

It may not only be the mRNA construct that is concerning, but also what happens to the spike protein generated by the mRNA when it infects cells, or what might happen when mRNA, DNA, or protein fragments are involved as they surely are (see chapter 11.3.7) or if any of these molecules wind up in exosomes. Nevertheless, the whole mRNA/lipid nanoparticle platform is being quickly adopted for implementation of the development of new vaccines in humans and livestock, where the body has been hijacked to manufacture the proteins of infectious pathogens.

The overall consequences of the public health response to COVID-19 for society, quite apart from the health consequences, were widespread and may indeed be the most daunting long-term consequences of the pandemic. Some of these have included the social impacts on children, the elderly, and those with comorbid conditions. Members of society from the police, military, commercial airline pilots, medical staff, ferry workers, and many more have all been negatively affected. Insofar as the adverse effects of the vaccines, citizens and governments may have to contemplate how we continue to function as a society when a significant fraction of the population, some in essential occupations, become chronically ill.

Perhaps worse, what has and will happen to that fundamental feature of any society: trust. Trust in institutions, including political structures, the financial system, the medical and legal fields, and the mainstream media are the inevitable long-term casualties of the pandemic response, arguably vastly more severe in both short- and long-term consequences than the pandemic itself. In brief, all of these entities have suffered a justifiable loss of trust by a considerable fraction of the population. Inevitably, as more people and their friends and relatives are harmed by the medical measures imposed during the pandemic, the backlash will grow. As an aside, it is clear that the scientific fields that have been so badly manipulated during the pandemic, such as vaccinology, epidemiology, and immunology, have routinely failed to bring the scientific perspective needed to understand the disease and its potential treatments. These disciplines, previously considered as scientifically sound, have significant flaws with a huge number of fundamentals of each field shown to be based on unsupported assumptions.

This book has served to highlight only some of the deficiencies that presently abound in our institutions that perform biomedical research, develop and regulate new preventative and therapeutic treatments, and disseminate the findings to those engaged in health care. These institutions include academia, industry, government, and the media.

COVID-19 pandemic parallels to the film *V for Vendetta* were posed in the preface of this volume. The point was made that citizens at large, with their complacency and willingness to defer to authorities, were at fault for the society that transpired. Now that the dust has begun to settle down on the whole COVID-19 affair and greater clarity is possible, we can recognize that a lot of work will be needed to restore these institutions before such trust can be earned once more.

This book has largely dealt with the actual, versus assumed, science of COVID-19. We hope that it will be a useful resource for politicians, health-care professionals, lawyers, and media reporters that seek to restore the integrity and effectiveness of our institutions before the next opportunistic pandemic is declared. We particularly hope that it will help non-scientists understand these issues. In order to help, we have tried to clarify the more complex aspects by defining terms and creating a glossary. Lastly, as noted previously, the damage done to our social institutions, medical, political, legal, etc. may turn out to be vastly more perilous to our collective future than the disease itself.

It is the hope of the diverse authors of this book that our efforts here will serve to alert and educate the public for the future. Our conviction is that only from true knowledge will come the ability and the resolve to prevent a recurrence of the last four years so that our children will never again have to face such a collective assault on their freedom through ignorance, fear, and greed. In the next volume from the CCCA, we will delve more deeply into the politics of COVID-19.

Author Profiles

Dr. Philip Britz-McKibbin

Full Professor in the Department of Chemistry and Chemical Biology at McMaster University BSc in Chemistry (University of Toronto); PhD in Analytical Chemistry (University of British Columbia)

Dr. Britz-McKibbin undertook a Japan Society for Promotion of Science PDF position in Japan (Hyogo University, 2001–2003) prior to starting his academic position at McMaster University. His research group is an affiliate member of The Metabolomics Innovation Centre (TMIC)—Canada's national metabolomics laboratory. His research interests in bio-analytical chemistry, separation science, mass spectrometry, and metabolomics include the design of novel analytical strategies to identify and quantify unknown metabolites of clinical significance in complex biological samples via untargeted profiling. Dr. Britz-McKibbin's laboratory aims to discover objective biomarkers that support early detection and prevention of chronic diseases with emphasis on improved newborn screening programs for cystic fibrosis. His research interests include the development of high throughput screening methods for large-scale epidemiological studies to better understand the roles of modifiable dietary habits and chemical exposures on human health outcomes. He has authored more than 130 scientific publications.

Glenn Chan

Patient-Advocate, BAA in Radio and Television Arts (Ryerson University)
Mr. Chan was injured by his second shot of Pfizer-BioNTech BNT162b2 in June 2021. He could not walk more than five minutes without experiencing a flaring of symptoms. In addition, he lost his ability to multi-task and lacked the cognitive capacity to engage in computer programming. As he faced limited access to health care in Ontario, he adopted the *Dallas Buyers Club* approach and obtained access to treatment options. Fortunately, he was lucky enough to recover most of his health. Having gone through the lived experience of vaccine injury, he has applied his Python data analysis skills to patient-led surveys that investigated the Post-COVID Vaccination Syndrome from which he suffered. In addition to patient-led research, he maintains resources for the vaccine injured at LongHaulWiki.com.

Dr. Claudia Chaufan

Associate Professor in the School of Health Policy and Management at York University MD (National University of Buenos Aires); BA in Community Studies and Journalism (University of California Santa Cruz); MA and PhD in Sociology/ Philosophy (University of California Santa Cruz)

Dr. Chaufan was trained as a physician in Argentina, and after a decade in medical practice, and upon earning her PhD in Sociology/Philosophy at the University of California, transitioned to an academic career in the social sciences. She is an associate professor of Health Policy and Global Health at York University. She previously held the positions of graduate program director in health and as a Fulbright Scholar in Public/Global Health. She has published widely in her field of expertise with over fifty-two research articles and commentaries in peer-review journals, five books, and four book chapters, and serves as an editorial board member and ad-hoc reviewer of leading refereed journals. As a sociologist specialized in health, illness, and the institutions of medicine/public health, and informed by her training in medicine, she works in the tradition of critical social, health, and policy studies. She teaches and researches comparative health policy, the geopolitics of global health, medicalization, and social control, and critical pedagogy in higher education. Her research engages the implications of expert health narratives for perceptions of disease risk, practices of stigmatization, strategies of legitimation, and policies of exclusion. Her current projects include the politics of sanctions policy, the geopolitics of Anti-Asian racism, and medical social control in the COVID-19 era. She is also an active member of the Canadian Academics for Covid Ethics.

Dr. Stefan Eberspaecher

Chiropractor (clinical practice), Project Manager for development of an interdisciplinary clinic in Ottawa BSc in Psychology (University of Guelph); Doctor of Chiropractic degree (Canadian Memorial Chiropractic College)

Dr. Eberspaecher has extensive experience implementing health-care programs in developing nations, including working with local health-care systems, governments, and communities. His peer-reviewed publications focus on the development and implementation of sustainable, evidence-based models of care for musculoskeletal conditions. He recently served as a member of the Peer Review Group for the World Health Organization's Rehab 2030 packages for Low Back Pain, Osteoarthritis, Rheumatoid Arthritis, and Fractures. After seeing the extreme psychological and physical toll the public health measures and the associated barrage of propaganda were taking on his patients and the broader community, he became active with the Canadian Citizens Care Alliance in 2021.

Dr. L. Maria Gutschi

Research Pharmacist, Drug Assessor, Hospital Pharmacy Manager, Antimicrobial Stewardship BScPhm (University of Toronto); Doctor of Pharmacy (Wayne State University)

Dr. Gutschi is an expert pharmacotherapeutic specialist with extensive experience in evidence-based medicine, critical care, antimicrobial therapy, mentoring, and teaching pharmaceutical care. She has been involved in pharmaceutical drug assessment and formulary management, and the preparation of educational materials and research reports for the Canadian Pharmacist Association and for regulatory agencies. She has been employed as a scientific officer for the Patented Medicines Prices Review Board in Canada, and as a clinical pharmacist for the Canadian Forces Health Service Centre, Canada Chemists, and the North West Company at Hawkesbury District and General Hospital.

Dr. Ondrej Halgas

Lead Protein Scientist at Liven Proteins BSc and MSc in Biochemistry (Comenius University in Bratislava); PhD in Structural Biology and Biomedical Research (University of Toronto)

Dr. Halgas is pursuing postdoctoral training at the University of Toronto and is a lead scientist at the biotech start-up company Liven Proteins. He has been involved in numerous international collaborative projects in areas of cancer and infectious diseases (particularly prion diseases and tropical diseases—trypanosomiases). His protein structure of a novel anti-cancer target with a drug that is being tested in numerous clinical trials was featured on the cover of prestigious scientific journal *Cancer Cell.* He has been very active since early 2021 in promoting early COVID-19 treatment, particularly the use of repurposed medications in Slovakia and Canada.

Dr. John Hardie

Retired, Oral Pathologist, Bachelor of Dental Surgery (University of Glasgow); MSc in General and Anatomic Pathology, (University of Western Ontario); PhD Thesis: "AIDS, Dentistry and the Illusion of Infection Control," Mellen University; Fellow of the Royal College of Dentists Canada

Dr. Hardie completed the necessary fellowship examinations to qualify as a consultant in Oral Pathology and Oral Medicine, which resulted in positions as the head of dentistry at the Ottawa Civic Hospital and Vancouver General Hospital. He served in a similar capacity at hospitals and health trusts in Saudi Arabia and Northern Ireland. In 1983, he became aware of the developing controversies associated with HIV/AIDS and published the first paper in the world to discuss the effect of systemic immunodeficiency on oral and dental diseases.

From the mid-1980s to the mid-1990s he was a spokesperson on HIV/AIDS for the Canadian Dental Association and represented Canada on this topic at meetings of the Centers for Disease Control and Prevention in Atlanta, Georgia. For the past thirty years, he has lectured throughout the world on the transmission of infectious diseases within clinical environments and related topics. He has published more than two hundred articles on oral diseases, and infection prevention and control. In 2000, Dr. Hardie was commissioned by the Royal College of Dental Surgeons of Ontario to prepare "A Literature Review, Recommendations and Guidelines Regarding Infection Control in the Dental Office." Although he has retired from clinical practice, he remains interested in the transmission of infectious diseases and has continued to publish in this area.

Dr. York N. Hsiang

Retired, Full Professor in the Department of Surgery at the University of British Columbia MB; ChB in General and Vascular Surgery (University of British Columbia); MHSc in Healthcare and Epidemiology (University of British Columbia); FRCSC

Dr. Hsiang completed a research fellowship at Harbor-University of California Los Angeles and later undertook a mini-endovascular fellowship at the Cleveland Clinic to develop an endovascular program at the University of British Columbia. He is now professor emeritus of surgery and was the former head of vascular surgery at the University of British Columbia and consultant surgeon at the Vancouver General Hospital, Vancouver, BC. Born in Taiwan, educated in the United States, New Zealand, and Canada, Dr. Hsiang has diverse interests in vascular engineering, vascular biology, lasers, and clinical epidemiology. He has extensively published over 127 research articles in these areas. Dr. Hsiang was also the director of surgical research in the UBC Department of Surgery and has a special clinical interest in Wound Care. He is a distinguished fellow member of the Society for Vascular Surgery, past president of the Western Vascular Surgery Society, and the past president of the Canadian Society for Science and Ethics in Medicine.

Dr. Niel A. Karrow

Full Professor in Department of Animal Biosciences at the University of Guelph BSc (University of Guelph); MSc in Toxicology (University of Waterloo); PhD in Immunotoxicology (University of Waterloo)

Dr. Karrow completed a post-doctoral fellowship in the Department of Pharmacology and Toxicology, Medical College of Virginia–Virginia Commonwealth University, which involved serving as study director for several immunotoxicity studies conducted for the National Institute of Health Sciences (NIEHS). Dr. Karrow completed a second post-doctoral fellowship in immunogenetics in the Department of Pathobiology, University of Guelph, and joined the Department of Animal Biosciences at the University of Guelph in 2002, where he now holds full professor status. Dr. Karrow also holds adjunct professor status in Sichuan Agricultural University, China, and is a chaired professor at Yangzhou University, China. Dr. Karrow's research interests focus on the immunoregulation, immunotoxicology, and immunogenetics of livestock and fish species. This includes identifying genetic markers associated with inflammatory diseases, assessing the effects of maternal stress on the developing fetal neuroendocrine-immune system, immunonutrition, and the immunotoxicity of microbial toxins. Dr. Karrow lectures in senior-level undergraduate courses in the areas of comparative immunology and animal health and has over 228 scientific research publications.

Dr. Anna E. Kreynes

Molecular biologist and independent researcher Hon. BSc (University of Toronto); MSc in Microbial Diversity and Evolution (University of British Columbia); PhD in Plant Molecular Biology and Biochemistry (Dept. of Botany and Dept. of Land and Food Systems; University of British Columbia)

Dr. Anna Evgenya Kreynes (formally Anna Evgenyevna Gangaeva) works as a consultant in the cannabis industry. Her current interests lie in researching medicinal plants and understanding how traditional medicines can be studied using modern biochemical and molecular tools, and applied in complementary and alternative medicine to treat chronic illness.

Dr. Bonnie Mallard

Full Professor of Immuno-Genetics in the Department of Pathology at the University of Guelph; Chief Executive Officer of ImmunoCeutica Inc. BSc, MSc in Quantitative Genetics and Immunology (University of Guelph); PhD in Immunogenetics (University of Guelph)

Dr. Mallard has published over a hundred full-length publications in referred journals and has presented hundreds of abstracts and oral presentations at scientific meetings. She has also published several book chapters on genetic regulation of the immune system and is a highly experienced university lecturer in immunology and medical genetics. She has held over $50 million in research funding over her career and has been the recipient of numerous prizes including among others: the Pfizer Award for Research; the prestigious Canada's Governor General's Award for Innovation (2017); the University of Guelph Innovation of the Year Award (2018) and the Lifetime Achievement Award (2018); the YMCA Women of Distinction Award (2018); and she was the 2020–21 winner of the prestigious NSERC Synergy Prize.

Dr. Bernard Massie

Retired, Independent biotech consultant; Associate Professor of Microbiology and Immunology at the Université de Montréal PhD in Microbiology (University of Montreal)

Following his PhD training, Dr. Massie undertook a three-year post-doctoral study at McGill University studying DNA tumor viruses. Dr. Massie joined the National Research Council of Canada (NRC) in 1985 as a research scientist in the Virology Group. He was appointed leader of the Animal Cell Engineering Group in 1992 and then the R&D director of the Antibody and Bioprocessing Department of Human Health Therapeutics in 2006. His work focused initially on viral expression vectors (adenovirus, baculovirus, and lentivirus) and their application to protein production and gene delivery. He has also dedicated a significant portion of his career to the development of integrated bioprocesses from vector construction and cell engineering to large-scale culture, for industrial production of therapeutic antibodies and other biotherapeutics such as adenovirus vaccines. He became the acting director general of the Therapeutics in Human Health Center from 2016 to 2019 at the NRC. His responsibilities were managing resource allocation, strategic planning, and budgeting of several R&D departments leading teams deployed in goal-oriented research programs in partnership with biopharma industry. He has published over 138 peer-reviewed papers and has twelve issued patents. Many of his technologies have been licensed to industry and, over the years, he was involved in numerous industrial projects generating several million dollars in revenue. Concurrently, he was also an associate professor at the Department of Microbiology and Immunology of Université de Montréal from 1998 to 2019. Since 2016, he has been a member of the Scientific Advisory Board of C3i (dedicated to the commercialization of cell and gene therapy for cancer immunotherapy), from 2019–2022, on the SAB of CQDM (a research consortium that funds the development of innovative tools and technologies that will accelerate the discovery and development of safer and more effective drugs) and from 2021, on the SAB of BioDF (dedicated to the development of platform enabling technologies for the production of added-value products from wastes and greenhouse gases). He recently served in 2023 as a commissioner on the National Citizen Inquiry on the Government's responses to COVID-19 pandemic in Canada.

Dr. Kanji Nakatsu

Professor emeritus, Pharmacology–Queen's University MSc in Pharmacology (University of Alberta); PhD in Pharmacology (University of British Columbia)

Dr. Nakatsu completed his post-doctoral studies at Stanford University and subsequently joined the faculty in the Department of Pharmacology at Queen's University in 1973. He retired in 2017 after forty-four years of teaching graduate and undergraduate students in the Life Sciences, medical and nursing students, and conducting an active research program that included the study of agonists and inhibitors of adenosine receptors and development of heme oxygenase inhibitors. He has authored around two hundred scientific research publications. Dr. Nakatsu also serves as a co-chair of the Therapeutics Committee at the CCCA and previously served as a president of the Pharmacology Society of Canada.

Dr. Meryl Nass

Medical Doctor BSc Biology (Massachusetts Institute of Technology), MD (University of Mississippi), Residency and Board Certified in Internal Medicine (University of Mississippi Medical Center)

Dr. Nass has been a practicing physician since 1986, was involved in investigations of the use of anthrax as a bioweapon during the Zimbabwe civil war in 1992, and has consulted for American and foreign agencies on chem/biowarfare and development of anthrax vaccines. Dr. Nass's medical license was suspended in 2022 for allegedly providing "misinformation" about COVID-19 and for treating her patients with ivermectin and hydroxychloroquine. She has provided expert testimony to various governmental organizations in the United States, including the US Congress. Dr. Nass helped to edit three of Robert F. Kennedy Jr.'s books: *The Real Anthony Fauci*, *Letter to Liberals*, and *The Wuhan Conspiracy*. She has also written and spoken about the growing power of the WHO and founded DoorToFreedom.org to stop the Great Reset and the WHO sovereignty grab.

Dr. Susan Natsheh

Retired, Pediatrician BSc Biology (Queen's University), BMedSc (Memorial University of Newfoundland), MD (Memorial University of Newfoundland), Clinical Fellow, Pediatric GI (GI/Nutrition) (University of Toronto at Hospital for Sick Children), Clinical Residency (Queen's University)

Dr. Natsheh was an associate professor at Dalhousie University and a staff pediatrician at Saint John Regional Hospital., where she was also a creator for the **B**alanced **L**ifestyles and **A**ctivitie**S** **T**reatment (BLAST) Program. She has served as a member of the Dr. David Stephen Foundation Board and the YMCA Owen Sound Board. She has published and presented in the gastroenterology field. She recently served as a panel member of the Citizen's Hearing June 2022, which was an independent inquiry into Canada's response to COVID-19, and was a coauthor of a synopsis of the over sixty testimonies that were offered at the Citizen's Hearing. She is also the senior editor of the CCCA website and newsletter and co-chair of the CCCA External Communications Committee.

Dr. Philip R. Oldfield

Retired, Clinical Biochemist, Immunologist BSc in Biochemistry (University of Sussex); DPhil (University of Sussex)

Dr. Oldfield has over thirty years of post-graduation pharmaceutical and biopharmaceutical industrial research experience, specializing in ligand binding and hybridization assay techniques and clinical immunology. In the last decade, he had worked as an independent scientific/regulatory consultant, both writing and reviewing technical reports, clinical protocols, and NDA submissions as well as giving presentations at numerous major scientific conferences related to therapeutics, clinical immunology, and prion disease. He is a fellow of the Royal Society of Chemistry, an associate member of the Royal College of Pathologists (until the end of 2020), and a member of the American Association of Pharmaceutical Scientists (until the end of 2022). Dr. Oldfield chaired the (AAPS) Ligand Binding Assay Bioanalytical Focus Group in 2008 that was involved in scientific and regulatory discussions with members of the focus group, the US Food & Drug Administration, as well as other regulatory authorities resulting in the publication of White Papers, setting the standards for industry. Through linkages with local universities, he was involved in supervising postgraduate students, lecturing students, and was a founder committee member of the Drug Development Program at McGill University. He has published twenty-four peer-reviewed scientific papers (including three White Papers), two book chapters, and authored around 1500 confidential scientific reports in support of regulatory submissions for the US Food and Drug Administration and the European Medicines Agency.

Dr. Steven Pelech (Co-chair of SMAC)

Full Professor in the Department of Medicine at the University of British Columbia; President & Chief Scientific Officer of Kinexus Bioinformatics Corporation BSc (Hon) and PhD in Biochemistry (University of British Columbia)

Dr. Pelech undertook his post-doctoral training at the University of Dundee with Sir Philip Cohen, and at the University of Washington in Seattle with Nobel laureate Dr. Edwin Krebs. He was one of the founding scientists of the immunology-based institute, The Biomedical Research Centre, at the University of British Columbia (UBC), a founder and president of Kinetek Pharmaceuticals Inc. from 1992 to 1998, and the founder, president, and chief scientific officer of Kinexus Bioinformatics Corporation from 1999 to the present. Kinetek was engaged in the development of drugs that inhibit protein kinases, primarily for oncology application and diabetes. Kinexus has produced over 1600 antibodies against cell regulatory proteins and employs these in novel high throughput methods to monitor cell communication systems in biological specimens from over two thousand academic and industrial clients in over thirty-five countries. Dr. Pelech has authored over 260 scientific publications in peer-reviewed journals and book chapters about cell communication systems important for immune function and implicated in the pathology of cancer, diabetes, neurological, and immunology-related diseases. Over the last three years, he has led a clinical study with over four and a half thousand participants to monitor their antibody levels to the SARS-CoV-2 virus. His accolades include the 1993 Martin F. Hoffman Award for Research at UBC, and the 1993 Merck Frosst Canada Prize from the Canadian Society of Biochemistry and Molecular Biology. He was also the 2001 distinguished lecturer for the Faculty of Medicine at UBC for the basic sciences. Dr. Pelech was one of the founders of the CCCA, and also serves as its vice-president.

Dr. Wendi Roscoe

Full Professor in the Department of Health Science at Fanshawe College, London, Ontario BSc (Hon) in Genetics; BEd (University of Western Ontario); PhD in Physiology (University of Western Ontario); Holistic Nutritionist

Dr. Roscoe's PhD research was focused on neuroinflammation in a mouse model of multiple sclerosis. She has published in several peer-reviewed journals, such as *Journal of Neuroimmunology* and *Journal of Neuroscience Research*. Dr. Roscoe has been teaching physiology, biology, anatomy, and nutrition courses at the university and college level since 2004, and is currently teaching biology and physiology at Fanshawe College. She is the author of the textbook *Human Biology, Anatomy, and Physiology for the Health Sciences*. She is also a registered holistic nutritionist, graduating from the Canadian School of Natural Nutrition, in 2017. She is a very active producer and poster of over seventy-one educational videos on health and fitness at https://dr-wendihealth.com/ and https://www.youtube.com/channel/UCYHEJh7g4ZIWwW8v2MBhEtw/videos. Recently, she spent nine months at Griffith University on Australia's Gold Coast researching active learning and flipped classroom teaching methods in higher education health-care programs.

Dr. Christopher A. Shaw (Co-chair of SMAC)

Full Professor in the Department of Ophthalmology and Visual Sciences at the University of British Columbia with cross appointments to the Department of Pathology and the Program in Experimental Medicine and the Program in Neuroscience. BSc in Biological Sciences (University of California Irvine); MSc in Medical Physiology (Hebrew University); PhD Neurobiology (Hebrew University)

Dr. Shaw spent eight years at Dalhousie University (Psychology), first as a post-doctoral fellow and then as a research associate, before beginning his affiliation with the University of British Columbia in 1988. His research focuses on Lou Gehrig's disease (ALS) using several models of the disease to explore the possible environmental or genetic triggers of the disease, the various stages in disease development, and emerging treatment options. A second main theme, related to the first, is to examine the role of aluminum in various neurological diseases, including autism spectrum disorder. He is the author of over 160 peer-reviewed articles, numerous book chapters and edited books, and has authored two books on neurological diseases and one on vaccine controversies.

Dr. David J. Speicher

Assistant Professor of Biology and Health Sciences a Redeemer University MSc (Hons) Clinical Microbiology, PhD Virology (Griffith University, Australia)

Dr. Speicher is a molecular virologist who has conducted research in Australia, India, Kenya, Cambodia, and Canada (including McMaster University, St. Joseph's Healthcare Hamilton, and the University of Guelph). His research expertise has touched on saliva as a diagnostic fluid, oral cancers, and sexually transmitted diseases. During the COVID-19 pandemic, Dr. Speicher examined the government's early pandemic response and served as laboratory and R&D director of Multiplex Genomics, a COVID-19 PCR testing facility. He confirmed the adulteration of the Pfizer and Moderna COVID-19 modRNA vaccines by showing the high level of plasmid DNA and the presence of the SV40 promoter and enhancer. This work has been discussed worldwide, including the US Senate and European Parliament, and was instrumental in Florida State Surgeon General Dr. Joseph Lapado calling for a halt to the COVID-19 modRNA vaccines.

Glossary of Terms and Definitions

Absolute efficacy (or safety) *(see also Relative efficacy and safety)*: A measure of how much an intervention, such as a vaccine, lowers the risk of contracting the disease for which the vaccine is developed. For example, in a study with a hundred vaccinated and a hundred control patients, one person may develop the disease versus ten in the control group so the absolute efficacy is 9 percent.

ACE2 (Angiotensin-converting enzyme-2): A molecule found on the surface of certain cells in a variety of animals, including humans, mice, civets, and others. ACE2 severs as the entry point for coronaviruses. The human version of ACE2 is hACE2. It is primarily found on the surface of cells and tissues throughout the human body, including the nose, mouth, and lungs. In the lungs, hACE2 is highly abundant on type 2 pneumocytes, an important cell type present in chambers within the lung called alveoli, where oxygen is absorbed and waste carbon dioxide is released. This is the primary entry point for SARS-CoV-2 into human cells.

After Action Report: A summary and critique of some event in which the participants discuss things that worked well, as well as things that did not, and both with the view to improve performance at a future event of the same nature.

Amino acids: Small molecules composed of carbon, nitrogen, hydrogen, and sometimes sulfur or oxygen.

Alveoli: A structure in the lungs where oxygen is absorbed and waste carbon dioxide is released.

Bacteria: A member of a large group of unicellular microorganisms that have cell walls but lack organelles and an organized nucleus, including some that can cause disease.

Betacoronavirus: One of the four subclassifications of coronaviruses. Typically found in bats and rodents. This viral genus includes SARS, MERS, SARS-CoV-2, and others.

Biosafety Level 1 (BSL1): Designed for work on microbes not known to cause disease in healthy adults that present minimal potential hazards to laboratory personnel and the environment. Work can be performed on an open laboratory bench or table.

Biosafety Level 2 (BSL2): For work with microbes that pose moderate hazards to laboratory personnel and the environment. The microbes are typically indigenous and associated with diseases of varying severity. Personal protective equipment includes laboratory coats and gloves. Work can be performed in the open or in a biological safety cabinet. Commonly compared to the level of safety observed in a dentist's office.

Bio Safety Level 3 (BSL3): For work with microbes that are either indigenous or exotic that can cause serious or potentially lethal disease through typically respiratory transmission (i.e., inhalation). Researchers should be under medical surveillance and potentially immunized for the microbes with which they work. Respirators may be required, in addition to standard personal protective equipment. Work must be performed within a biological safety cabinet. Exhaust air from the cabinet cannot be recirculated and the laboratory must have sustained directional airflow by drawing air into the laboratory from clean areas toward potentially contaminated areas.

Biosafety Level 4 (BSL4): This is the highest level of biological safety. The microbes in a BSL-4 laboratory are dangerous and exotic, posing a high risk of aerosol-transmitted infections. Infections caused by these microbes are frequently fatal and without treatment or vaccines. Researchers must change clothing prior to entering the lab, shower upon exiting, and decontaminate all materials before exiting. All work with microbes must be performed in a Class III biological safety cabinet or while wearing a full body, air-supplied, positive pressure suit. The laboratory must be in a separate building or in a restricted zone, and must have dedicated supply and exhaust air, as well as vacuum lines and decontamination systems.

Blinded and double blinded study: A "blinded" study is one where the study participants or the experimenters do not know which group is the experimental versus control group. A "double blinded" study is one in which neither group knows the members of either experimental or control group until the data are de-coded for analysis.

Carbohydrates: Large molecules made up of chains of sugars.

CGG Double Codon "CGG-CGG": This group of six nucleotides (a group of three nucleotides is also known as a codon) is half of the twelve nucleotides that create the furin cleavage site of the COVID-19 spike protein. The CGG double codon is relatively rare in coronaviruses, and SARS-CoV-2 is the only coronavirus in its family to have one.

Chinese Academy of Sciences: The national academy for natural sciences in the People's Republic of China (PRC). It reports to the State Council of the PRC.

Chimeric Virus: An artificial, man-made virus, created by joining two or more viral fragments.

Cochrane Collaboration: The Cochrane Collaboration is a British international organization, ostensibly created to evaluate medical research findings to provide guidance, ideally evidence-based, for health-care providers. Once considered to be a foundation of rigorous analysis of medical studies, this status has come into question due to allegations of corporate influence.

Coronavirus: An RNA virus that causes disease in mammals and birds. In humans, the range in severity varies from similar to the common cold and mild coronavirus infection with SARS-CoV-2 with variable levels of severity. The coronavirus family also includes more severe illnesses such as MERS.

Corresponding Author: The point of contact for editors and outside readers who have questions about an academic paper. Typically, the corresponding author is also the senior author, i.e., the head of the laboratory where the research was conducted and often acquired the funding that allowed the research to happen.

Chain of Infection: The steps needed for a pathogen such as a virus or bacterium to cause a disease state.

Chromosome: A chromosome is defined as a long DNA molecule with part or all of the genetic material of an organism. In most humans, there are twenty-three pairs of chromosomes that contain both genes and other DNA, the latter often termed "dark" DNA, which is about 97 percent of all DNA.

Cytokine: Cytokines are signaling proteins that help control inflammation in the body, either labeled as pro- or anti-inflammatory.

D-dimer: A D-dimer is a protein fragment that the body makes when a blood clot dissolves in the body. The test for this in blood measures the levels of this protein.

Deoxynucleotides: Small molecules that are nucleotides lacking one oxygen atom.

Disease: An upset of structure and function in an organism that is associated with distinctive signs and symptoms. Note that exposure to a pathogen does not necessarily result in disease.

Disinformation: Information that is deliberately created to be false and used to promote particular narratives. *See misinformation.*

DNA (deoxyribonucleic acid): Large molecules made up of chains of deoxynucleotides.

Differences between DNA and RNA include the following:

Sugar moiety: DNA, deoxyribose; RNA, ribose which has an additional hydroxyl molecule (-OH). DNA is a double-stranded molecule, while RNA is a single-stranded molecule.

Base pairing: DNA uses the bases adenine, thymine, cytosine, and guanine; RNA uses adenine, uracil, cytosine, and guanine. Uracil differs from thymine in that it lacks a methyl group in its ring structue.

Endocytosis: The cellular process by which substances are brought into the cell.

Endoplasmic Reticulum (ER): A cellular organelle to which mRNA binds to initiate the creation of a particular protein.

Endotoxin: A toxic molecule produced by bacteria that is released when the bacterium disintegrates.

Exosome: Exosomes are secreted cellular organelles of small, single-membrane, secreted organelles of approximately 30 to 200 nm in diameter. They typically contain proteins, lipids, nucleic acids, and glycoconjugates. Some consider them to be the structures otherwise considered to be viruses. The evidence supporting this view is controversial and not widely accepted by mainstream medicine.

Fomite: An object such as a book, a mask, or an instrument that is not by itself harmful, but is able to harbor pathogens and thus might serve as a source for the transmission of an infectious agent.

Furin cleavage site: An amino acid sequence in the spike protein of SARS-CoV-2 that increases how infectious the virus is to humans. SARS-CoV-2 is the only betacoronavirus to have this structure.

Gain-of-Function (GoF) research: "Research that improves the ability of a pathogen to cause disease" according to the US Department of Health and Human Services. Various countries engage in this sort of research ostensibly to prevent another country from using some GoF organism as a weapon.

Gene: A gene is considered to be the basic unit of heredity consisting of a sequence of nucleotides in DNA that is transcribed by messenger RNA to produce a protein.

Genetics System: A method in molecular genetics that is used to help understand the function(s) of a gene by analyzing the phenotypic effects caused by genetically engineering specific nucleic acid sequences within the gene. It can be used to create chimeric viruses virtually indistinguishable from natural viruses.

Glia, or glial cells: Support cells within the central nervous system (CNS) that serve various functions. For example, astrocytes buffer various ions and sequester substances such as glutamate, the latter a major nervous system neurotransmitter. Oligodendrocytes of various types are cells that insulate axons (the long projections form neurons) to speed up transmission. Oligodendrocytes also have support functions. Microglia are the CNS immune cells that destroy pathogens and infected neurons.

Glycosylation: The addition of one or more sugar (glucose) molecules to a molecular structure, such as a protein or some other biological molecule. For example, the addition of a glycose molecule to a steryl (sometimes written as sterol) backbone changes aspects of the steryl's activity.

Host: Describes a person or animal characterized by having pathogens.

Infection: The invasion and multiplication of pathogens in body tissues.

Infectious diseases: Diseases caused by pathogens that are transmitted directly between hosts or indirectly via a vector or the environment. They are often referred to as communicable diseases. Note that exposure to a pathogen does not necessarily result in disease based on how much pathogen the person is exposed to, as well as on the immune health of that person.

Infectivity: A measure of the probability that a pathogen will induce an infection.

Lipids: Molecules comprised primarily of carbon and hydrogen, which are not soluble in water. Cells use lipids and proteins to construct the external envelope of the cell, as well as membranous structures inside the cell.

MERS (Middle East Respiratory Syndrome): A viral respiratory disease caused by MERS-CoV, a betacoronavirus. First identified as the cause of a 2012 outbreak.

mRNA (messenger RNA): A type of RNA in the cell that attaches to an organelle called a ribosome to produce a particular protein.

Meta-analysis: A meta-analysis is a statistical analysis that combines the results of multiple scientific studies (especially randomized control trials). It is considered to be the highest level of medical validity.

Microbiome (microbiota): The microorganisms, symbiotic and pathogenic, living in and on all vertebrates in various organs; much of it in the gastrointestinal system.

Misinformation: Information that is deemed to be false; disinformation is information deemed to be deliberately false and designed to sway people to a particular viewpoint.

Natural immunity: A form of immunity acquired after exposure to a pathogen that results in infection with the actual disease. This is distinguished from vaccine-induced immunity, which is acquired through the introduction of a killed or weakened form of the disease organism through an injected vaccine, typically into skeletal muscle. Some vaccines currently used and in development use an inhalation route of delivery. Of note, the mRNA vaccines produced to combat COVID-19 do not provide prolonged immunity from disease.

Natural Virus: A virus found in nature, i.e., "wild type."

Nuremberg Code: The Code came into existence in 1947 as a response to Nazi experimentation on prisoners and those in the various concentration camps. In summary:

> The judgment by the war crimes tribunal at Nuremberg laid down 10 standards to which physicians must conform when carrying out experiments on human subjects in a new code that is now accepted worldwide.
>
> This judgment established a new standard of ethical medical behavior for the post World War II human rights era. Among other requirements, this document enunciates the requirement of *voluntary informed consent* of the human subject. The principle of voluntary informed consent protects the right of the individual to control his own body.
>
> This code also recognizes that the risk must be weighed against the expected benefit, and that unnecessary pain and suffering must be avoided.

This code recognizes that doctors should avoid actions that injure human patients.

The principles established by this code for medical practice now have been extended into general codes of medical ethics. (https://www.cirp.org/library/ethics/nuremberg/)

Nucleotides: Small molecules composed of carbon, oxygen, and nitrogen.

Oncology: The branch of science that studies cancers, their causes, and treatment.

Pathogen: Any disease-producing microorganism. A simple classification consists of living entities such as parasites (helminths, protozoa), fungi and bacteria, and non-living entities such as viruses and prions. COVID-19, as described in this book, is thought to be caused by the virus SARS-CoV-2.

Pathogenicity: The quality of production or the ability to produce pathologic (abnormal) changes or disease.

Pathogenicity vs. Virulence: Relative terms dependent on a variety of circumstances that might convert a microorganism from a non-pathogenic state to a pathogenic one and might confer highly virulent characteristics on a pathogen normally considered to be of low virulence.

The presence of a pathogen of sufficient pathogenicity and virulence to induce disease in a susceptible host are necessary elements of the Chain of Infection.

Placebo: A drug or substance that is inert in that it is not expected to have any effect on an individual. In scientific experiments, a placebo is included as a control versus the drug or substance that is expected to alter biological activity. For example, in COVID-19 vaccine trials, some companies stated that the vaccines were tested against injections of saline. In drug trials, such as with ivermectin for treatment of COVID-19, the control was the existing standard of treatment that was also included with the patients with ivermectin.

Phosphorylation: The addition of a phosphorus ion to part of a biological molecule, typically a protein. The enzymes that perform this function are called kinases. The removal of the phosphorus ion is termed dephosphorylation and is performed by enzymes called phosphatases.

Phylogenetic Analysis: The study of the evolutionary development of a species or a group of organisms or a particular characteristic of an organism. It is used to identify the relationship between different viruses in the same family and their origins.

Polysaccharide: A carbohydrate consisting of a chain of sugar molecules bonded together.

Primary Author: The first listed author of an academic paper; often the person who contributes the most to that paper in terms of the experiments, writing, and analysis.

Pro-drug: A molecule that is inactive until metabolized by the body to make it active as a drug.

Praxis: Events in the real world versus those in theory.

Proteins: Large molecules made up of chains of amino acids.

Protease: An enzyme that cuts proteins. In relation to SARS-CoV-2, the protease is often TMPRSS2.

Pseudo-uridine: An alternative nucleotide for uridine used in the synthesis of mRNA "vaccines" that imparts major changes in the mRNA such as significantly increasing stability after injection, but carries the risk of protein mutation by ribosomal frame-shifting.

Randomized Control Trial (RCT): A study in which the participants are randomly assigned to either the experimental or control groups to prevent the introduction of uncontrolled variables. It is considered to be the most rigorous form of any medical study and is used to evaluate the performance of a drug or procedure.

RBD (Receptor-Binding Domain): The specific short region in a spike protein of a virus that binds the virus to a specific receptor on the host cell.

Receptor: A membrane-bound protein structure to which extracellular molecules, such as other molecules, can bind to elicit a cellular response. For example, the ACE2 receptor is one site where SARS-CoV-2 viruses attach.

Relative efficacy (or safety): A measure of how much an intervention, such as a vaccine, lowers the risk of contracting the disease for which the vaccine is developed. For example, in a study with a hundred vaccinated and a hundred control patients, one person may develop the disease versus ten in the control group, so the relative efficacy is almost 90 percent. *For comparison, see Absolute efficacy.*

Ribosome: Intracellular organelles comprised of RNA and proteins where proteins are synthesized.

RNA (ribonucleic acid): Large molecules made up of chains of nucleotides as in DNA with the exception of uracil (U) in place of thymidine(T). *See DNA for other differences.*

RNA polymerase: An enzyme that catalyzes the chemical reactions to synthesize RNA from a DNA template.

SARS (Severe Acute Respiratory Syndrome): A viral respiratory disease caused by SARS-CoV, a betacoronavirus. It was first identified as the cause of a 2002–2003 epidemic.

SARS-CoV-2: The betacoronavirus that has been linked to COVID-19.

Spike protein: Protein structures on the surface of a virus responsible for anchoring the virus to the host cell's surface and enabling the injection of the virus's genetic material into the host cell. Spike proteins are characteristic of the coronavirus family and were the desired product of the mRNA platform vaccines by making the recipient's own cells produce the modified spike protein to evoke immunity to SARS-CoV-2.

Sugars: Small molecules such as glucose, fructose, and ribose that comprise carbon, oxygen, and hydrogen. Sugars are water soluble.

Upper respiratory tract: These structures involved are the nose and nasal passages, paranasal sinuses, the pharynx, and the portion of the larynx above the vocal cords.

Wuhan Institute of Virology (WIV): A research institute in Wuhan, China focused on virology. It consists of at least two facilities: the Wuhan National Biosafety Laboratory and the Wuhan Institute of Virology Headquarters. According to still emerging evidence, the original SARS-CoV-2 virus may have originated in this facility.

WIV Headquarters: The older WIV facility, located in Wuchang District, Wuhan near the Wuhan Branch of the Chinese Academies of Science.

WIV1: The first novel coronavirus isolated by WIV researchers from bat fecal samples in 2013. WIV is a SARS-like coronavirus. The other coronaviruses studied at WIV include: **WIV16**, the second coronavirus isolated by WIV researchers isolated from a single bat fecal sample in 2016. WIV16 is a SARS-like coronavirus. **Rs4874** is the third coronavirus isolated by WIV researchers isolated from a single bat fecal sample in 2017. Rs4874 is a SARS-like coronavirus. **ID4491/RaTG13** is a SARS-like coronavirus collected in 2013 in a mining cave. It shares 96.1 percent nucleotide similarity to SARS-CoV-2.

Vaccine: Historically, vaccines have been defined as preparations of biological materials, typically weakened/killed or partial forms of the pathogen or its toxins. These formulations are intended to provide active (acquired) immunity for a period of time to prevent infection in the vaccinated individual and to prevent onward transmission of the pathogen to other people. Vaccines often contain adjuvants such as aluminum compounds to enhance the immune response, as well as various molecules added for stability and to control bacterial overgrowth in multiuser vials. In the latter case, the ethyl mercury compound Thimerosal has typically been used. It should be noted that during the early stages of the COVID-19 pandemic, the CDC changed the definition of vaccine from "a product that stimulates a person's immune system to produce immunity to a specific disease" to "a preparation that is used to stimulate the body's immune response against diseases." (See, https://www.miamiherald.com/news/coronavirus/article254111268.html#storylink=cpy.)

With this change, there has been speculation that the change of definition was meant to accommodate the inability of mRNA vaccines to prevent disease infection or transmission.

Vector: An animal or human carrier in whose body a pathogenic organism develops and multiplies prior to being transmitted to a new host. *Anopheles* mosquitoes are an example of an animal that can carry malarial parasites from person to person.

Viability: In context to pathogens, the term refers to the ability of the pathogen to reproduce itself.

Virulence: The degree of pathogenicity of a pathogen indicated by the severity of the disease produced and its ability to invade tissues of the host.

Virus: Small biological structures that can infect various species, including humans. Examples include the virus responsible for COVID-19 and the numerous variants of the initial Wuhan strain. Viruses are not considered to be "alive" but can propagate by infecting the cells of various species (including other viruses) to replicate using the machinery in the infected cells. Typically, viruses are pathological to the infected species and are usually brought under control by that species immune response. Successful viruses are infectious without being pathological and tend to mutate to that state. There are some people, including some in medicine, who deny that viruses exist.

Water: The universal solvent for living organisms on Earth.

WHO (World Health Organization): The body of the United Nations (UN) responsible to the UN for issues of global health.

World Economic Forum (WEF): An organization sited in Davos, Switzerland and headed by Klaus Schwab, the son of a prominent Nazi during the Third Reich. Schwab has declared in various forums the concept of a "Great Reset" designed to transform human society. Participants in the WEF's annual meetings include a number of corporations, representatives of various governments, and a number of billionaires.

Zoonosis and zoonotic: An infectious disease caused by some pathogen in one species that can jump to another species. Initial claims for the origin of COVID-19 were that the disease in animals such as bats or pangolins jumped to infect humans.

Endnotes

Preface

1 Curie, Marie. Retrieved from www.brainyquote.com/quotes/marie_curie_389010.

Foreword

1 All quotations are from the book itself.

Chapter 1

1 Coronaviridae Study Group of the International Committee on Taxonomy of Viruses. (2020) The species *Severe acute respiratory syndrome-related coronavirus*: Classifying 2019-nCoV and naming it SARS-CoV-2. *Nat Microbiol* 5(4):536–44. doi:10.1038/s41564–020-0695-z.

2 (2023) WHO chief declares end to COVID-19 as a global health emergency. *United Nations News*. Retrieved from news.un.org/en/story/2023/05/1136367.

3 Rancourt, D., Hickey, J. (2023) Quantitative evaluation of whether the Nobel-Prize-winning COVID-19 vaccine actually saved millions of lives. Correlation Report. October 8, 2023. Retrieved from denisrancourt.ca/uploads_entries/1696822761794_2023–10-08-Correlation-Whether-Nobel-vaccine-saved-millions-of-lives.pdf.

4 Kiderlin, S. (2023) The richest 1% of people amassed almost two-thirds of new wealth created in the last two years, Oxfam says. CNBC. Retrieved from www.cnbc.com/2023/01/16/richest-1percent-amassed-almost-two-thirds-of-new-wealth-created-since-2020-oxfam.html.

5 Lowery, T. (2022) The world's 10 richest men doubled their fortunes during COVID-19, and 6 other factors on wealth inequality. *Global Citizen*. Retrieved from www.globalcitizen.org/en/content/oxfam-inequality-report-2022-billionaires-covid-19/.

Chapter 2

1 Hill, T. (Producer) (2022) Fauci defends "I am the science" speech, Vows not to fully retire. Retrieved from www.youtube.com/watch?v=877w94ndqLk.

2 Capurro, G., Jardine, C.G., Tustin, J., Driedger, M. (2021) Communicating scientific uncertainty in a rapidly evolving situation: A framing analysis of Canadian coverage in early days of COVID-19. *BMC Public Health* 21(1):2181. doi:10.1186/s12889–021-12246-x.

3 Cernic, M. (2018) *Ideological constructs of vaccination*. Vega Press, Ltd.

4 D'Augustino, T. (2017) What makes a good scientist? Retrieved from www.canr.msu.edu/news/what_makes_a_good_scientist.
5 Oreskes, N. (2021) If you say "science is right," You're wrong. *Scientific American*. Retrieved from www.scientificamerican.com/article/if-you-say-science-is-right-youre-wrong.
6 Vera, M. A., El-Khoury, J. M., Thorp, H., Tofel, R. J., Ross, J. S., et al. (2022) Public misinformation and science communication in times of public health crises. *Clinical Chemistry* 68(8):1008–14. doi:10.1093/clinchem/hvac088.
7 Bradford, A. (2022) What is a scientific theory? Retrieved from www.livescience.com/21491-what-is-a-scientific-theory-definition-of-theory.html.
8 (2023) Dictionary.com. Retrieved from www.dictionary.com/.

Chapter 3

1 Statista. (2022) Death rate for other and unspecified infectious and parasitic diseases and their sequelae in Canada from 2000 to 2020. Retrieved from www.statista.com/statistics/434404/death-rate-for-infectious-and-parasitic-diseases-in-canada/.
2 Statistics Canada. (2023) Table 13–10-0394–01 Leading causes of death, total population, by age group. Retrieved from www150.statcan.gc.ca/t1/tbl1/en/tv.action?pid=1310039401.
3 Health Canada. (2023) Opioid- and stimulant-related harms in Canada. Retrieved from health-infobase.canada.ca/substance-related-harms/opioids-stimulants/.
4 Sender, R., Fuchs, S., Milo, R. (2016) Are we really vastly outnumbered? Revisiting the ratio of bacterial to host-cells in humans. *Cell* 164(3):337–40. doi:10.1016/j.cell.2016.01.013.
5 Davis, C. D. (2016) The gut microbiome and its role in obesity. *Nutr Today* 51(4):167–74. doi:10.1097/NT.0000000000000167.
6 Goldman, B. (2020) Stanford scientists link ulcerative colitis to missing gut microbes. Stanford Medicine News Center. Retrieved from med.stanford.edu/news/all-news/2020/02/stanford-scientists-link-ulcerative-colitis-to-missing-gut-micro.html.
7 Ritchie, H. (2022) How many species are there? Retrieved from ourworldindata.org/how-many-species-are-there.
8 Woolhouse, M., Scott, F., Hudson, Z., Howey, R., Chase-Topping, M. (2012) Human viruses: Discovery and emergence. *Philos Trans R Soc Lond B Biol Sci* 367(1604):2864–71. doi:10.1098/rstb.2011.0354.
9 Racaniello, V. (2013) How many viruses on Earth? Retrieved from virology.ws/2013/09/06/how-many-viruses-on-earth/.
10 Mougari, S., Sahmi-Bounsiar, D., Levasseur, A., Colson, P., La Scola, B. (2019) Virophages of giant viruses: An update at eleven. *Viruses* 11(8):733. doi:10.3390/v11080733.
11 Pride, D. (2020) Viruses can help us as well as harm us. *Scientific American*. Retrieved from www.scientificamerican.com/article/viruses-can-help-us-as-well-as-harm-us/.
12 Wylie, K. M., Weinstock, G. M., Storch, G. A. (2012) Emerging view of the human virome. *Translational Res* 160(4):283–90. doi:10.1016/j.trsl.2012.03.006.
13 Marian, A. J. (2014) Sequencing your genome: What does it mean? *Methodist Debakey Cardiovasc J* 10(1):3–6. doi:10.14797/mdcj-10–1-3.
14 Salzberg, S. L. (2018) Open questions: How many genes do we have? *BMC Biol* 16(1):94. doi:10.1186/s12915–018-0564-x.

15 Joseph, A. (2023) Chapter 3. Water worlds in the solar system. Retrieved from www.sciencedirect.com/topics/earth-and-planetary-sciences/panspermia#I.
16 Campbell, A. (2001) The origins and evolution of viruses. *Trends Microbiol* 9(2):61. doi:10.1016/s0966–842x(00)01934-x.
17 Shulman, T. S. (1992) *The biologic and clinical basis of infectious diseases,* 4th edition. Toronto: W.B. Saunders.
18 Ibid.
19 Ibid.
20 Ibid.
21 Ibid.
22 Runnels, R. R. (1984) *Infection control in the wet finger environment.* Salt Lake City: Publishers Press.
23 Shulman, *The biologic and clinical basis of infectious diseases.*
24 Dobson, M. (2007) *Disease: The extraordinary stories behind history's deadliest killers.* London: Quercus.
25 Mordue, A. (2022) The betrayal of public health during the Covid Pandemic. Retrieved from dailysceptic.org/the-betrayal-of-public-health-during-the-covid-pandemic/.
26 U.S. Department of Health and Human Services. (2020) Update on the new coronavirus outbreak first identified in Wuhan, China. YouTube. Retrieved from youtube.com/watch?v=w6koHkBCoNQ&t=2642s.
27 Feuer, W., Higgins-Dunn, N. (2020) "Asymptomatic spread of coronavirus is very rare," WHO says. CNBC. www.cnbc.com/2020/06/08/asymptomatic-coronavirus-patients-arent-spreading-new-infections-who-says.html.
28 Tayyar, R., Kiener, M. A., Liang, J. W., Contreras, G., Rodriguez-Nava, G., et al. (2023) Low infectivity among asymptomatic patients with a positive severe acute respiratory coronavirus virus 2 (SARS-CoV-2) admission test at a tertiary care center, 2020–2022. *Infect Control Hosp Epidemiol* 25:1–3. doi:10.1017/ice.2023.210.

Chapter 4

1 Munywoki, P. K., Koech, D. C., Agoti, C. N., Bett, A., Cane, P. A., et al. (2015) Frequent asymptomatic respiratory syncytial virus infections during an epidemic in a rural Kenyan household cohort. *J Infect Dis* 212(11):1711–18. doi:10.1093/infdis/jiv263.
2 Bylsma, L. C., Suh, M., Movva, N., Fryzek, J. P., Nelson, C. B. (2022) Mortality among US infants and children under 5 years of age with respiratory syncytial virus and bronchiolitis: A systematic literature review. *J Infect Dis* 226(Suppl 2):S267–81. doi:10.1093/infdis/jiac226.
3 Al-Hakim, A. (2022) What is RSV? Here's what to know about the virus as cases surge in Canada. Retrieved from globalnews.ca/news/9228518/canada-respiratory-syncytial-virus-rsv-what-is-it/.
4 Tam, J., Papenburg, J., Fanella, S., Asner, S., et al. (2019) Pediatric Investigators Collaborative Network on Infections in Canada study of respiratory syncytial virus-associated deaths in pediatric patients in Canada, 2003–2013. *Clin Infect Dis* 68(1):113–19. doi:10.1093/cid/ciy413.
5 Harding, A. (2008) Research shows why 1960s RSV shot sickened children. Reuters. Retrieved from www.reuters.com/article/us-rsv-shot-idUSTRE4BM4SH20081223.
6 (2023) U.S. FDA approves ABRYSVO™, Pfizer's vaccine for the prevention of respiratory syncytial virus (RSV) in older adults. Retrieved from www.pfizer.com/news/press-release/press-release-detail/us-fda-approves-abrysvotm-pfizers-vaccine-prevention.

7 Walsh, E. E., Marc, G. O., Zareba, A. M., Falsey, A. R., Jiang, Q. J., et al. (2023) Efficacy and safety of a bivalent RSV Prefusion F vaccine in older adults. *N Engl J Med* 388(16):1465–77. doi:10.1056/NEJMoa2213836.

8 Kampmann, B., Madhi, S. A., Munjal, I., Simões, E. A. F., Pahud, B. A. (2023) MATISSE Study Group. Bivalent prefusion F vaccine in pregnancy to prevent RSV illness in infants. *N Engl J Med* 388(16):1451–64. doi:10.1056/NEJMoa2216480.

9 (2021) Prospective study for the use of Palivizumab (Synagis®) in high-risk children in Germany. Retrieved from clinicaltrials.gov/ct2/show/NCT01155193.

10 Graci, J. D., Cameron, C. E. (2006) Mechanisms of action of ribavirin against distinct viruses. *Rev Med Virol* 16 (1):37–48. doi:10.1002/rmv.483.

11 DeLaire, M. (2022) "We are so overwhelmed": Children's hospitals across Canada stretched as RSV cases, flu-like illnesses spike. Retrieved from www.ctvnews.ca/health/we-are-so-overwhelmed-children-s-hospitals-across-canada-stretched-as-rsv-cases-flu-like-illnesses-spike-1.6139599.

12 Paramo, M. V., Abu-Raya B., Reicherz F., Xu R. Y., Bone J. N., et al. (2022) Comparative analysis of pediatric Respiratory Syncytial Virus epidemiology and clinical severity before and during the COVID-19 pandemic in British Columbia, Canada. medRxiv (preprint). doi:10.1101/2022.11.18.22282477.

13 (2022) Types of influenza viruses. Retrieved from www.cdc.gov/flu/about/viruses/types.htm.

14 Liang, S. T., Liang, L. T., Rosen, J. M. (2021) COVID-19: A comparison to the 1918 influenza and how we can defeat it. *Postgrad Med J* 97(1147):273–74. doi:10.1136/postgradmedj-2020–139070.

15 Yang, W., Petkova, E., Shaman, J. (2014) The 1918 influenza pandemic in New York City: Age-specific timing, mortality, and transmission dynamics. *Influenza Other Respir Viruses* 8(2):177–88. doi:10.1111/irv.12217.

16 Barry, J. M. (2004) The site of origin of the 1918 influenza pandemic and its public health implications. *J Transl Med* 2(1):3. doi:10.1186/1479–5876-2–3.

17 Kung, H. C., Jen, K. F., Yuan, W. C., Tien, S. F., Chu, C. M. (1978) Influenza in China in 1977: Recurrence of influenza virus A subtype H1N1. *Bull World Health Organ* 56(6):913–18.

18 Nakajima, K., Desselberger, U., Palese, P. (1978) Recent human influenza A (H1N1) viruses are closely related genetically to strains isolated in 1950. *Nature* 274(5669):334–39. doi:10.1038/274334a0.

19 Rozo, M., Gronvall, G. K. (2015) The reemergent 1977 H1N1 strain and the gain-of-function debate. *mBio* 6(4). doi:10.1128/mBio.01013–15.

20 Okoli, G. N., Racovitan, F., Abdulwahid, T., Righolt, C. H., Mahmud, S. M., et al. (2021) Variable seasonal influenza vaccine effectiveness across geographical regions, age groups and levels of vaccine antigenic similarity with circulating virus strains: A systematic review and meta-analysis of the evidence from test-negative design studies after the 2009/10 influenza pandemic. *Vaccine* 39(8):1225–40. doi:10.1016/j.vaccine.2021.01.032.

21 Centers for Disease Control and Prevention, N. C. f. I. a. R. D. N. (2023) Vaccine effectiveness: How well do flu vaccines work? Retrieved from www.cdc.gov/flu/vaccines-work/vaccineeffect.htm.

22 Public Health Agency of Canada. (2021) Flu Watch annual report: 2019–2020 influenza season. Retrieved from www.canada.ca/en/public-health/services/publications/diseases-conditions/fluwatch/2019–2020/annual-report.html.

23 Nwosu, A., Lee, L., Schmidt, K., Buckrell, S., Sevenhuysen, C., Bancej, C. (2021) National Influenza Annual Report, Canada, 2020–2021, in the global context. *Can Commun Dis Rep* 47(10):405–13. doi:10.14745/ccdr.v47i10a02.

24 Ibid.

25 Ibid.

26 Public Health Agency of Canada. (2022) Flu Watch. December 11–December 31, 2022. Retrieved from www.canada.ca/content/dam/phac-aspc/documents/services/publications/diseases-conditions/fluwatch/2022–2023/weeks-50–52-december-11-december-31–2022/weeks-50–52-december-11-december-31–2022.pdf.

27 Tenforde, M. W., Weber, Z. A., Yang, D. H., DeSilva, M. B., Dascomb, K., et al. (2023) Influenza vaccine effectiveness against influenza-A-associated emergency department, urgent care, and hospitalization encounters among U.S. adults, 2022–2023. *J Infect Dis* jiad542. doi:10.1093/infdis/jiad542.

28 (2023) Seasonal influenza, avian influenza and pandemic influenza. Retrieved from ipac-canada.org/influenza-resources.

29 Dattani, S., and Spooner, F. (2022) How many people die from the flu? OurWorldInData.org. Retrieved from ourworldindata.org/influenza-deaths.

30 (2020) 430,000 people have traveled from China to U.S. since coronavirus surfaced. Retrieved from www.nytimes.com/2020/04/04/us/coronavirus-china-travel-restrictions.html.

31 Escobar, L. E., Molina-Cruz, A., Barillas-Mury, C. (2020) BCG vaccine protection from severe coronavirus disease 2019 (COVID-19). *Proc Natl Acad Sci USA* 117(30):17720–26. doi:10.1073/pnas.2008410117; Gonzalez-Perez, M., Sanchez-Tarjuelo, R., Shor, B., Nistal-Villan, E., Ochando, J. (2021) The BCG vaccine for COVID-19: First verdict and future directions. *Front Immunol* 12:632478. doi:10.3389/fimmu.2021.632478.

32 Gong, W., An, H., Wang, J., Cheng, P., Qi, Y. (2022) The natural effect of BCG vaccination on COVID-19: The debate continues. *Front Immunol* 13:953228. doi:10.3389/fimmu.2022.953228.

33 Weiss, S. R., Leibowitz, J. L. (2011) Coronavirus pathogenesis. *Adv Virus Res* 81:85–164. doi:10.1016/b978–0-12–385885-6.00009–2.

34 Machemer, T. (2021) Over 20,000 years ago, a coronvirus epidemic left marks in human DNA. *Smithsonian Magazine*. Retrieved from www.smithsonianmag.com/smart-news/over-20000-years-ago-coronavirus-epidemic-left-marks-human-dna-180978088/.

35 Zhou, P., Yang, X. L., Wang, X. G., Hu, B., Zhang, L., et al. (2020) A pneumonia outbreak associated with a new coronavirus of probable bat origin. *Nature* 579:270–73. doi:10.1038/s41586–020-2012–7.

36 Padhan, K., Parvez, M. K., Al-Dosari, M. S. (2021) Comparative sequence analysis of SARS-CoV-2 suggests its high transmissibility and pathogenicity. *Future Virol* 16(3):245–54. doi:10.2217/fvl-2020–0204.

37 Vlasak, R., Luytjes, W., Spaan, W., Palese, P. (1988) Human and bovine coronaviruses recognize sialic acid-containing receptors similar to those of influenza C viruses. *Proc Natl Acad Sci USA* 85(12):4526–29. doi:10.1073/pnas.85.12.4526; Huang, X., Dong, W., Milewska, A., Golda, A., Qi, Y., et al. (2015) Human coronavirus HKU1 spike protein uses O-acetylated sialic acid as an attachment receptor determinant and employs hemagglutinin-esterase protein as a receptor-destroying enzyme. *J Virol* 89(14):7202–13. doi:10.1128/JVI.00854–15.

38 Yeager, C. L., Ashmun, R. A., Williams, R. K., Cardellichio, C. B., Shapiro, L. H., et al. (1992) Human aminopeptidase N is a receptor for human coronavirus 229E. *Nature* 357(6377):420–22. doi:10.1038/357420a0.

39 Hofmann, H., Pyrc, K., van der Hoek, L., Geier, M., Berkhout, B., et al. (2005) Human coronavirus NL63 employs the severe acute respiratory syndrome coronavirus receptor for cellular entry. *Proc Natl Acad Sci USA* 102(22):7988–93. doi:10.1073/pnas.0409465102.

40 Anderson, E. M., Goodwin, E. C., Verma, A., Arevalo, C. P., Bolton, M. J., et al. (2021) Seasonal human coronavirus antibodies are boosted upon SARS-CoV-2 infection but not associated with protection. *Cell* 184(7):1858–64. doi:10.1016/j.cell.2021.02.010.

41 Sagar, M., Reifler, K., Rossi, M., Miller, N. S., Sinha, P., et al. (2021) Recent endemic coronavirus infection is associated with less-severe COVID-19. *J Clin Invest* 131(1). doi:10.1172/jci143380.

42 World Health Organization: Summary of probable SARS cases with onset of illness from 1 November 2002 to 31 July 2003. July 24, 2015 Meeting Report. WHO. Retrieved from www.who.int/csr/sars/country/table2004_04_21/en/.

43 World Health Organization: SARS: Cumulative number of reported probable cases. WHO. Retrieved from www.who.int/csr/sars/country/en/.

44 Rae, R., Zeng, A. (2023) SARS in Canada. The Canadian Encyclopedia. Retrieved from www.thecanadianencyclopedia.ca/en/article/sars-severe-acute-respiratory-syndrome.

45 Marra, M. A., Jones, S. J., Astell, C. R., Holt, R. A., Brooks-Wilson, A., et al. (2003) The Genome sequence of the SARS-associated coronavirus. *Science* 300(5624):1399–1404. doi:10.1126/science.1085953.

46 (2003) SARS-associated coronavirus (SARS-CoV) sequencing. Retrieved from www.cdc.gov/sars/lab/sequence.html.

47 Parashar, U. D., Anderson, L. J. (2004) Severe acute respiratory syndrome: Review and lessons of the 2003 outbreak. *Int J Epidemiol* 33(4):628–34. doi:10.1093/ije/dyh198.

48 Seto, W. H., Tsang, D., Yung, R. W., Ching, T. Y., Ng, T. K., et al. (2003) Effectiveness of precautions against droplets and contact in prevention of nosocomial transmission of severe acute respiratory syndrome (SARS). *Lancet* 361(9368):1519–20. doi:10.1016/s0140–6736(03)13168–6.

49 World Health Organization. (2004) 2004-China. Retrieved from www.who.int/emergencies/disease-outbreak-news/item/2004_04_23-en.

50 Song, H. D., Tu, C. C., Zhang, G. W., Wang, S. Y., Zheng, K., et al. (2005) Cross-host evolution of severe acute respiratory syndrome coronavirus in palm civet and human. *Proc Natl Acad Sci USA* 102(7):2430–35. doi:10.1073/pnas.0409608102.

51 Hu, B., Zeng, L.-P., Yang, X.-L., Ge, X.-Y., Zhang, W., et al. (2017) Discovery of a rich gene pool of bat SARS-related coronaviruses provides new insights into the origin of SARS coronavirus. *PLOS Pathog* 13(11):e1006698. doi:10.1371/journal.ppat.1006698; Cyranoski, D. (2017) Bat cave solves mystery of deadly SARS virus—and suggests new outbreak could occur. *Nature* 552(7683):15–16. doi:10.1038/d41586–017-07766–9; Lau, S. K. P., Fan, R. Y. Y., Luk, H. K. H., Zhu, L., Fung, J., et al. (2018) Replication of MERS and SARS coronaviruses in bat cells offers insights to their ancestral origins. *Emerg Microbes Infect* 7:209. doi:10.1038/s41426–018-0208–9.

52 Li, W., Moore, M. J., Vasilieva, N., Sui, J., Wong, S. K., et al. (2003) Angiotensin-converting enzyme 2 is a functional receptor for the SARS coronavirus. *Nature* 426(6965):450–54. doi:10.1038/nature02145.

53 Padhan, K., Parvez, M. K., Al-Dosari, M. S., Comparative sequence analysis of SARS-CoV-2 suggests its high transmissibility and pathogenicity.
54 World Health Organization. (2020) Middle East respiratory syndrome coronavirus (MERS-CoV). Retrieved from www.who.int/emergencies/mers-cov/en/.
55 Widagdo, W., Raj, V. S., Schipper, D., Kolijn, K., van Leenders, G. J. L. H., et al. (2016) Differential expression of the Middle East Respiratory Syndrome coronavirus receptor in the upper respiratory tracts of humans and dromedary camels. *J Virol* 90(9): 4838–42. doi:10.1128/JVI.02994–15.
56 Raj, V. S., Mou, H., Smits, S. L., Dekkers, D. H., Müller, M. A., et al. (2013) Dipeptidyl peptidase 4 is a functional receptor for the emerging human coronavirus-EMC. *Nature* 495(7440):251–54. doi:10.1038/nature12005.
57 Padhan, K., Parvez, M. K., Al-Dosari, M. S., Comparative sequence analysis of SARS-CoV-2 suggests its high transmissibility and pathogenicity.
58 Millet, J. K., Whittaker, G. R. (2014) Host cell entry of Middle East respiratory syndrome coronavirus after two-step, furin-mediated activation of the spike protein. *Proc Natl Acad Sci USA* 111(42):15214–19. doi:10.1073/pnas.1407087111.
59 Braun, E., Sauter, D. (2019) Furin-mediated protein processing in infectious diseases and cancer. *Clin Transl Immunology* 8(8):e1073. doi:10.1002/cti2.1073.
60 Hoffmann, M., Kleine-Weber, H., Schroeder, S., Krüger, N., Herrler, T., et al. (2020) SARS-CoV-2 cell entry depends on ACE2 and TMPRSS2 and is blocked by a clinically proven protease inhibitor. *Cell* 181(2):271–80.e278. doi:10.1016/j.cell.2020.02.052.
61 Millet, J. K., Whittaker, G. R., Host cell entry of Middle East respiratory syndrome coronavirus after two-step, furin-mediated activation of the spike protein.

Chapter 5

1 Zhou, P., Yang, X.-L., Wang, X.-G., Hu, B., Zhang, L., et al. (2020) A pneumonia outbreak associated with a new coronavirus of probable bat origin. *Nature* 579(7798):270–73. doi:10.1038/s41586–020-2012–7.
2 Zhu, N., Zhang, D., Wang, W., Li, X., Yang, B., et al. (2020) China novel coronavirus investigating and research team. A novel coronavirus from patients with pneumonia in China, 2019. *N Engl J Med* 382(8):727–33. doi:10.1056/NEJMoa2001017.
3 Cantutu-Castelvetri, L., Ojha, R., Pedro, L. D., Djannatian, M., Franz, J., et al. (2020) Neuropilin-1 facilitates SARS-CoV-2 cell entry and infectivity. *Science* 370(6518):856–60. doi:10.1126/science.abd298.
4 Moutal, A., Martin, L. F., Boinon, L., Gomez, K., Ran, D., et al. (2021) SARS-CoV-2 spike protein co-opts VEGF-A/neuropilin-1 receptor signaling to induce analgesia. *Pain* 162(1):243–52. doi:10.1097/j.pain.0000000000002097.
5 Mobini, S., Chizari, M., Mafakher, L., Rismani, E., Rismani, E. (2021) Structure-based study of immune receptors as eligible binding targets of coronavirus SARS-CoV-2 spike protein. *J Mol Graph Model* 108:107997. doi:10.1016/j.jmgm.2021.107997.
6 Oliveira, A. S. F., Ibarra, A. A., Bermudez, I., Casalino, L., Gaieb, Z., et al. (2020) Simulations support the interaction of the SARS-CoV-2 spike protein with nicotinic acetylcholine receptors and suggest subtype specificity. bioRxiv (preprint) 2020.07.16.206680. doi:10.1101/2020.07.16.206680.

7 Scheim, D. E., Vottero, P., Santin, A. D., Hirsh, A. G. (2023) Sialylated glycan bindings from SARS-CoV-2 Spike protein to blood and endothelial cells govern the severe morbidities of COVID-19. *Int J Mol Sci* 24(23):17039. doi:10.3390/ijms242317039.

8 Tipnis, S. R., Hooper, N. M., Hyde, R., Karran, E., Christie, G., Turner, A. J. (2000) A human homolog of angiotensin-converting enzyme. Cloning and functional expression as a captopril-insensitive carboxypeptidase. *J Biol Chem* 275(43):33238–43. doi:10.1074/jbc.M002615200.

9 Bosso, M., Thanaraj, T. A., Abu-Farha, M., Alanbaei, M., Abubaker, J., Al-Mulla, F. (2020) The two faces of ACE2: The role of ACE2 receptor and its polymorphisms in hypertension and COVID-19. *Mol Ther Methods Clin Dev* 18:321–27. doi:10.1016/j.omtm.

10 Gaddam, R. R., Chambers, S., Bhatia, M. (2014) ACE and ACE2 in inflammation: A tale of two enzymes. *Inflamm Allergy Drug Targets* 13(4):224–34. doi:10.2174/187152811366614071316450 6.

11 Lonsdale, J., Thomas, J., Salvatore, M., Phillips, R., Lo, E., et al. (2013) The Genotype-Tissue Expression (GTEx) project. *Nat. Genet* 45:580–85. doi:10.1038/ng.2653.

12 Thul, P. J., and Lindskog, C. (2018) The human protein atlas: A spatial map of the human proteome. *Protein Sci* 27:233–44. doi:10.1002/pro.3307.

13 Brunetti, N. S., Davanzo, G. G., de Moraes, D., Ferrari, A. J. R., Souza, G. F., et al. (2023) SARS-CoV-2 uses CD4 to infect T helper lymphocytes. *Elife* 12:e84790. doi:10.7554/eLife.84790.

14 Wang, Y., Lenoch, J., Kohler, D., DeLiberto, T. J., Tang, C. Y., et al. (2023) SARS-CoV-2 exposure in Norway rats (*Rattus norvegicus*) from New York City. *mBio* 14(2):0362122. doi:10.1128/mbio.03621–22.

15 Chandler, J. C., Bevins, S. N., Ellis, J. W., Linder, T. J., Tell, R. M., et al. (2021) SARS-CoV-2 exposure in wild white-tailed deer (*Odocoileus virginianus*). *Proc Natl Acad Sci USA* 118(47):e2114828118. doi:10.1073/pnas.2114828118.

16 Caserta, L. C., Martins, M., Butt, S. L., Hollingshead, N. A., Covaleda, L. M., et al. (2023) White-tailed deer (*Odocoileus virginianus*) may serve as a wildlife reservoir for nearly extinct SARS-CoV-2 variants of concern. *PNAS USA* 120(6):e2215067120. doi:10.1073/pnas.2215067120.

17 Hammer, A. S., Quaade, M. L., Rasmussen, T. B., Fonager, J., Rasmussen, M., et al. (2021) SARS-CoV-2 Transmission between mink (*Neovison vison*) and humans, Denmark. *Emerg Infect Dis* 27(2):547–51. doi:10.3201/eid2702.203794.

18 Bosco-Lauth, A. M., Root, J. J., Porter, S. M., Walker, A. E., Guilbert, L., et al. (2021) Peridomestic mammal susceptibility to severe acute respiratory syndrome coronavirus 2 Infection. *Emerg Infect Dis* 27(8):2073–80. doi:10.3201/eid2708.210180.

19 Koopmans, M. (2021) SARS-CoV-2 and the human-animal interface: Outbreaks on mink farms. *Lancet Infect Dis* 21(1):18–19. doi:10.1016/S1473–3099(20)30912–9.

20 Hale, V. L., Dennis, P. M., McBride, D. S., Nolting, J. M., Madden, C., et al. (2022) SARS-CoV-2 infection in free-ranging white-tailed deer. *Nature* 602(7897):481–86. doi:10.1038/s41586–021-04353-x.

21 Penn State University (2021) Over 80% of deer in study test positive for COVID—They may be a reservoir for the virus to continue to circulate. *SciTech Daily*. Retrieved from scitechdaily.com/over-80-of-deer-in-study-test-positive-for-covid-they-may-be-a-reservoir-for-the-virus-to-continually-circulate/.

22 Cui, S., Liu, Y., Zhao, J., Peng, X., Lu, G., et al. (2022) An updated review on SARS-CoV-2 infection in animals. *Viruses* 14(7):1527. doi:10.3390/v14071527.

23 Hale et al., SARS-CoV-2 infection in free-ranging white-tailed deer.

24 Ibid.

25 Bosco-Lauth et al., Peridomestic mammal susceptibility to severe acute respiratory syndrome coronavirus 2 Infection.

26 Scheim et al., Sialylated glycan bindings from SARS-CoV-2 Spike protein.

27 Beumer, J., Geurts, M.H., Lamers, M.M., Puschhof, J., Zhang, J., *et al.* (2021) A CRISPR/Cas9 genetically engineered organoid biobank reveals essential host factors for coronaviruses. *Nat Commun.* 12(1):5498. doi:10.1038/s41467–021-25729–7.

28 Mykytyn, A.Z., Breugem, T.I., Riesebosch, S., Schipper, D., van den Doel, P.B., et al. (2021) SARS-CoV-2 entry into human airway organoids is serine protease-mediated and facilitated by the multibasic cleavage site. Elife. 10:e64508. doi:10.7554/eLife.64508.

29 Lamers, M.M., Mykytyn, A.Z., Breugem, T.I., Wang, Y., Wu, D.C., *et al.* (2021) Human airway cells prevent SARS-CoV-2 multibasic cleavage site cell culture adaptation. Elife. 10:e66815. doi:10.7554/eLife.66815.

30 Hoffmann, M., Hofmann-Winkler, H., Smith, J.C., Krüger, N., Arora, P., et al. (2021) Camostat mesylate inhibits SARS-CoV-2 activation by TMPRSS2-related proteases and its metabolite GBPA exerts antiviral activity. *EBioMedicine.* 65:103255. doi:10.1016/j.ebiom.2021.103255.

31 Wei, C., Shan, K. J., Wang, W., Zhang, S., Huan, Q., Qian, W. (2021) Evidence for a mouse origin of the SARS-CoV-2 Omicron variant. *J Genet Genomics* 48(12):1111–21. doi:10.1016/j.jgg.2021.12.003.

32 Zhou, T., Gilliam, N. J., Li, S., Spandau, S., Osborn, R. M., et al. (2023) Generation and functional analysis of defective viral genomes during SARS-CoV-2 infection. *mBio* 14(3):e0025023. doi:10.1128/mbio.00250–23.

33 Shapira, T., Vimalanathan, S., Rens, C., Pichler, V., Peña-Díaz, S., et al. (2022) Inhibition of glycogen synthase kinase-3-beta (GSK3β) blocks nucleocapsid phosphorylation and SARS-CoV-2 replication. *Mol Biomed* 3(1):43. doi:10.1186/s43556–022-00111–1.

34 Yadav et al., Role of structural and non-structural proteins and therapeutic targets of SARS-CoV-2 for COVID-19.

35 El-Kamand, S., Du Plessis, M.-D., Breen, N., Johnson, L., Beard, S., et al. (2022) A distinct ssDNA/RNA binding interface in the Nsp9 protein from SARS-CoV-2. *Proteins* 90(1):176–85. doi:10.1002/prot.26205.

36 Zheng, Y., Deng, J., Han, L., Zhuang, M.W., Xu, Y., et al. (2022) SARS-CoV-2 NSP5 and N protein counteract the RIG-I signaling pathway by suppressing the formation of stress granules. *Sig Transduct Target Ther* 7:22. doi:10.1038/s41392–022-00878–3.

37 Mathieu, E., Ritchie, H., Rodés-Guirao, L., Appel, C., Giattino, C., et al. (2020) Coronavirus pandemic (COVID-19). OurWorldInData.org. Search for Canada. Retrieved from ourworldindata.org/covid-cases.

38 CanCOGen. (2022) Sequencing Update. Retrieved from mailchi.mp/b44efcbca5ff/cancogen-briefing-note-dinformation-sur-rcangco.

39 Colson, P., Parola, P., Raoult, D. (2022) The emergence, dynamics and significance of SARS-CoV-2 variants. *New Microbes New Infect* 45:100962. doi:10.1016/j.nmni.2022.100962.

40 Government of Canada (2023) COVID-19 epidemiology update: Testing and variants. Retrieved from health-infobase.canada.ca/covid-19/testing-variants.html.

41 Wu, F., Zhao, S., Yu, B., Chen, Y.M., Wang, W., et al. (2020) A new coronavirus associated with human respiratory disease in China. *Nature* 579(7798):265–69. doi:10.1038/s41586–020-2008–3.

42 Wrapp, D., Wang, N., Corbett, K. S., Goldsmith, J. A., Hsieh, C. L., et al. (2020) Cryo-EM structure of the 2019-nCoV spike in the prefusion conformation. *Science* 367(6483):1260–63. doi:10.1126/science.abb2507.

43 Ledford, H. (2021) How severe are Omicron infections? *Nature* 600(7890):577–78. doi:10.1038/d41586–021-03794–8.

44 Africa Center for Disease Control and Prevention (2023) COVID-19 vaccination. Africa Center for Disease Control and Prevention. Retrieved from africacdc.org/covid-19-vaccination/.

45 Mathieu, E., Ritchie, H., Rodés-Guirao, L., Appel, C., Giattino, C., et al. (2020) Coronavirus pandemic (COVID-19). OurWorldInData.org. Search for Canada. Retrieved from ourworldindata.org/covid-deaths.

46 Dion, P. (2021) Reductions in life expectancy directly associated with COVID-19 in 2020. Statistics Canada. Retrieved from www150.statcan.gc.ca/n1/pub/91f0015m/91f0015m2021002-eng.htm.

47 Katella, K. (2023) What to know about EG.5 (Eris)—the latest coronavirus strain. Yale Medicine. Retrieved from www.yalemedicine.org/news/covid-eg5-eris-latest-coronavirus-strain.

48 Lewnard, J. A., Hong, V. X., Patel, M. M., Kahn, R., Lipsitch, M., Tartof, S. Y. (2022) Clinical outcomes associated with SARS-CoV-2 Omicron (B.1.1.529) variant and BA.1/BA.1.1 or BA.2 subvariant infection in Southern California. *Nat Med* 28(9): 1933–43. doi:10.1038/s41591–022-01887-z.

49 Kaku, Y., Okumura, K., Padilla-Blanco, M., Kosugi, Y., Uriu, K., et al. (2024) Genotype to phenotype Japan (G2P-Japan) Consortium; Zahradnik, J., Ito, J., Sato, K. Virological characteristics of the SARS-CoV-2 JN.1 variant. *Lancet Infect Dis* 24(2):e82. doi:10.1016/S1473–3099(23)00813–7.

50 Focosi, D., Maggi, F. (2022) Recombination in coronaviruses, with a focus on SARS-CoV-2. *Viruses* 14(6):1239. doi:10.3390/v14061239.

51 Turakhia, Y., Thornlow, B., Hinrichs, A., McBroome, J., Ayala, N., et al. (2022) Pandemic-scale phylogenomics reveals the SARS-CoV-2 recombination landscape. *Nature* 609(7929):994–97. doi:10.1038/s41586–022-05189–9.

52 Baric, R. S., Fu, K., Schaad, M. C., Stohlman, S. A. (1990) Establishing a genetic recombination map for murine coronavirus strain A59 complementation groups. *Virology* 177(2):646–56. doi:10.1016/0042–6822(90)90530–5.

53 Holmes, E. C., Rambaut, A. (2004) Viral evolution and the emergence of SARS coronavirus. *Philos Trans R Soc Lond B Biol Sci* 359(1447):1059–65. doi:10.1098/rstb.2004.1478.

54 Corman, V. M., Ithete, N. L., Richards, L. R., Schoeman, M. C., Preiser, W., et al. (2014) Rooting the phylogenetic tree of Middle East respiratory syndrome coronavirus by characterization of a conspecific virus from an African bat. *J Virol* 88(19):11297–303. doi:10.1128/JVI.01498–14.

55 Tanaka, A., Miyazawa, T. (2023) Unnaturalness in the evolution process of the SARS-CoV-2 variants and the possibility of deliberate natural selection. *Zenodo*. doi:10.5281/zendo.8216373.

56 Shrestha, L. B., Foster, C., Rawlinson, W., Tedla, N., Bull, R. A. (2022) Evolution of the SARS-CoV-2 omicron variants BA.1 to BA.5: Implications for immune escape and transmission. *Rev Med Virol* 32(5):e2381. doi:10.1002/rmv.2381.

57 Tanaka and Miyazawa, Unnaturalness in the evolution process of the SARS-CoV-2 variants.

58 Ibid.

59 Ibid.

60 Karim, F., Moosa, M. Y. S., Gosnell, B. I., Cele, S., Giandhari, J., Pillay, S., et al. (2021) Persistent SARS-CoV-2 infection and intra-host evolution in association with advanced HIV infection. medRxiv (preprint). doi:10.1101/2021.06.03.21258228.

61 Wei et al., Evidence for a mouse origin of the SARS-CoV-2 Omicron variant.

62 Stolberg, S. G., Mueller, B., Zimmer, C. (2023) The origins of the Covid pandemic: What we know and don't know. *New York Times*. Retrieved from www.nytimes.com /article/covid-origin-lab-leak-china.html.

63 Temmam, S., Vongphayloth, K., Baquero, E., Munier, S., Bonomi, M., et al. (2022) Bat coronaviruses related to SARS-CoV-2 and infectious for human cells. *Nature* 604(7905):330–36. doi:10.1038/s41586–022-04532–4.

64 Mohammed, M. E. A. (2021) The percentages of SARS-CoV-2 protein similarity and identity with SARS-CoV and BatCoV RaTG13 proteins can be used as indicators of virus origin. *J Proteins Proteom* 12(2):81–91. doi:10.1007/s42485–021-00060–3.

65 Temmam, S., Vongphayloth, K., Baquero, E., Munier, S., Bonomi, M., et al. Bat coronaviruses related to SARS-CoV-2 and infectious for human cells.

66 Segreto, R., Deigin, Y. (2021) The genetic structure of SARS-CoV-2 does not rule out a laboratory origin. *BioEssays* 43(3):2000240. doi:10.1002/bies.202000240.

67 Ambati, B. K., Varshney, A., Lundstrom, K., Palú, G., Uhal, B. D., et al. (2022) MSH3 homology and potential recombination link to SARS-CoV-2 furin cleavage site. *Frontiers in Virology* 2:834808. doi:10.3389/fviro.2022.834808.

68 Ambati, B. K., Varshney, A., Lundstrom, K., Palú, G., Uhal, B. D., et al. (2022) Corrigendum: MSH3 homology and potential recombination link to SARS-CoV-2 furin cleavage site. *Frontiers in Virology* 2:884169. doi:10.3389/fviro.2022.884169.

69 Bruttel, V., Washburne, A., VanDongen, A. (2023) Endonuclease fingerprint indicates a synthetic origin of SARS-CoV-2. bioRxiv (preprint) 2022.2010.2018.512756. doi:10.1101/2022.10.18.512756.

Chapter 6

1 von Bartheld, C. S., Wang, L. (2023) Prevalence of olfactory dysfunction with the Omicron variant of SARS-CoV-2: A systematic review and meta-analysis. *Cells* 12(3): 430. doi1:10.3390/cells12030430.

2 Chen, G., Wu, D., Guo, W., Cao, Y., Huang, D., et al. (2019) Clinical and immunological features of severe and moderate coronavirus disease. *J Clin Invest* 130(5):2620–29. doi:10.1172/JCI137244.

3 Laverty, M., Salvadori, M. I., Squires, S. G., Ahmed, M. A., Eisenbeis, L., et al. (2021) Multisystem inflammatory syndrome in children in Canada. *Can Commun Dis Rep* 47(11):461–65. doi:10.14745/ccdr.v47i11a03.

4 Patel, P., DeCuir, J., Abrams, J., Campbell, A. P., Godfred-Cato, S., Belay, E. D. (2021) Clinical characteristics of multisystem inflammatory syndrome in adults: A systematic review. *JAMA Netw Open* 4(9):e2126456. doi:10.1001/jamanetworkopen.2021.26456.

5 Varatharajah, N. (2020) COVID-19 clot: What is it? Why in the Lung? Extracellular histone, "auto-activation" of prothrombin, emperipoiesis, megakaryocytes, "self-association" of Von Willebrand factor and beyond. *Preprints* 2020070516. doi:10.20944/preprints 202007.0516.v1.

6 Knight, R., Walker, V., Ip, S., Cooper, J. A., Bolton, T., et al. (2022) Association of COVID-19 with major arterial and venous thrombotic diseases: A population-wide cohort study of 48 million adults in England and Wales. *Circulation* 146(12):892–906. doi:10.1161/circulationaha.122.060785.

7 Mann, K. G., Brummel-Ziedins, K. E. (2018) Normal coagulation. In *Rutherford's Vascular Surgery* (7th ed., Vol 1, pp. 518–40). Philadelphia: Saunders/Elsevier.

8 Lapner, S. T., Kearon, C. (2013) Diagnosis and management of pulmonary embolism. *Br Med J* 346:f757. doi:10.1136/bmj.f757.

9 Liebman, H. A., Weitz, I. C. (2018) Hypercoagulable states. In *Rutherford's Vascular Surgery*. (7th ed., Vol 1, pp 588–99). Philadelphia: Saunders/Elsevier.

10 Weaver, F. A. (2018) Bleeding and Clotting. In *Rutherford's Vascular Surgery* (7th Edition, p 533). Philadelphia: Saunders/Elsevier.

11 Mann, K. G., Brummel-Ziedins, K. E. (2018) Normal coagulation. In *Rutherford's Vascular Surgery*.

12 Marik, P. E., Iglesias, J., Varon, J., Kory P. (2021) A scoping review of the pathophysiology of COVID-19. *Int J Immunopath and Pharmacol* 35:20587384211048026. doi:10.1177/20587384211048026.

13 Lei, Y., Zhang, J., Schiavon, C. R., He, M., Chen, L., et al. (2021) SARS-CoV-2 spike protein impairs endothelial function via down regulation of ACE2. *Circ Res* 128(9):1323–26. doi:10.1161/circresaha.121.318902.

14 Raghavan, S., Kenchappa, D. B., Leo, M. D. (2021) SARS-CoV-2 spike protein induces degradation of junctional proteins that maintain endothelial barrier integrity. *Front Cardiovasc Med* 8:687783. doi:10.3389/fcvm.2021.687783.

15 Venter, C., Bezuidenhout, J. A., Laubscher, G. J., Lourens, P. J., Steenkamp, J., et al. (2020) Erythrocyte, platelet, serum ferritin, and P-selectin pathophysiology implicated in severe hypercoagulation and vascular complications in COVID-19. *Int J Mol Sci* 21(21):8234. doi:10.3390/ijms21218234.

16 Borczuk, A. C., Salvatore, S. P., Seshan, S. V., Patel, S. S., Bussel, J. B., et al. (2020) COVID-19 pulmonary pathology: A multi-institutional autopsy cohort from Italy and New York City. *Modern Pathology* 33(11):2156–68. doi:10.1038/s41379–020-00661–1.

17 Lodigani, C., Iapichino, G., Carenzo, L., Cecconi, M., Ferrazzi, P., et al. (2020) Venous and arterial thromboembolic complications in COVID-19 patients admitted to an academic hospital in Milan, Italy. *Thromb Res* 191:P9–14. doi:10.1016/j.thromres.2020.04.024.

18 Xie, Y., Xu, E., Bowe, B., Al-Aly, Z. (2022) Long-term cardiovascular outcomes of COVID-19. *Nat Med* 28(3):583–90. doi:10.1038/s41591–022-01689–3.

19 Hemasian, H., Ansari, B. (2020) First case of COVID-19 with cerebral venous thrombosis: A rare and dreaded case. *Revue Neurol* 176(6):521–23. doi:10.1016/j.neurol.2020.04.013.

20 Thompson, A., Morgan, C., Smith, P., Jones, C., Ball, H., et al. (2020) Cerebral venous sinus thrombosis associated with COVID-19. *Prac Neurol* 21(1):75–76. doi:10.1136/practneurol-2020–002678.

21 Chen, C., Shi, P. F., Qian, S. X. (2022) Acute mesenteric ischemia in patients with COVID-19: Review of the literature. *J Natl Med Assoc* 14(1):47–55. doi:10.1016/j.jnma.2021.12.003.

22 NIH COVID-19 Treatment Guidelines PNEL. (2023) Coronavirus Disease 2019 (COVID-19) Treatment Guidelines: Antithrombotic therapy in patients with COVID-19. Retrieved from www.COVID19treatmentguidelines.nih.gov/therapies/antithrombotic-therapy/.

23 Chou, S. H., Beghi, E., Helbok, R., Moro, E., Sampson, J., et al. (2021) Global incidence of neurological manifestations among patients hospitalized with COVID-19. A report for the GCS-NeuroCOVID Consortium and the ENERGY Consortium. *JAMA Network Open* 4(5):e2112131. doi:10.1001/jamanetworkopen2021.12131.

24 Ousseiran, Z. H., Fares, Y., Chamoun, W. T. (2023) Neurological manifestations of COVID-19: A systematic review and detailed comprehension. *Int J Neurosci* 133(7):754–69. doi:10.1080/00207454.2021.

25 Veleri, S. (2021) Neurotropism of SARS-CoV-2 and neurological diseases of the central nervous system in COVID-19 patients. *Exp Brain Res* 240(1):9–25. doi:10.1007/s00221–021-06244-z.

26 Joshi, D., Gyanpuri, V., Pathak, A., Chaurasia, R. N., Mishra, V. N., et al. (2022) Neuropathic pain associated with COVID-19: A systematic review of case reports. *Curr Pain Headache Rep* 26(8):595–603. doi:10.1007/s11916–022-01065–3.

27 Favas, T. T., Dev, P., Chaurasia, R. N., Chakravarty, K., Mishra, R., et al. (2020) Neurological manifestations of COVID-19: A systematic review and meta-analysis of proportions. *Neurological Sciences* 41(12):3437–70. doi:10.1007/s10072–020-04801-y.

28 Fotuhi, M., Mian, A., Meysami, S., Raji, C. A. (2020) Neurobiology of COVID-19. *J Alzheimer's Dis* 76(1):3–19. doi:10.3233/JAD-200581.

29 Helms, J., Kremer, S., Merdji, H., Clere-Jehl, R., Schenck, M., et al. (2020) Neurologic features in severe SARS-CoV-2 infection. *N Engl J Med* 382(23):2268–70. doi:10.1056/NEJMc2008597.

30 Liotta, E. M., Batra, A., Clark, J. R., Shlobin, N. A., Hoffman, S. C., et al. (2020) Frequent neurologic manifestations and encephalopathy-associated morbidity in Covid-19 patients. *Ann Clin Trans Neurol* 7(11):2221–30. doi:10.1002/acn3.51210.

31 Najjar, S., Najjar, A., Chong, D. J., Pramanik, B. K., Kirsch C., et al. (2020) Central nervous system complications associated with SARS-CoV-2 infection: Integrative concepts of pathophysiology and case reports. *J Neuroinflammation* 17(1):231. doi:10.1186/s12974–020-01896–0.

32 Nepal, G., Rehrig, J. H., Shrestha, G. S., Shing, Y. K., Yadav, J. K., et al. (2020) Neurological manifestations of COVID-19: A systematic review. *Critical Care* 24(1): 421. doi:10.1186/s13054–020-03121-z.

33 Singh, A. K., Bhushan, B., Maurya, A., Mishra, G., Singh, S. K., Awasthi, R. (2020) Novel coronavirus disease 2019 (COVID-19) and neurodegenerative disorders. *Dermatologic Therapy* 33(4):e13591. doi:10.1111/dth.13591.

34 Nazari, S., Azari, J. A., Mirmoeeni, S., Sadeghian, S., Heidari, M. E., et al. (2021) Central nervous system manifestations in COVID-19 patients: A systematic review and meta-analysis. *Brain Behav* 11(5), e02025. doi:10.1002/brb3.2025

35 Ongur, D., Perlis, R., Goff, D. (2020) Psychiatry and COVID-19. *JAMA* 324(12):1149–50. doi:10.1001/jama.2020.14294.

36 Taquet, M., Luciano, S., Geddes, J.R., Harrison, P. J. (2021) Bidirectional associations between COVID-19 and psychiatric disorder: Retrospective cohort studies of 62 354 COVID-19 cases in the USA. *Lancet Psychiatry* 8(2):130–40. doi:10.1016/S2215–0366(20)30462.

37 Baig, A. M. (2020) Deleterious outcomes in long-hauler COVID- 19: The effects of SARS-CoV-2 on the CNS in chronic COVID syndrome. *ACS Chem Neurosci* 11(24):4017–20. doi:10.1021/acschemneuro.0c00725.

38 Kempuraj, D., Selvakumar, G. P., Ahmed, M. E., Raikwar, S. P., Thangavel, R., et al. (2020) COVID-19, mast cells, cytokine storm, psychological stress, and neuroinflammation. *Neuroscientist* 26(5–6):402–14. doi:10.1177/1073858420941476; Taquet et al., Bidirectional associations between COVID-19 and psychiatric disorder.

39 Levin, S. N., Venkatesh, S., Nelson, K. E., Li, Y., Aguerre, I., et al. (2021) Manifestations and impact of the COVID-19 pandemic in neuroinflammatory diseases. *Ann Clin Transl Neurol* 8(4):918–28. doi:10.1002/acn3.51314.

40 Theoharides, T. Could SARS-CoV-2 spike protein be responsible for long-COVID syndrome? *Mol Neurobiol* 59(3):1850–61. doi:10.1007/s12035–021-02696–0.

41 Theoharides, T., Kempuraj. Role of SARS-CoV2 spike protein-induced activation of microglia and mast cells in pathogenesis of Neuro-COVID. *Cells* 12(5):688. doi:10.3390/cells12050688.

42 Theoharides, T. Could SARS-CoV-2 spike protein be responsible for long-COVID syndrome?; Seneff, S., Nigh, G., Kyriakopoulos, A.M., McCullough P.A. (2022) Innate immune suppression by SARS-CoV-2 mRNA vaccinations: The role of G-quadruplexes, exosomes, and MicroRNAs. Food Chem Toxicol. 164:113008 doi:10.1016/j.fct.2022.113008.

43 Dosch, S. F., Mahajan, S. D., Collins, A. R. (2009) SARS coronavirus spike protein-induced innate immune response occurs via activation of the NF-kappaB pathway in human monocyte macrophages *in vitro*. *Virus Res* 142(1–2):19–27. doi:10.1016/j.virusres.2009.01.005.

44 Theoharides, T. C., Conti, P. (2020) COVID-19 and multisystem inflammatory syndrome, or is it mast cell activation syndrome? *J Biol Regul Homeost Agents* 34(5):1633–36. doi:10.23812/20-EDIT3.

45 Barhoumi, T., Alghanem, B., Shaibah, H., Mansour, F. A., Alamri, H. S., et al. (2021) SARS-CoV-2 coronavirus spike protein-induced apoptosis, inflammatory, and oxidative stress responses in THP-1-like-macrophages: Potential role of angiotensin-converting enzyme inhibitor (Perindopril). *Front Immunol* 20(12):728896. doi:10.3389/fimmu.2021.728896.

46 Robles, J.P., Zamora, M., Adan-Castro, E., Siqueiros-Marquez, L., Martinez de la Escalera, G., Clapp, C. (2022) The spike protein of SARS-CoV-2 induces endothelial inflammation through integrin α5β1 and NF-κB signaling. *J Biol Chem.* 298(3):101695. doi:10.1016/j.jbc.2022.101695.

47 DeOre, B. J., Tran, K. A., Andrews, A. M., Ramirez, S. H., Galie, P. A. (2021) SARS-CoV-2 Spike protein disrupts blood-brain barrier integrity via RhoA activation. *J Neuroimmune Pharmacol* 16(4):722–28. doi:10.1007/s11481–021-10029–0.

48 Rhea, E. M., Logsdon, A. F., Hansen, K. M., Williams, L. M., Reed, M. J., et al. (2021) The S1 protein of SARS-CoV-2 crosses the blood-brain barrier in mice. *Nature Neurosci* 24(3):368–78. doi:10.1038/s41593–020-00771–8.

49 Kim, E. S., Jeon, M. T., Kim, K. S., Lee, S., Kim, S., Kim, D. G. (2021) Spike proteins of SARS-CoV-2 induce pathological changes in molecular delivery and metabolic function in the brain endothelial cells. *Viruses* 13(10):021. doi:10.3390/v13102021.

50 Xia, H., Lazartigues, E. (2008) Angiotensin-converting enzyme 2 in the brain: Properties and future directions. *J Neurochem* 107(6):1482–94. doi:10.1111/j.1471–4159.2008.05723.x.

51 Fertig, T. E., Chitoiu, L., Marta, D. S., Ionescu, V. S., Cismasiu, V. B., et al. (2022) Vaccine mRNA can be detected in blood at 15 days post-vaccination. *Biomedicines* 10(7):1538. doi:10.3390/biomedicines10071538.

52 Röltgen, K., Nielsen, S. C. A., Silva, O., Younes, S. F., Zaslavsky, M., et al. (2022) Immune imprinting, breadth of variant recognition, and germinal center response in human SARS-CoV-2 infection and vaccination. *Cell* 185(6):1025–40.e14. doi: 10.1016/j.cell.2022.01.018.

53 Castruita, J. A. S., Schneider, U. V., Mollerup, S., Leineweber, T. D., Weis, N., et al. (2023) SARS-CoV-2 spike mRNA vaccine sequences circulate in blood up to 28 days after COVID-19 vaccination. *APMIS* 131(3):128–32. doi:10.1111/apm.13294.

54 Ogata, A. F., Cheng, C. A., Desjardins, M., Senussi, Y., Sherman, A. C., et al. (2022) Circulating severe acute respiratory syndrome coronavirus 2 (SARS-CoV-2) vaccine antigen detected in the plasma of mRNA-1273 vaccine recipients. *Clin Infect Dis* 74(4):715–18. doi:10.1093/cid/ciab465.

55 Rong, Z., Mai, H., Kapoor, S., Puelles, V. G., Czogalla, J., et al. (2023) SARS-CoV-2 spike protein accumulation in the skull-meninges-brain axis: Potential implications for long-term neurological complications in post-COVID-19. bioRxiv [Preprint]. doi:10.1101/2023.04.04.535604.

56 Mörz, M. (2022) A case report: Multifocal necrotizing encephalitis and myocarditis after BNT162b2 mRNA vaccination against COVID-19. *Vaccines* (Basel) 10(10):1651. doi:10.3390/vaccines10101651.

57 Health Info Database (2023) COVID-19: Longer-term symptoms among Canadian adults—Highlight. Retrieved from health-infobase.canada.ca/covid-19/post-covid-condition/.

58 Davis, H. E., McCorkell, L., Vogel, J. M., Topol, E. J. (2023) Long COVID: Major findings, mechanisms and recommendations. *Nat Rev Microbiol* 21:133–46. doi:10.1038/s41579–022-00846–2.

59 Ayoubkhani, D., Bosworth, M. K., King, A., Pouwels, K. B., Glickman, M., et al. (2022) Risk of Long COVID in people infected with severe acute respiratory syndrome coronavirus 2 after 2 doses of a coronavirus disease 2019 vaccine: Community-based, matched cohort study, *Open Forum Infectious Diseases* 9(9):ofac464. doi:10.1093/ofid/ofac464.

60 CDC. (2022) Long COVID—household pulse survey—COVID-19. CDC. Retrieved from www.cdc.gov/nchs/covid19/pulse/long-covid.htm.

61 Williamson, A. E., Tydeman, F., Miners, A., Pyper, K., Martineau, A. R. (2022) Short-term and long-term impacts of COVID-19 on economic vulnerability: A population-based longitudinal study (COVIDENCE UK). *BMJ Open* 12(8):e065083. doi:10.1136/bmjopen-2022–065083.

62 Ziauddeen, N., Gurdasani, D., O'Hara, M. E., Hastie, C., Roderick, P., et al. (2022) Characteristics and impact of Long Covid: Findings from an online survey. *PLOS One* 17(3):e0264331. doi:10.1371/journal.pone.0264331.

63 Public Health Agency of Canada. (2023) Post COVID-19 condition (long COVID). Retrieved from www.canada.ca/en/public-health/services/diseases/2019-novel-coronavirus-infection/symptoms/post-covid-19-condition.html.

64 Lambert, N., El-Azab, S.A., Ramrakhiani, N. S., Barisano, A., Yu, L., et al. (2022) The other COVID-19 survivors: Timing, duration, and health impact of post-acute sequelae of SARS-CoV-2 infection. *J Clin. Nurs* 10.1111/jocn.16541. doi:10.1111/jocn.16541.

65 Girl to Mom. (2021) Heidi's eulogy. Retrieved from web.archive.org/web/20210920221136/girltomom.com/a-prayer/heidis-eulogy.

66 r/medicine. (2021) Reddit. A new study finds that most "Long COVID" symptoms are not independently associated with evidence of prior SARS-CoV-2 infection (except loss of sense of smell), but is associated with belief in having had COVID. Retrieved from www.reddit.com/r/medicine/comments/qsbav1/comment/hke8ado/?context=8&depth=9.

67 Bisaccia, G., Ricci, F., Recce, V., Serio, A., Iannetti, G., et al. (2021) Post-acute sequelae of COVID-19 and cardiovascular autonomic dysfunction: What do we know? *J. Cardiovascular Dev Dis 8*(11):156. doi:10.3390/jcdd8110156.

68 Diexer, S., Klee, B., Gottschick, C., Xu, C., Broda, A., et al. (2023) Association between virus variants, vaccination, previous infections, and post-COVID-19 risk. *Int J Infect Dis* 136:14–21. doi:10.1016/j.ijid.2023.08.019.

69 Schieffer, E. Schieffer, B. (2022) The rationale for the treatment of long-Covid symptoms—A cardiologist's view. *Front. Cardiovasc. Med* 9:992686. doi:10.3389/fcvm.2022.992686.

70 Long COVID or post-COVID conditions. Retrieved from web.archive.org/save/www.cdc.gov/coronavirus/2019-ncov/long-term-effects/index.html.

71 Tsuchida, T., Hirose, M., Inoue, Y., Kunishima, H., Otsubo, T., Matsuda, T. (2022) Relationship between changes in symptoms and antibody titers after a single vaccination in patients with Long COVID. *J Med Virol* 94(7):3416–20. doi:10.1002/jmv.27689.

72 Asadi-Pooya, A. A., Nemati, M., Shahisavandi, M., Nemati, H., Karimi, A., et al. (2024) How does COVID-19 vaccination affect long-COVID symptoms? *PLoS One* 19(2):e0296680. doi:10.1371/journal.pone.0296680.

73 Del Franco, H., Carvallo, C., Roberto, H. (2022) Ivermectin in Long-Covid patients: A retrospective study. *J. Biomed Res Clin Invest* 2(1):1008. doi:10.31546/2633–8653.1008.

74 Xie, Y., Choi, T., Al-Aly, Z. (2022) Nirmatrelvir and the risk of post-acute sequelae of COVID-19. medRxiv (Preprint). doi:10.1101/2022.11.03.22281783.

75 Peluso, M. J., Ryder, D., Flavell, R., Wang, Y., Levi, J., et al. (2023) Multimodal molecular imaging reveals tissue-based T Cell activation and viral RNA persistence for up to 2 years following COVID-19. medRxiv (preprint) 2023.07.27.23293177. doi:10.1101/2023.07.27.23293177.

76 Bramante, C. T., Buse, J. B, Liebovitz, D. M., Nicklas, J. M., Puskarich, M. A., et al. (2023) Outpatient treatment of COVID-19 and incidence of post-COVID-19 condition over 10 months (COVID-OUT): A multicentre, randomised, quadruple-blind, parallel-group, phase 3 trial. *Lancet Infect Dis* 8:S1473–3099(23)00299–2. doi:10.1016/S1473–3099(23)00299–2.

77 Statistics Canada. (2023) Between April and August 2022, 98 percent of Canadians had antibodies against COVID-19 and 54 percent had antibodies from a previous infection.

Retrieved from www150.statcan.gc.ca/n1/daily-quotidien/230327/dq230327b-eng.htm.

78 COVID-19 epidemiology update: Summary. (2023) Health Infobase. Public Health Agency of Canada. Retrieved from health-infobase.canada.ca/src/data/Covidlive/epidemiological-summary-of-Covid-19-cases-in-Canada-Canada.ca.pdf.

79 Klann, J.G., Strasser, Z.H., Hutch, M.R., Kennedy, C.J., Marwaha, J.S., et al.; Consortium for Clinical Characterization of COVID-19 by EHR (4CE). (2022) Distinguishing admissions specifically for COVID-19 from incidental SARS-CoV-2 admissions: National retrospective electronic health record study. *J Med Internet Res.* 24(5):e37931. doi:10.2196/37931; Carrigg, D. (2022) Majority of new COVID-19 hospitalizations in B.C. among people admitted for other reasons. *The Vancouver Sun.* Retrieved from https://vancouversun.com/news/local-news/majority-of-new-covid-19-hospitalizations-among-people-admitted-for-other-reasons.

80 Lewnard, J.A., Hong, V.X., Patel, M.M., Kahn, R., Lipsitch, M. Tartof, S.Y. (2022) Clinical outcomes associated with SARS-CoV-2 Omicron (B.1.1.529) variant and BA.1/BA.1.1 or BA.2 subvariant infection in southern California. *Nat Med.* 28(9):1933–1943. doi:10.1038/s41591–022-01887-z.

81 (2023) Mortality Analysis. John Hopkins University of Medicine Coronavirus Resource Center. Retrieved from https://coronavirus.jhu.edu/data/mortality.

82 (2023) COVID-19 epidemiology update: Summary. Health Infobase. Public Health Agency of Canada. Retrieved from https://health-infobase.canada.ca/src/data/Covidlive/epidemiological-summary-of-Covid-19-cases-in-Canada-Canada.ca.pdf.

Chapter 7

1 Gordon, S. (2008) Elie Metchnikoff: Father of natural immunity. *Eur J Immunol* 38(12):3257–64. doi:10.1002/eji.200838855.

2 Yu, X., Tsibane, T., McGraw, P., House, F.S., Keefer, C.J., et al. (2008) Neutralizing antibodies derived from the B-cells of 1918 influenza pandemic survivors. *Nature* 455(7212):532–36. doi:10.1038/nature07231.

Chapter 8

1 Coronavirus disease (COVID-19): Contact tracing. World Health Organization. (2021) Retrieved from www.who.int/news-room/questions-and-answers/item/coronavirus-disease-covid-19-contact-tracing.

2 Sparks, D., and Mayo Clinic staff writers. (2020) Contact tracing and COVID-19: What is it and how does it work? Mayo Clinic. Retrieved from newsnetwork.mayoclinic.org/discussion/contact-tracing-and-covid-19-what-is-it-and-how-does-it-work.

3 Ibid.

4 Ibid.

5 Fetzer, T., Graeber, T. (2021) Measuring the scientific effectiveness of contact tracing: Evidence from a natural experiment. *Proc Natl Acad Sci USA* 118(33):e2100814118. doi:10.1073/pnas.2100814118; (2020) CCDR: Volume 46 Issue 11/12, November 5, 2020: Oral Health in Canada. Public Health Agency of Canada. Retrieved from https://www.canada.ca/en/public-health/services/reports-publications/canada-communicable-disease-report-ccdr/monthly-issue/2020–46/issue-11–12-november-5–2020.html.

6 COVID-19 for health professionals: Transmission. (2021) Public Health Agency of Canada. Retrieved from www.canada.ca/en/public-health/services/diseases/2019-novel-coronavirus-infection/health-professionals/transmission.html.

7 Public Health Agency of Canada. COVID-19 for health professionals: Diagnostic testing. (2021).

8 Ibid.

9 Ibid.

10 Ibid.

11 Mayo Clinic Staff. (2022) COVID-19 diagnostic testing. Mayo Clinic. Retrieved from www.mayoclinic.org/tests-procedures/covid-19-diagnostic-test/about/pac-20488900.

12 Udugama, B. P., Kadhiresan, H. N., Kozlowski, A., Malekjahani, M., Osborne, V. Y. C., et al. (2020) Diagnosing COVID-19: The disease and tools for detection. *ACS Nano* 14(4):3822–3835. doi:10.1021/acsnano.0c02624.

13 Bullard, J., Dust, K., Funk, D., Strong, J. E., Alexander, D., et al., (2020) Predicting infectious SARS-CoV-2 from diagnostic samples. *Clin. Infect. Dis* 71(10):2663–66. doi:10.1093/cid/ciaa638.

14 Bridle, B. W. (2022) Fundamentally flawed COVID-19 "Science": The misinformation that crushed constitutional freedoms of healthy/asymptomatic people. COVID Chronicles. Retrieved from viralimmunologist.substack.com/p/fundamentally-flawed-covid-19-science.

15 Panbio™ COVID-19 Ag rapid test device. (2023) Abbott. Retrieved from www.globalpointofcare.abbott/ca/en/product-details/panbio-covid-19-ag-antigen-test-ca.html.

16 Interim guidance for the detection of SARS-CoV-2 with the Abbott Panbio COVID-19 antigen rapid test. (2021) Public Health Agency of Canada. Retrieved from www.canada.ca/en/public-health/services/reports-publications/canada-.

17 SARS-CoV-2 antibody testing (COVID-19 serology). (2023) BC Centre for Disease Control, Provincial Health Services Authority. Retrieved from www.bccdc.ca/health-professionals/clinical-resources/covid-19-care/covid-19-testing/antibody-testing-(serology).

18 CanCOGeN: Canadian COVID-19 Genomics Network. (2021) Genome Canada. Retrieved from www.genomecanada.ca/en/cancogen Estimated COVID-19 burden.

19 Between April and August 2022, 98 percent of Canadians had antibodies against COVID-19 and 54 percent had antibodies from a previous infection. (2023) Statistic Canada. Retrieved from www150.statcan.gc.ca/n1/daily-quotidien/230327/dq230327b-eng.htm.

20 Action to beat coronavirus. (2020) Centre for Global Health research, Angus Reid Forum Inc. Retrieved from www.abcstudy.ca/.

21 Tang, X., Sharma, A., Pasic, M., Brown, P., Colwill, K., et al. (2022) Assessment of SARS-CoV-2 seropositivity during the first and second viral waves in 2020 and 2021 among Canadian adults. *JAMA Netw. Open* 5(2):e2146798. doi:10.1001/jamanetworkopen.2021.46798.

22 (2021) Interactive data visualizations of COVID-19: Count of total cases of COVID-19 in Canada as of August 19, 2021. Retrieved from web.archive.org/web/20210820134648/health-infobase.canada.ca/covid-19/?stat=num&measure=total#a2.

23 (2022) Estimated COVID-19 burden. Retrieved from www.cdc.gov/coronavirus/2019-ncov/cases-updates/burden.html.

24 Statistics Canada. Between April and August 2022, 98 percent of Canadians had antibodies against COVID-19 and 54 percent had antibodies from a previous

infection. (2023) Retrieved from www150.statcan.gc.ca/n1/daily-quotidien/230327/dq230327b-eng.htm.

25 COVID-19 antibody blood test panel. (2023) LifeLabs. Retrieved from www.lifelabs.com/test/covid19-antibody/.

26 Pısıl, Y., Shida, H., Miura, T. (2021) A neutralization assay based on pseudo-typed lentivirus with SARS CoV-2 spike protein in ACE2-expressing CRFK cells. *Pathogens* 10(2):153. doi:10.3390/pathogens10020153.

27 Majdoubi, A., Michalski, C., O'Connell, S. E., Dada, S., Narpala, S., et al. (2021) A majority of uninfected adults show pre-existing antibody reactivity against SARS-CoV-2. *JCI Insight* 6(8): e14631. doi:10.1172/jci.insight.146316.

28 Tools for COVID-19 research. Meso Scale (2023) Diagnostics. Retrieved from www.mesoscale.com/en/products_and_services/assay_kits/covid-19.

29 Majdoubi et al., A majority of uninfected adults show pre-existing antibody reactivity against SARS-CoV-2.

30 Members of the CITF Secretariat. (2023) Most Canadians have acquired antibodies against SARS-CoV-2. Retrieved from www.covid19immunitytaskforce.ca/most-canadians-have-acquired-antibodies-against-sars-cov-2/.

31 Health Canada, Interactive data visualizations of COVID-19.

32 Canadian Blood Services COVID-19 Seroprevalence Brief Report #19A (2022): February 1–15, 2022 Survey. Retrieved from www.covid19immunitytaskforce.ca/wp-content/uploads/2022/04/covid-19-report-feb-2022-march-2022.pdf.

33 Spotlight on CITF-funded research. COVID-19 Immunity Task Force. (2023) Retrieved from us2.campaign-archive.com/?u=45f45be60b2c411f213c404a2&id=cae24a1167

34 Ibid.

35 Personal communication: Mr. Michael Kuzmickas, Chief Executive Officer, Ichor Blood Services.

36 Parsons, P. (2022) Health expert urges caution after blood-testing firm claims "pandemic is over" in Alberta hamlet. Canadian Broadcasting Corporation News. Retrieved from www.cbc.ca/news/canada/edmonton/private-covid-19-antibody-tests-la-crete-alberta-1.6307357.

37 Pelech, S. (2023) The COVID-19 pandemic—What really happened. Canadian Covid Care Alliance. Retrieved from www.canadiancovidcarealliance.org/wp-content/uploads/2023/06/2023MAY3_Pelech-NCI-Presentation.pdf.

38 Skowronski, D., Kaweski, S. E., Irvine, M. A., Kim, S., Chuang, E. S. Y., et al. (2022) Serial cross-sectional estimate of vaccine and infection-induced SARS-CoV-2 seroprevalence in children and adults, British Columbia, Canada: March 2020 to August 2022. *CMAJ* 194(47):E1599-E1609. doi:10.1503/cmaj.221335.

39 Mallapaty, S. (2022) Most US kids have caught the coronavirus, antibody survey finds. *Nature* 605(7909):207. doi:10.1038/d41586–022-01231-y.

40 Clarke, K. E. N., Jones, J. M., Deng, Y., Nycz, E., Lee, A., et al. (2022) Seroprevalence of infection-induced SARS-CoV-2 antibodies—United States, September 2021–February 2022. *MMWR Morb Mortal Wkly Rep* 71(17):606–8. doi:10.15585/mmwr.mm7117e3.

41 Office for National Statistics. (2022) COVID-19 school infection survey, antibody data, England. Retrieved from www.ons.gov.uk/peoplepopulationandcommunity/healthandsocialcare/conditionsanddiseases/datasets/covid19schoolsinfectionsurveyantibodydataengland.

42 Immunity Diagnostics Inc. (2020) To unravel the secrets of the immune system. Retrieved from web.archive.org/web/20221202165035/www.immunity-dx.com/.
43 Ichor Blood Services. (2023) T-Detect™ T cell COVID-19 testing is now available in Canada as of March 7th. Retrieved from ichorblood.ca/tcell.
44 The COVID vaccine study. (2023) Control Group Wiki. Retrieved from www.vcgwiki.com/the-covid-vaccine-study.
45 Verkerk, R., Kathrada, N., Plothe, C., Lindley, K. (2022) Self-selected COVID-19 "unvaccinated" cohort reports favorable health outcomes and unjustified discrimination in global survey. *Int J Vacc Theor Prac Res* 2(2):321–54. doi:10.56098/ijvtpr.v2i2.43.
46 Gazit, S., Shlezinger, R., Perez, G., Lotan, R., Peretz, A., et al. (2022) Severe Acute Respiratory Syndrome Coronavirus 2 (SARS-CoV-2) naturally acquired immunity versus vaccine-induced immunity, reinfections versus breakthrough infections: A retrospective cohort study. *Clin Infect Dis* 75(1):e545–51. doi:10.1093/cid/ciac262.
47 Hall, V. J., Foulkes, S., Charlett, A., Atti, A., Monk, E. J. M., et al.; SIREN Study Group. (2021) SARS-CoV-2 infection rates of antibody-positive compared with antibody-negative health-care workers in England: a large, multicentre, prospective cohort study (SIREN). *Lancet* 397(10283):1459–69. doi:10.1016/S0140–6736(21)00675–9.
48 Wang, Z., Muecksch, F., Schaefer-Babajew, D., Finkin, S., Viant, C., et al. (2021) Naturally enhanced neutralizing breadth against SARS-CoV-2 one year after infection. *Nature* 595(7867):426–31. doi:10.1038/s41586–021-03696–9.
49 Gallais, F., Gantner, P., Bruel, T., Velay, A., Planas, D., et al. (2021) Evolution of antibody responses up to 13 months after SARS-CoV-2 infection and risk of reinfection. *EBioMedicine* 71:103561. doi:10.1016/j.ebiom.2021.103561.

Chapter 9

1 Bostock, J. (1855) Translated Book XXXIII. The natural history of metals. Chapter 40. *Natural History of Pliny, the Elder*.
2 Black, W. (2020) Plague doctors: Separating medical myths from facts. *Live Science*. Retrieved from www.livescience.com/plague-doctors.html.
3 Clark, D. (2020) San Francisco had the 1918 flu under control. And then it lifted the restrictions. NBC News. Retrieved from www.nbcnews.com/politics/politics-news/san-francisco-had-1918-flu-under-control-then-it-lifted-n1191141.
4 Lee, S.-A., Grinshpun, S. A., Reponen, T. (2008) Respiratory performance offered by N95 respirators and surgical masks: Human subject evaluation with NaCl aerosol representing bacterial and viral particle size range. *Ann Occup Hyg* 52:177–85. doi:10.1093/annhyg/men005.
5 Zhu, N., Zhang, D., Wang, W., Li, X., Yang, B., et al. (2019) A novel coronavirus from patients with pneumonia in China, 2019. *N Engl J Med*. doi:10.1056/NEJMoa2001017.
6 (2006) The Canadian pandemic influenza plan for the health sector. Retrieved from www.longwoods.com/articles/images/Canada_Pandemic_Influenza.pdf, see page 227.
7 (2015) Surveillance annex: Canadian pandemic influenza preparedness: Planning guidance for the health sector. Retrieved from www.canada.ca/en/public-health/services/flu-influenza/canadian-pandemic-influenza-preparedness-planning-guidance-health-sector/surveillance-annex.htm.

8 (2020) Tam: Current evidence doesn't support public needing masks. Retrieved from www.youtube.com/watch?app=desktop&v=_edxN5kkBtc.

9 Thomson Reuters. (2020) Wear a mask while having sex with someone new, Canada's top doctor suggests. Canadian Broadcasting Corporation News. Retrieved from www.cbc.ca/news/health/wear-a-mask-while-having-sex-1.5709698.

10 (2020) Message from Dr. Bonnie Henry provincial health officer. Retrieved from optometrybc.com/notices/news-stories/message-from-dr-bonnie-henry-provincial-health-officer/.

11 (2020) Dr. Bonnie Henry: Masks don't work. Retrieved from rumble.com/vt4za6-dr-bonnie-henry-masks-dont-work.html.

12 McElroy, J. (2020) B.C.'s mask mandate an about-face in a province struggling to replicate its 1st wave success. Canadian Broadcasting Corporation News. Retrieved from www.cbc.ca/news/canada/british-columbia/covid-masks-bc-mandate-november-2020–1.5809260.

13 (2022) B.C. takes next step in balanced plan to lift COVID-19 restrictions. Retrieved from news.gov.bc.ca/releases/2022HLTH0081–000324.

14 Chan, C. (2022) "Heavy hand" of mask mandate not needed in B.C.: Dr. Bonnie Henry. *Vancouver Sun*. Retrieved from vancouversun.com/news/local-news/bc-health-officials-respiratory-illnesses-calls-mask-requirements.

15 Wyton, M. (2023) B.C. ends mask mandate in health-care facilities and proof of vaccination for long-term care visitors. Canadian Broadcasting Corporation News. Retrieved from www.cbc.ca/news/canada/british-columbia/henry-dix-respiratory-update-april-2023–1.6804003#.

16 Lindsay, B., Pawson, C. (2023) New masking rules for health care settings in B.C. coming into force Oct 3, officials confirm. Canadian Broadcasting Corporation News. Retrieved from www.cbc.ca/news/canada/british-columbia/bc-enhanced-masking-health-care-settings-1.6980600.

17 Roche, D. (2021) Fauci said masks "not really effective in keeping out virus," email reveals. *Newsweek*. Retrieved from www.newsweek.com/fauci-said-masks-not-really-effective-keeping-out-virus-email-reveals-1596703.

18 (2023) Did Fauci say not to wear masks? Retrieved from www.cnn.com/factsfirst/politics/factcheck_e58c20c6–8735-4022-a1f5–1580bc732c45.

19 World Health Organization. (2020) Advice on the use of masks in the community, during home care and in healthcare settings in the context of the novel coronavirus (2019-nCoV) outbreak: Interim guidance, 29 January 2020 [Internet]. Geneva: World Health Organization. Retrieved from apps.who.int/iris/handle/10665/330987.

20 Ghebreyesus, T. A. (2020) WHO Director-General's opening remarks at the media briefing on COVID-19—5 June 2020. World Health Organization. Retrieved from www.who.int/director-general/speeches/detail/who-director-general-s-opening-remarks-at-the-media-briefing-on-covid-19—5-june-2020.

21 Chu, D. K., Akl, E. A., Duda, S., Solo, K., Yaacoub, S., et al. (2020) Physical distancing, face masks, and eye protection to prevent person-to-person transmission of SARS-CoV-2 and COVID-19: A systematic review and meta-analysis. *Lancet* 395:1973–87. doi:10.1016/S0140–6736(20)31142–9.

22 Jefferson, T., Jones, M., Ansari, L. A. A., Bawazeer, G., Beller, E., et al. (2020) Physical interventions to interrupt or reduce the spread of respiratory viruses. Part 1-Face masks, eye protection and person distancing: Systematic review and meta-analysis. medRxiv (preprint). doi:10.1101/2020.03.30.20047217.

23 Oran, D. P., Topol, E. J. (2020) Prevalence of asymptomatic SARS-CoV-2 infection: A narrative review. *Ann Intern Med* 10.7326/M20–3012. doi:10.7326/M20–3012.

24 (2020) Covid-19: How the virus gets in and how to block it: Aerosols, droplets, masks, face shields, & More. Retrieved from www.youtube.com/watch?v=Cio3rh6ta3w.

25 Dau, N.Q., Peled, H., Lau, H., Lyou, J., Skinner, C. (2020) Why N95 should be the standard for all COVID-19 inpatient care. *Ann Intern Med* 173(9):749–51. doi: 10.7326/M20–2623.

26 Escandon, K., Rasmussen, A. L., Bogoch, I. I., Murray, E. J., Escandon, K., et al. (2021) COVID-19 false dichotomies and a comprehensive review of the evidence regarding public health, COVID-19 symptomatology, SARS-CoV-2 transmission, mask wearing, and reinfection. *BMC Infect Dis* 21:710. doi.10.1186/s12879–021-06357–4.

27 Bridle, B. W. (2022) Fundamentally flawed COVID-19 "Science": The misinformation that crushed constitutional freedoms of healthy/asymptomatic people. COVID Chronicles. Retrieved from viralimmunologist.substack.com/p/fundamentally-flawed-covid-19-science.

28 Rancourt, D. G. (2020) Face masks, lies, damn lies, and public health officials: A growing body of evidence. Technical Report. doi:10.13140/RG2.2.25042.58569 Retrieved from www.rcreader.com/file/denis-rancourt-face-masks-lies-damn-lies-and-public-healthofficials-growing-body-evidence#overlay-context=commentary/masks-dont-work-covid-a-review-of-science-relevant-to-covide-19-social-policy.

29 Xie, X., Li, Y., Chwang, A. T., Ho, P. L., Seto, W. H. (2007) How far droplets can move in indoor environments—revisiting the Wells evaporation-falling curve. *Indoor Air* 17(3):211–25. doi:10.1111/j.1600–0668.2007.00469.x.

30 Ibid.

31 Carraturo, F., Del Giudice, C., Morelli, M., Cerullo, V., Libralato, G., et al. (2020) Persistence of SARS-CoV-2 in the environment and COVID-19 transmission risk from environmental matrices and surfaces. *Environ Pollut* 265(Pt B):115010. doi:10.1016/j.envpol.2020.115010.

32 (2018) Chemicals and materials: How do particulates enter the respiratory system? Retrieved from www.ccohs.ca/oshanswers/chemicals/how_do.html.

33 Du, W., Iacoviello, F., Fernandez, T., et al. (2021) Microstructure analysis and image-based modelling of face masks for COVID-19 virus protection. *Commun Mater* 2:69 (2021). doi:10.1038/s43246–021-00160-z.

34 Ibid.

35 Ibid.

36 Lee, H. P., Wang, D. Y. (2011) Objective assessment of increase in breathing resistance of N95 respirators on human subjects. *Ann Occup Hyg* 55:917–21. doi:10.1093/annhyg/mer065.

37 Roberge, R., Bayer, E., Powell, J., Coca, A., Roberge, M., Benson, S. (2010) Effect of exhaled moisture on breathing resistance of N95 filtering facepiece respirators. *Ann Occup Hyg* 54:671–77. doi:10.1093/annhyg/meq042.

38 Du, Iacoviello, Fernandez, et al., Microstructure analysis and image-based modelling of face masks for COVID-19 virus protection.

39 Business Insider. (2015) From 1860 to 1916 the British Army required every soldier to have a mustache. Today I Found Out. Retrieved from www.businessinsider.com/from-1860–1916-the-british-army-required-every-soldier-to-have-a-mustache-2015–10.

40 Harvey, I. (2015) Reason behind Hitler's rectangular moustache established. War History Online. Retrieved from www.warhistoryonline.com/war-articles/reason-behind-hitlers-rectangular-moustache-established.html?.
41 Konda, A., Prakash, A., Moss, G. A., Schmoldt, M., Grant, G. D., Guha, S. (2020) Aerosol filtration efficiency of common fabrics used in respiratory cloth masks. *ACS Nano* 14(5):6339–47. doi:10.1021/acsnano.0c03252.
42 Parlin, A. F., Stratton, S. M., Culley, T. M., Guerra, P. A. (2020) A laboratory-based study examining the properties of silk fabric to evaluate its potential as a protective barrier for personal protective equipment and as a functional material for face coverings during the COVID-19 pandemic. *PLOS One* 15(9):e0239531. doi:10.1371/journal.pone.0239531.
43 Data & Science. Centers for Disease Control and Prevention. Retrieved from web.archive.org/web/20230101004812/www.cdc.gov/coronavirus/2019-ncov/science/science-briefs/masking-science-sars-cov2.html#previous.
44 Leffler, C. T., Ing, E., Lykins, J. D., Hogan, M. C., McKeown, C. A., Grzybowski, A. (2020) Association of country-wide coronavirus mortality with demographics, testing, lockdowns, and public wearing of masks. *Am J Trop Med Hyg* 103(6):2400–2411. doi:10.4269/ajtmh.20–1015.
45 Chernozhukov, V., Kasahara, H., Schrimpf. (2020) Causal impact of masks, policies, behavior on early covid-19 pandemic in the U.S. *J. Econometrics* 220(1):23–62. doi:10.1016/j.jeconom.2020.09.003.
46 Li, Y., Liang, M., Gao, L., Ahmed, M. A., Uy, J. P., Cheng, C. (2020) Face masks to prevent transmission of COVID-19: A systematic review and meta-analysis. *Journal of Infection Control* 49(7):900–906. doi:10.1016/j.ajic.2020.12.007.
47 Liang, M., Gao, L., Cheng, C., Zhou, Q., Uy, J.P., et al. (2020) Efficacy of face mask in preventing respiratory virus transmission: A systematic review and meta-analysis. *Travel Med Infect Dis* 36, 101751. doi:10.1016/j.tmaid.2020.101751.
48 Moher, D., Shamseer, L., Clarke, M., et al. (2015) Preferred reporting items for systematic review and meta-analysis protocols (PRISMA-P) 2015 statement. *Systematic Reviews* 4(1):1. doi:10.1186/2046–4053-4–1
49 Evidence-based medicine (EBM) toolkit » Learn EBM » "What is GRADE?" at the website "BMJ Best Practice." Retrieved from bestpractice.bmj.com/info/toolkit/learn-ebm/what-is-grade/.
50 Guyatta, G. H., Oxman, A., Kunz, R., Brozek, J., Alonso-Coello, P., et al. (2011) GRADE guidelines 6. Rating the quality of evidence—imprecision. *J Clin Epid* 64(12):P1283–93. doi:10.1016/j.jclinepi.2011.01.012.
51 Khalil, M. M., Alam, M. M., Arefin, M. K., Chowdhury, M. R., Huq, M. R., et al. (2020) Role of personal protective measures in prevention of COVID-19 spread among physicians in Bangladesh: A multicenter cross-sectional comparative study. *SN Compr Clin Med* 2(10):1733–39. doi:10.1007/s42399–020-00471–1.
52 Ibid.
53 Abaluck, J., Kwong, L. H., Styczynski, A., Haque, A., Kabir, A., et al. (2021) Impact of community masking on COVID-19: A cluster-randomized trial in Bangladesh. *Science* 375(6577). doi:10.1126/science.abi9069.
54 Leung, N. H. L., Chu, D. K. W., Shiu, E. Y. C., Chan, K. H., McDevitt, J. J., et al. (2020) Respiratory virus shedding in exhaled breath and efficacy of face masks. *Nat Med* 26(5):676–80. doi:10.1038/s41591–020-0843–2.

55 Spiegel, M., Tookes, H. (2021) Business restrictions and COVID-19 fatalities. *The Review of Financial Studies* 34(11):5266–5308. doi:10.1093/rfs/hhab069.

56 Alexander, P. E. (2021) More than 170 comparative studies and articles on mask ineffectiveness and harms. Retrieved from brownstone.org/articles/studies-and-articles-on-mask-ineffectiveness-and-harms/.

57 Alexander, P. E. (2021) More than 400 studies on the failure of compulsory COVID interventions (lockdowns, restrictions, closures). Retrieved from brownstone.org/articles/more-than-400-studies-on-the-failure-of-compulsory-covid-interventions/.

58 Sickbert-Bennett, E. E., Samet, J. M., Clapp, P. W., Chen, H., Berntsen, J., et al. (2020) Filtration efficiency of hospital face mask alternatives available for use during the COVID-19 pandemic. *JAMA Internal Medicine* 11:11. doi:10.1001/jamainternmed.2020.4221.

59 Hunter, P. R., Colón-Gonález, F. J., Brainard, J., Rushton S. (2021) Impact of non-pharmaceutical interventions against COVID-19 in Europe in 2020: A quasi-experimental non-equivalent group and time series design study. *Euro Surveill* 26(28):pii=2001401. doi:10.2807/1560–7917.ES.2021.26.28.2001401.

60 Lyu, W., Wehby, G. L. (2020) Community use of face masks and COVID-19: Evidence from a natural experiment of state mandates in the US. *Health Aff* (Millwood) 39(8):1419–25. doi:10.1377/hlthaff.2020.00818.

61 Liu, I. T., Prasad, V., Darrow, J. J. (2021) Evidence for community cloth face masking to limit the spread of SARS-CoV-2: A critical review, CATO Institute. Working Paper 64. Retrieved from www.cato.org/working-paper/evidence-community-cloth-face-masking-limit-spread-sars-cov-2-critical-review.

62 Barasheed, O., Almasri, N., Badahdah, A. M., Heron, L., Taylor, J., et al. (2014) Pilot randomized controlled trial to test effectiveness of facemasks in preventing influenza-like illness transmission among Australian Hajj pilgrims in 2011. *Infect Disord Drug Targets* 14(2):110–16. doi:10.2174/1871526514666141021112855.

63 Aiello, A. E., Perez, V., Coulborn, R. M., Davis, B. M., Uddin, M., Monto, A. S. (2012) Facemasks, hand hygiene, and influenza among young adults: A randomized intervention trial. *PLOS One* 7(1):e29744. doi:10.1371/journal.pone.0029744.

64 Cowling, B. J., Chan, K. H., Fang, V. J., Cheng, C. K., Fung, R. O., et al. (2009) Facemasks and hand hygiene to prevent influenza transmission in households: A cluster randomized trial. *Ann Intern Med* 151(7):437–46. doi:10.7326/0003–4819-151–7-200910060–00142.

65 MacIntyre, C. R., Cauchemez, S., Dwyer, D. E., Seale, H., Cheung, P., et al. (2009) Face mask use and control of respiratory virus transmission in households. *Emerg Infect Dis* 15(2):233–41. doi:10.3201/eid1502.081167.

66 Dugre, N., Ton, J., Perry, D., Garrison, S., Falk, J., et al. (2020) Masks for prevention of viral respiratory infections among health care workers and the public: PEER umbrella systematic review. *Can Fam Physician* 66(7):509–17. Retrieved from www.ncbi.nlm.nih.gov/pmc/articles/pmc7365162/.

67 Aggarwal, N., Dwarakanathan, V., Gautam, N., Ray, A. (2020) Facemasks for prevention of viral respiratory infections in community settings: A systematic review and meta-analysis. *Indian J Public Health* d64(Suppl):S192–200. doi:10.4103/ijph.ijph_470_20.

68 MacIntyre, C. R., Wang, Q., Cauchemez, S., Seale, H., Dwyer, D. E., et al. (2011) A cluster randomized clinical trial comparing fit-tested and non-fit-tested N95 respirators

to medical masks to prevent respiratory virus infection in health care workers. *Influenza Other Respir Viruses* 5:170–79. doi:10.1111/j.1750–2659.2011.00198.x.

69 MacIntyre, C. R., Wang, Q., Seale, H., Yang, P., Shi, W., et al. (2013) A randomized clinical trial of three options for N95 respirators and medical masks in health workers. *Am J Respir Crit Care Med* 187:960–66. doi:10.1164/rccm.201207–1164OC.

70 MacIntyre, C. R., Chughtai, A. A. (2015) Facemasks for the prevention of infection in healthcare and community settings. *BMJ* 350:h694. doi:10.1136/bmj.h694.

71 MacIntyre, C. R., Tham, C. D., Seale, H., Chughtai, A. (2020) COVID-19, shortage of masks and the use of cloth masks as a last resort. *BMJ Open* 5(4) Retrieved from bmjopen.bmj.com/content/5/4/e006577.responses#covid-19-shortages-of-masks-and-the-use-of-cloth-masks-as-a-last-resort.

72 MacIntyre, C. R., Zhang, Y., Chughtai, A. A., Seale, H., Zhang, D., et al. (2016) Cluster randomized controlled trial to examine medical mask use as source control for people with respiratory illness. *BMJ Open* 6(12):e012330. doi:10.1136/bmjopen-2016–012330.

73 MacIntyre, C. R., Chughtai, A. A. (2020) A rapid systematic review of the efficacy of face masks and respirators against coronaviruses and other respiratory transmissible viruses for the community, healthcare workers and sick patients. *Int J Nurs Stud* 108:103629. doi:10.1016/j.ijnurstu.2020.103629.

74 Rancourt, Face masks, lies, damn lies, and public health officials.

75 Jefferson, T., Dooley, L., Ferroni, E., Al-Ansary, L. A., van Driel, M. L., et al. (2023) Physical interventions to interrupt or reduce the spread of respiratory viruses. *Cochrane Database of Systematic Reviews* Issue 1. Art. No.: CD006207. doi:10.1002/14651858.CD006207.pub6 Retrieved from www.cochranelibrary.com/cdsr/doi/10.1002/14651858.CD006207.pub6/full?utm_source=mp-fotoscapes.

76 Høeg, T. B., Haslam, A., Prasad, V. (2023) An analysis of studies pertaining to masks in *Morbidity and Mortality Weekly Report*: Characteristics and quality of studies from 1978 to 2023. *Am J Med.* doi:10.1016/j.amjmed.2023.08.026 Retrieved from www.amjmed.com/article/S0002–9343(23)00580–6/fulltext#articleInformation.

77 Ibid.

78 Tufekci, Z. (2023) Here's why the science is clear that masks work. *New York Times.* Retrieved from www.nytimes.com/2023/03/10/opinion/masks-work-cochrane-study.html.

79 (2023) Statement on "Physical interventions to interrupt or reduce the spread of respiratory viruses" review. Retrieved from www.cochrane.org/news/statement-physical-interventions-interrupt-or-reduce-spread-respiratory-viruses-review.

80 Heneghan, C., Jefferson, T. (2023) Cochrane Scandal: We found no evidence masks worked—and that had to be silenced. *Daily Sceptic.* Retrieved from dailysceptic.org/2023/09/15/cochrane-scandal-we-found-no-evidence-masks-worked-and-that-had-to-be-silenced/.

81 Suess, T., Remschmidt, C., Schink, S. B., Schweiger, B., Nitsche, A., et al. (2012) The role of facemasks and hand hygiene in the prevention of influenza transmission in households: Results from a cluster randomised trial; Berlin, Germany, 2009–2011. *BMC infect Dis* 12:26. doi:10.1186/1471–2334-12–26.

82 Larson, E. L., Ferng, Y.-H., Wong-McLoughlin, J., Wang, S., Haber, M., Morse, S. S. (2010) Impact of nonpharmaceutical interventions on URIs and influenza in crowded, urban households. *Public Health Rep* 125(2):178–91. doi:10.1177/003335491012500206.

83 Canini, L., Andréoletti, L., Ferrari, P., D'Angelo, R., Blanchon, T., et al. (2010) Surgical mask to prevent influenza transmission in households: A cluster randomized trial. *PLOS One* 5(11):e13998. doi:10.1371/journal.pone.0013998.

84 Simmerman, J. M., Suntarattiwong, P., Levy, J., Jarman, R. G., Kaewchana, S., et al. (2011) Findings from a household randomized controlled trial of hand washing and face masks to reduce influenza transmission in Bangkok, Thailand. *Influenza and Other Respiratory Viruses* 5(4):256–67. doi:10.1111/j.1750–2659.2011.00205.x.

85 Ibid.

86 Uchida, M., Kaneko, M., Hidaka, Y., Yamamoto, H., Honda, T., et al. (2016) Effectiveness of vaccination and wearing masks on seasonal influenza in Matsumoto City, Japan, in the 2014/2015 season: An observational study among all elementary schoolchildren. *Prev Med Rep* 5:86–91. doi:10.1016/j.pmedr.2016.12.002.

87 Sandlund, J., Duriseta, R., Ladhani, S. N., Stuart, K., Noble, J., Høeg, T. B. (2023) Child mask mandates for COVID-19: a systematic review. *Arch Dis Child* 0:1–7. doi:10.1136/archdischild-2023–326215.

88 Ibid.

89 Data & Science. Centers for Disease Control and Prevention.

90 Ibid.

91 Georgi, C., Haase-Fielitz, A., Meretz, D., Gäsert, L., Butter, C. (2020) Einfluss gängiger gesichtsmasken auf physiologische parameter und belastungsempfinden unter arbeitstypischer körperlicher anstrengung. *Deutsches Ärzteblatt* 674–75. doi:10.3238/arztebl.2020.0674.

92 Fikenzer, S., Uhe, T., Lavall, D., Rudolph, U., Falz, R., et al. (2020) Effects of surgical and FFP2/N95 face masks on cardiopulmonary exercise capacity. *Clin Res Cardiol* 109: 1522–30. doi:10.1007/s00392–020-01704-y.

93 Data & Science. Centers for Disease Control and Prevention.

94 Ibid.

95 World Health Organization. (2020) Advice on the use of masks in the context of COVID-19: Interim guidance [Internet]. Geneva: World Health Organization. Retrieved from apps.who.int/iris/bitstream/handle/10665/332293/WHO-2019-nCov-IPC_Masks-2020.4-eng.pdf.

96 Matusiak, Ł., Szepietowska, M., Krajewski, P., Białynicki-Birula, R., Szepietowski, J. C. (2020) Inconveniences due to the use of face masks during the COVID-19 pandemic: A survey study of 876 young people. *Dermatol Ther* 33(4) e13567. doi:10.1111/dth.13567.

97 Szepietowski, J. C., Matusiak, Ł., Szepietowska, M., Krajewski, P. K., Białynicki-Birula, R. (2020) Face mask induced itch: A self-questionnaire study of 2,315 responders during the COVID-19 pandemic. *Acta Derm Venereol* 2020;100(10):adv00152. doi:10.2340/00015555–3536.

98 Lan, J., Song, Z., Miao, X., Li, H., Li, Y., et al. (2020) Skin damage among health care workers managing Coronavirus Disease-2019. *J Am Acad Dermatol* 82:1215–16. doi:10.1016/j.jaad.2020.03.014.

99 Xie, H., Han, W., Xie, Q., Xu, T., Zhu, M., Chen, J. (2022) Face mask—A potential source of phthalate exposure for human. *J Hazard Mater* 422:126848. doi:10.1016/j.jhazmat.2021.126848.

100 Hua, W., Zuo, Y., Wan, R., Xiong, L., Tang, J., et al. (2020) Short-term skin reactions following use of N95 respirators and medical masks. *Contact Dermat* 83:115–21. doi:10.1111/cod.13601.

101 Badri, F. M. A. (2017) Surgical mask contact dermatitis and epidemiology of contact dermatitis in healthcare workers. *Curr Allergy Clin Immunol* 30:183–88.
102 Rebmann, T., Carrico, R., Wang, J. (2013) Physiologic and other effects and compliance with long-term respirator use among medical intensive care unit nurses. *Am J Infect Control* 41(12):1218–23. doi:10.1016/j.ajic.2013.02.017.
103 Rosner, E. (2020) Adverse effects of prolonged mask use among healthcare professionals during COVID-19. *J Infect Dis Epidemiol* 6(3):130. doi:10.23937/2474–3658/1510130.
104 Foo, C. C. I., Goon, A. T. J., Leow, Y., Goh, C. (2006) Adverse skin reactions to personal protective equipment against Severe Acute Respiratory Syndrome—A descriptive study in Singapore. *Contact Dermat* 55:291–94. doi:10.1111/j.1600–0536.2006.00953.x.
105 Chen, X., Ran, L., Liu, Q., Hu, Q., Du, X., Tan, X. (2020) Hand hygiene, mask-wearing behaviors and its associated factors during the COVID-19 epidemic: A cross-sectional study among primary school students in Wuhan, China. *Int J Environ Res Public Health* 17(8):2893. doi:10.3390/ijerph17082893.
106 Allison, M. A., Guest-Warnick, G., Nelson, D., Pavia, A. T., Srivastava, R., et al. (2010) Feasibility of elementary school children's use of hand gel and facemasks during influenza season. *Influenza Other Respir Viruses* 4(4):223–29. doi:10.1111/j.1750–2659.2010.00142.x.
107 Stebbins, S., Downs, J. S., Vukotich, C. J. Jr. (2009) Using nonpharmaceutical interventions to prevent influenza transmission in elementary school children: Parent and teacher perspectives. *J Public Health Manag Pract* 15(2):112–17. doi:10.1097/01.phh.0000346007.66898.67.
108 Strachan, D. P. (1989) Hay fever, hygiene, and household size. *British Medical Journal* 299:1259. doi:10.1136/bmj.299.6710.1259.
109 Weiss, S. T. (2002) Eat dirt—the hygiene hypothesis and allergic diseases. *New England Journal of Medicine* 347:930–31. doi:10.1056/NEJMe020092.
110 Luksamijarulkul, P., Aiempradit, N., Vatanasomboon, P. (2014) Microbial contamination on used surgical masks among hospital personnel and microbial air quality in their working wards: A hospital in Bangkok. *Oman Med. J* 29:346–50. doi:10.5001/omj.2014.92.
111 Chughtai, A. A., Stelzer-Braid, S., Rawlinson, W., Pontivivo, G., Wang, Q., et al. (2019) Contamination by respiratory viruses on outer surface of medical masks used by hospital healthcare workers. *BMC Infect. Dis* 19:491. doi:10.1186/s12879–019-4109-x.
112 Monalisa, A. C., Padma, K. B., Manjunath, K., Hemavathy, E., Varsha, D. (2017) Microbial contamination of the mouth masks used by post-graduate students in a private dental institution: An *in-vitro* study. *IOSR J Dent Med Sci* 16:61–67.
113 Liu, Z., Chang, Y., Chu, W., Yan, M., Mao, Y., et al. (2018) Surgical masks as source of bacterial contamination during operative procedures. *J Orthop Transl* 14:57–62. doi:10.1016/j.jot.2018.06.002.
114 Liu, C., Li, G., He, Y., Zhang Z., Ding, Y. (2020) Effects of wearing masks on human health and comfort during the COVID-19 pandemic. *IOP Conf Ser Earth Environ Sci* 531:012034. doi:10.1088/1755–1315/531/1/012034.
115 Muley, P. (2020) "Mask mouth"—A novel threat to oral health in the COVID era—Dr Pooja Muley. Dental Tribune South Asia 2020. Retrieved from in.dental-tribune.com/news/mask-mouth-a-novel-threat-to-oral-health-in-the-covid-era/.
116 Heider, C. A., Álvarez, M. L., Fuentes-López, E., González, C. A., León, N. I., et al. (2020) Prevalence of voice disorders in healthcare workers in the universal masking COVID-19 era. *Laryngoscope* 131(4):E1227–33. doi:10.1002/lary.29172.

117 Asadi, S., Cappa, C. D., Barreda, S., Wexler, A. S., Bouvier, N. M., Ristenpart, W. D. (2020) Efficacy of masks and face coverings in controlling outward aerosol particle emission from expiratory activities. *Sci Rep* 10:15665. doi:10.1038/s41598–020-72798–7.
118 Ibid.
119 Ibid.
120 Brody, B. (2021) Hypercapnia (Hypercarbia). WebMD. Retrieved from www.webmd.com/lung/copd/hypercapnia-copd-related.
121 Lubrano, R., Bloise, S., Testa, A., Marcellino, A., Dilillo, A., et al. (2021) Assessment of respiratory function in infants and young children wearing face masks during the COVID-19 pandemic. *JAMA Netw Open* 4(3):e210414. doi: 10.1001/jamanetwork open.2021.0414.
122 Shaw, K. A., Butcher, S., Ko, J. B., Absher, A., Gordon, J., et al. (2021) Wearing a surgical face mask has minimal effect on performance and physiological measures during high-intensity exercise in youth ice-hockey players: A randomized cross-over trial. *Int J Environ Res Public Health* 18(20):10766. doi:10.3390/ijerph182010766.
123 Roberge, R. J., Kim, J. H., Benson, S.M. (2012) Absence of consequential changes in physiological, thermal and subjective responses from wearing a surgical mask. *Respir Physiol Neurobiol* 181(1):29–35.
124 Kisielinski, K., Giboni, P., Prescher, A., Klosterhalfen, B., Graessel, D., et al. (2021) Is a mask that covers the mouth and nose free from undesirable side effects in everyday use and free of potential hazards? *Int J Environ Res Public Health* 18(8):4344. doi:10.3390/ijerph18084344.
125 Roberge, R. J., Kim, J.-H., Powell, J. B. (2014) N95 respirator use during advanced pregnancy. *Am J Infect Control* 42:1097–1100. doi:10.1016/j.ajic.2014.06.025.
126 Johnson, A. T. (2016) Respirator masks protect health but impact performance: A Review. *J Biol Eng* 10:4. doi:10.1186/s13036–016-0025–4.
127 Prousa, D. (2020) Studie zu psychischen und psychovegetativen Beschwerden mit den aktuellen Mund-Nasenschutz-Verordnungen. *PsychArchives*. doi:10.23668/psycharchives.3135.
128 Matuschek, C., Moll, F., Fangerau, H., Fischer, J. C., Zänker, K., et al. (2020) Face masks: Benefits and risks during the COVID-19 Crisis. *Eur. J. Med. Res* 25:32. doi:10.1186/s40001–020-00430–5.
129 Forgie, S. E., Reitsma, J., Spady, D., Wright, B., Stobart, K. (2009) The "Fear Factor" for surgical masks and face shields, as perceived by children and their parents. *Pediatrics* 124:e777–81. doi:10.1542/peds.2008–3709.
130 Schwarz, S., Jenetzky, E., Krafft, H., Maurer, T., Martin, D. (2021) Corona children studies "Co-Ki": First results of a Germany-wide registry on mouth and nose covering (mask) in children. *Monatsschrift Kinderheilkde* 1–10. doi:10.1007/s00112–021-01133–9.
131 Prousa, Studie zu psychischen und psychovegetativen Beschwerden mit den aktuellen Mund-Nasenschutz-Verordnungen.
132 World Health Organization (WHO) (2020) Shortage of personal protective equipment endangering health workers worldwide. Retrieved from www.who.int/news-room/detail/03–03-2020-shortage-of-personal-protective-equipment-endangering-health-workers-worldwide.
133 Lu, M. (2021) 1.6 billion disposable masks entered our oceans in 2020. *Visual Capitalist*. Retrieved from www.visualcapitalist.com/1–6-billion-disposable-masks-entered-our-oceans-in-2020/.

134 Fadare, O. O., Okoffo, E. D. (2020) COVID-19 face masks: A potential source of microplastic fibers in the environment. *Sci. Total Environ* 737:140279. doi:10.1016/j.scitotenv.2020.140279.

135 Klemeš, J. J., Fan, Y. V., Jiang, P. (2020) The energy and environmental footprints of COVID-19 fighting measures—PPE, disinfection, supply chains *Energy* 217:118701. doi:10.1016/j.rser.2020.109883.

136 Klemeš, J. J., Fan, Y. V., Tan, R. R., Jiang, P. (2020) Minimising the present and future plastic waste, energy and environmental footprints related to COVID-19. *Renew Sustain Energy Rev* 127: 109883. doi:10.1016/j.rser.2020.109883.

Chapter 10

1 Sun, D., Gao, W., Hu, H., Zhou, S. (2022) Why 90% of clinical drug development fails and how to improve it? *Acta Pharm Sin B* 12(7):3049–62. doi:10.1016/j.apsb.2022.02.002.

2 How long do clinical research studies take? QPS Blog. (2020) Retrieved from 417studies.com/how-long-do-clinical-trials-take/.

3 DiMasi, J. A., Grabowski, H. G., Hansen, R. W. (2016) Innovation in the pharmaceutical industry: New estimates of R&D costs. *J Health Econ* 47:20–33. doi:10.1016/j.jhealeco.2016.01.012.

4 Staff desk. (2022) What is the most profitable pharmaceutical drug ever? Vakil Search. Retrieved from vakilsearch.com/blog/what-is-the-most-profitable-pharmaceutical-drug-ever/.

5 Pfizer. (2022) Financial performance. Retrieved from www.pfizer.com/sites/default/files/investors/financial_reports/annual_reports/2021/performance/.

6 Ibid.

7 Kolmar, C. (2023) 25+ incredible U.S. pharmaceutical statistics [2023]: Facts, data, trends and more. Zippia. Retrieved from www.zippia.com/advice/us-pharmaceutical-statistics/.

8 Mikulic, M. (2023) Pharmaceutical market: worldwide revenue 2001–2022. Retrieved from www.statista.com/statistics/263102/pharmaceutical-market-worldwide-revenue-since-2001/.

9 The worldwide pharmaceutical market from 2001 to 2022. (2023) Statista. College of Physicians of Philadelphia. Retrieved from historyofvaccines.org/vaccines-101/how-are-vaccines-made/vaccine-development-testing-and-regulation.

10 VAERS Vaccine Adverse Event Reporting System. (2023) CDC and FDA. Retrieved from vaers.hhs.gov/index.html.

11 McLachlan, S., Osman, M., Dube, K., Chiketero, P., Choi, Y., Fenton, N. E. (2021) Analysis of COVID-19 vaccine death reports from the Vaccine Adverse Events Reporting System (VAERS) Database Interim: Results and analysis. ResearchGate. doi:10.13140/RG.2.2.26987.26402.

12 Lazarus, R., Klompas, M. (2011) Harvard Pilgrim Study—Lazarus Final Report 2011. Grant Final Report ID R18 HS 017045. Retrieved from www.scribd.com/document/434088983/Lazarus-Final-Report-2011.

13 VigiAccess. World Health Organization. (2023) Retrieved from www.vigiaccess.org/.

14 Human regulatory: EudraVigilance (2023) European Medicines Agency. Retrieved from www.ema.europa.eu/en/human-regulatory/research-development/pharmacovigilance/eudravigilance.

15 Welcome to the Yellow Card reporting site. (2023) Medicines and Healthcare Products Regulatory Agency. Retrieved from yellowcard.mhra.gov.uk/.

16 Venning, G. R. (1982) Validity of anecdotal reports of suspected adverse drug reactions: The problem of false alarms. *Br Med J (Clin Res Ed)* 284(6311):249–52.

17 Canadian Adverse Events Following Immunization Surveillance System (CAEFISS). (2023) Public Health Agency of Canada. Retrieved from www.canada.ca/en/public-health/services/immunization/canadian-adverse-events-following-immunization-surveillance-system-caefiss.html.

18 Vaccine injury compensation program. Civil Division. (2023) U.S. Department of Justice. Retrieved from www.justice.gov/civil/vicp.

19 Brink, E. W., Hinman, A. R. (1989) The vaccine injury compensation act: The new law and you. *Contemp Pediatr* 6(3):28–32, 35–36, 39, 42.

20 Office of the Secretary (2020) Declaration under the Public Readiness and Emergency Preparedness Act for Medical Countermeasures against COVID-19. Department of Health and Human Services. Retrieved from www.govinfo.gov/content/pkg/FR-2020–03-17/pdf/2020–05484.pdf.

21 End of the Federal COVID-19 Public Health Emergency (PHE) Declaration. (2023) Centers for Disease Control and Prevention. Retrieved from www.cdc.gov/coronavirus/2019-ncov/your-health/end-of-phe.html.

22 Iannelli, V. (2017) Underreporting of side effects to VAERS. *Vaxopedia*. Retrieved from vaxopedia.org/2017/08/26/underreporting-of-side-effects-to-vaers/.

Chapter 11

1 About Edward Jenner. (2023) The Jenner Institute. Retrieved from www.jenner.ac.uk/about/edward-jenner#.

2 Variolation. (2023) Wikipedia. Retrieved from en.wikipedia.org/wiki/Variolation#

3 Castrodeza-Sanz, J., Sanz-Muñoz, I., Eiros, J. M. (2023) Adjuvants for COVID-19 vaccines. *Vaccines* (Basel) 11(5):902. doi:10.3390/vaccines11050902.

4 Khoshnood, S., Ghanavati, R., Shirani, M., Ghahramanpour, H., Sholeh, M., et al. (2022) Viral vector and nucleic acid vaccines against COVID-19: A narrative review. *Front Microbiol* 13:984536. doi:10.3389/fmicb.2022.984536.

5 Ibid.

6 Ibid.

7 Karikó, K., Buckstein, M., Ni, H., Weissman, D. (2005) Suppression of RNA recognition by Toll-like receptors: the impact of nucleoside modification and the evolutionary origin of RNA. *Immunity* 23(2):165–75. doi:10.1016/j.immuni.2005.06.008.

8 Bansal, S., Perincheri, S., Fleming, T., Poulson, C., Tiffany, B., et al. (2021) Cutting Edge: Circulating exosomes with COVID spike protein are induced by BNT162b2 (Pfizer–BioNTech) vaccination prior to development of antibodies: A novel mechanism for immune activation by mRNA Vaccines. *J Immunol* 207(10):2405–10. doi:10.4049/jimmunol.2100637.

9 Gutschi, L. M. (2022) Quality issues with mRNA Covid vaccine production. Bitchute. Retrieved from www.bitchute.com/video/muB0nrznCAC4/.

10 Comirnaty European Public Assessment Report. Dec 21, 2020. European Medicines Agency. Retrieved from www.ema.europa.eu/en/documents/assessment-report/comirnaty-epar-public-assessment-report_en.pdf.

11 Tinari, S. (2021) The EMA COVID-19 data leak, and what it tells us about mRNA instability. *BMJ* 372:n627. doi:10.1136/bmj.n627.

12 Rappaport Rolling Review Report overview LoQ-COVID-19 mRNA vaccine BioNTec, 2020. COVID Truths. (2021) Retrieved from www.covidtruths.co.uk/2021/04/ema-leaked-papers/.

13 (2020) Media Advisory. Health Canada authorizes first COVID-19 vaccine. Retrieved from www.canada.ca/en/health-canada/news/2020/12/health-canada-authorizes-first-covid-19-vaccine.html.

14 Moderna. Quarterly Report Pursuant to Section 13 or 15(d) of the Securities Exchange Act of 1934. Moderna, Ed.; Securities and Exchange Commission. (2020) Retrieved from www.sec.gov/Archives/edgar/data/1682852/000168285220000017/mrna-20200630.htm.

15 COMMISSION DIRECTIVE 2009/120/EC of 14 September 2009 Amending Directive 2001/83/EC of the European Parliament and of the Council on the Community Code Relating to Medicinal Products for Human Use as Regards Advanced Therapy Medicinal Products. Available online: eur-lex.europa.eu/eli/dir/2009/120/oj.

16 Guideline on the non-clinical studies required before first clinical use of gene therapy medicines. CHMP, Ed. European Medicines Agency. (2008) Vol. EMEA/CHMP/GTWP/125459/2006. Retrieved from www.ema.europa.eu/en/documents/scientific-guideline/guideline-non-clinical-studies-required-first-clinical-use-gene-therapy-medicinal-products_en.pdf.

17 Preclinical assessment of investigational cellular and gene therapy products. (2013) CBER, Ed.; U.S. Federal Drug Administration. Vol. FDA-2012-D-1038. Retrieved from www.fda.gov/regulatory-information/search-fda-guidance-documents/preclinical-assessment-investigational-cellular-and-gene-therapy-products.

18 Design and analysis of shedding studies for virus or bacteria-based gene therapy and oncolytic products. Research, C. f. B. E. a., Ed. US Federal Drug Administration. (2015) Retrieved from www.fda.gov/regulatory-information/search-fda-guidance-documents/design-and-analysis-shedding-studies-virus-or-bacteria-based-gene-therapy-and-oncolytic-products.

19 World Health Organization. (2005) WHO guidelines on non-clinical evaluation of vaccines TRS No 927. Vol. Annex 1. Retrieved from www.who.int/publications/m/item/nonclinical-evaluation-of-vaccines-annex-1-trs-no-927.

20 World Health Organization. (2022) Evaluation of the quality, safety and efficacy of messenger RNA vaccines for the prevention of infectious diseases: Regulatory considerations. Annex 3, TRS No 1039, WHO, Ed. Retrieved from www.who.int/publications/m/item/annex-3-mRNA-vaccines-trs-no-1039.

21 Oh, S. S. (2022) Cellular, Tissue, and Gene Therapy Advisory Committee Meeting. Review of Intramural Research Program—Gene Transfer and Immunogenicity Branch, March 10, 2022. US Food and Drug Administration. Retrieved from www.fda.gov/media/156771/download.

22 Viswanathan, S., Bubela, T. (2015) Current practices and reform proposals for the regulation of advanced medicinal products in Canada. *Regen Med* 10(5):647–63. doi:10.2217/rme.15.28.

23 FDA. (2020) Long term follow-up after administration of human gene therapy products: Guidance for industry. Retrieved from www.fda.gov/media/113768/download.

24 Banoun, H. (2023) mRNA: Vaccine or gene therapy? The safety regulatory issues. *Int J Mol Sci* 24(13):10514. doi:10.3390/ijms241310514.

25 Whitley, J., Zwolinski, C., Denis, C., Maughan, M., Hayles, L., et al. (2022) Development of mRNA manufacturing for vaccines and therapeutics: mRNA platform requirements and development of a scalable production process to support early phase clinical trials. *Transl Res* 242:38–55. doi:10.1016/j.trsl.2021.11.009.

26 Kim, S. C., Sekhon, S. S., Shin, W. R., Ahn, G., Cho, B. K., et al. (2022) Modifications of mRNA vaccine structural elements for improving mRNA stability and translation efficiency. *Mol Cell Toxicol* 18(1):1–8. doi:10.1007/s13273–021-00171–4.

27 Raab, D., Graf, M., Notka, F., Schödl, T., Wagner, R. (2010) The GeneOptimizer algorithm: Using a sliding window approach to cope with the vast sequence space in multiparameter DNA sequence optimization. *Syst Synth Biol* 4(3):215–25. doi:10.1007/s11693–010-9062–3.

28 Nobel Prize Assembly at the Karolinska Institute. (2023) The Nobel Prize in Physiology or Medicine 2023. Retrieved from www.nobelprize.org/prizes/medicine/2023/press-release/.

29 Sahin, U., Karikó, K., Türeci, Ö. (2014) mRNA-based therapeutics—developing a new class of drugs. *Nat Rev Drug Discov* 13(10):759–80. doi:10.1038/nrd4278.

30 Ibid.

31 Röltgen, K., Nielsen, S., Silva, O., Younes, S. F., Zaslavasky, M., et al. (2022) Immune imprinting, breadth of variant recognition, and germinal center response in human SARS-CoV-2 infection and vaccination. *Cell* 185(6):1025–40.e14. doi:10.1016/j.cell.2022.01.018.

32 Bansal, S., Perincheri, S., Fleming, T., Poulson, C., Tiffany, B., et al. (2021) Cutting edge: Circulating exosomes with COVID spike protein are induced by BNT162b2 (Pfizer-BioNTech) vaccination prior to development of antibodies: A novel mechanism for immune activation by mRNA vaccines. *J Immunol* 207(10):2405–10. doi:10.4049/jimmunol.2100637.

33 Röltgen, Nielsen, Silva, Younes, Zaslavasky, et al. Immune imprinting, breadth of variant recognition, and germinal center response in human SARS-CoV-2 infection and vaccination.

34 Seneff, S., Nigh, G., Kyriakopoulos, A.M., McCullough, P. (2022) Innate immune suppression by SARS-CoV-2 mRNA vaccinations: The role of G-quadruplexes, exosomes, and microRNAs. *Food Chem Toxicol* 164:113008. doi:10.1016/j.fct.2022.113008.

35 Patterson, B. K., Francisco, E. B., Yogendra, R., Long, E., Pise, A., et al. (2022) SARS-CoV-2 S1 protein persistence in SARS-CoV-2 negative post-vaccination individuals with Long Covid/PASC-like symptoms. Research Square (Preprint). Retrieved from www.researchsquare.com/article/rs-1844677/latest.

36 Magen, E., Mukherjee, S., Bhattacharya, M., Detroja, R., Merzon, E., et al. (2022) Clinical and molecular characterization of a rare case of BNT162b2 mRNA COVID-19.

37 Comirnaty European Public Assessment Report.

38 World Health Organization. (2021) WHO consultation on COVID-19 vaccine research: How can vaccine research further contribute to achieve the control of the pandemic everywhere? Retrieved from www.who.int/news-room/events/detail/2021/12/06/default-calendar/who-consultation-on-covid-19-vaccines-research-how-can-vaccine-research-further-contribute-to-achieve-the-control-of-the-pandemic-everywhere.

39 Krammer, F. (2021) Challenges to develop and assess variant-specific vaccines. Cdn.who.int. Retrieved from cdn.who.int/media/docs/default-source/blue-print/florian-krammer_3_anticipated-challenges_vrconsultation_6.12.2021.pdf.
40 ACIP Meeting (2022) September 1, 2022—Booster doses of Moderna; Prizer/BioNTech COVID-19 Omicron-modified. YouTube. Retrieved from www.youtube.com/watch?v=i34wDDfhRpg&t=2176s.
41 Rosa, S. S., Prazeres, D. M. F., Azevedo, A. M., Marques, M. P. C. (2021) mRNA vaccines manufacturing: Challenges and bottlenecks. *Vaccine* 39(16):2190–2200. doi:10.1016/j.vaccine.2021.03.038.
42 Ouranidis, A., Vavilis, T., Mandala, E., Davidopoulou, C., Stamoula, E., et al. (2022) mRNA therapeutic modalities design, formulation and manufacturing under Pharma 4.0 Principles. *Biomedicines* 10(1):50. doi:10.3390/biomedicines10010050.
43 Unchained Labs. (2023) Ultrafiltration and Diafiltration (UF/DF). Retrieved from www.unchainedlabs.com/ultrafiltration-diafiltration-uf-df/.
44 Rosa, S. S., Prazeres, D. M. F., Azevedo, A. M., Marques, M. P. C. (2021) mRNA vaccines manufacturing: Challenges and bottlenecks. *Vaccine* 39(16):2190–2200. doi:10.1016/j.vaccine.2021.03.038.
45 Josephson, Rapporteur's Rolling Review assessment report.
46 Banoun, H. (2022) Current state of knowledge on the excretion of mRNA and spike produced by anti-COVID-19 mRNA vaccines; possibility of contamination of the entourage of those vaccinated by these products. *Infect Dis Res* 3(4):22. doi:10.53388/IDR20221125022.
47 Josephson, Rapporteur's Rolling Review assessment report.
48 European Medicines Agency. (2005) ICH Topic Q 5 E. Comparability of Biotechnological/Biological products. Retrieved from www.ema.europa.eu/en/documents/scientific-guideline/ich-q-5-e-comparability-biotechnological/biological-products-step-5_en.pdf.
49 European Medicines Agency. (2007) Guideline on comparability of biotechnology-derived medicinal products after a change in the manufacturing process. Vol. EMEA/CHMP/BMWP/101695/2006. CHMP, Ed. European Medicines Agency. Retrieved from www.ema.europa.eu/en/documents/scientific-guideline/guideline-comparability-biotechnology-derived-medicinal-products-after-change-manufacturing-process_en.pdf.
50 Josephson, Rapporteur's Rolling Review assessment report.
51 Veronika, J. (2020) E-mail dated November 24, 2020, to Dr. Evdokia Korakianiti of the EMA. EMA Leaks\09.png. Retrieved from covidvaccinereactions.com/wp-content/uploads/2021/04/EMA-Docs-and-CVR-Edits.zip.
52 Polack, Thomas, Kitchin, Absalon, Gurtman, et al., C4591001 Clinical Trial Group.
53 Block, J. (2022) COVID-19: Researchers face wait for patient level data from Pfizer and Moderna vaccine trials. *BMJ* 378:o1731. doi:10.1136/bmj.o1731.
54 The Information Commissioner's Office. (2023) Internal review of FOI 23/510. Medicines and Healthcare Products Regulatory Agency. Retrieved from dailysceptic.org/wp-content/uploads/2023/09/IR-23–510.pdf.
55 Ibid.
56 Josephson, Rapporteur's Rolling Review assessment report.
57 Zhang, S., Liu, Y., Wang, X., Yang, L., Li, H., et al. (2020) SARS-CoV-2 binds platelet ACE2 to enhance thrombosis in COVID-19. *J Hematol Oncol* 13(1):120. doi:10.1186/s13045–020-00954–7.

58 Cappelletto, A., Allan, H. E., Cresente, M., Schneider, E., Bussani, R., et al. (2021) SARS-CoV-2 spike protein activates TMEM16F-mediated platelet pro-coagulant activity. BioRxiv (preprint). doi:10.1101/2021.12.14.472668d.
59 Li, T., Yang, Y., Li, Y., Wang, Z., Ma, F., et al. (2020) Platelets mediate inflammatory monocyte activation by SARS-CoV-2 spike protein. *J Clin Invest* 132(4):e150101. doi:10.1172/JCI150101.
60 Cox, D. (2021) Targeting SARS-CoV-2-platelet interactions in COVID-19 and vaccine-related thrombosis. *Front. Pharmacol* 12:708665. doi:10.3389/fphar.2021.708665.
61 Prasad, M., Lin, J. L., Gu, Y., Gupta, R., Macary, P., Schwarz, H. (2021) No cross-reactivity of anti-SARS-CoV-2 Spike protein antibodies with Syncytin-1. *Cell Mol Immunol* 18(11):2566–68. doi:10.1038/s41423–021-00773-x.
62 Mattar, C. N. Z., Koh, W., Seow, Y., Hoon, S., Venkatesh, A., et al. (2022) BNT162B2 COVID-19 mRNA vaccination did not promote substantial anti-syncytin-1 antibody production nor mRNA transfer to breast milk in an exploratory pilot study. *Ann Acad Med Singap* 51(5):309–12. doi:10.47102/annals-acadmedsg.2021447.
63 Pelech, S., Winkler, D. (2023) personal communication.
64 Baiersdörfer, M., Boros, G., Muramatsu, H., Mahiny, A., Vlatkovic, I., et al. (2019) A facile method for the removal of dsRNA contaminant from *in vitro*-transcribed mRNA. *Mol Ther Nucleic Acids* 15:26–35. doi:10.1016/j.omtn.2019.02.018.
65 Nelson, J., Sorensen, E. W., Mintri, S., Rabideau, A. E., Zheng, W., et al. (2020) Impact of mRNA chemistry and manufacturing process on innate immune activation. *Sci Adv* 6(26):eaaz6893. doi:10.1126/sciadv.aaz6893.
66 Milano, G., Gal, J., Creisson, A., Chamorey, E. (2021) Myocarditis and COVID-19 mRNA vaccines: A mechanistic hypothesis involving dsRNA. *Future Virol* 10.2217/fvl-2021–0280. doi:10.2217/fvl-2021–0280.
67 Kranz, L. M., Diken, M., Haas, H., Kreiter, S., Loquai, C., et al. (2016) Systemic RNA delivery to dendritic cells exploits antiviral defence for cancer immunotherapy. *Nature* 534(7607):396–401. doi:10.1038/nature18300.
68 Whitley, J., Zwolinski, C., Denis, C., Maughan, M., Hayles, L., et al. (2022) Development of mRNA manufacturing for vaccines and therapeutics: mRNA platform requirements and development of a scalable production process to support early phase clinical trials. *Transl Res* 242:38–55. doi:10.1016/j.trsl.2021.11.009.
69 Li, Y., Fujita, M., Boraschi, D. (2017) Endotoxin contamination in nanomaterials leads to the misinterpretation of immunosafety results. *Front Immunol* 8:472. doi:10.3389/fimmu.2017.00472.
70 Samsudin, F., Raghuvamsi, P., Petruk, G., Puthia, M., Petrlova, J., et al. (2023) SARS-CoV-2 spike protein as a bacterial lipopolysaccharide delivery system in an overzealous inflammatory cascade. *J Mol Cell Biol* 14(9):mjac058. doi:10.1093/jmcb/mjac058.
71 Munford, R. S. (2016) Endotoxemia-menace, marker, or mistake? *J Leukoc Biol* 100 (4):687–98. doi:10.1189/jlb.3RU0316–151R.
72 Cinquegrani, G., Spigoni, V., Iannozzi, N. T., Parello, V., Bonadonna, R. C., Dei Cas, A. (2022) SARS-CoV-2 spike protein is not pro-inflammatory in human primary macrophages: Endotoxin contamination and lack of protein glycosylation as possible confounders. *Cell Biol Toxicol* 38(4):667–78. doi:10.1007/s10565–021-09693-y.
73 Parhiz, H., Brenner, J. S., Patel, P. N., Papp, T. E., Shahnawaz, H., et al. (2022) Added to pre-existing inflammation, mRNA-lipid nanoparticles induce inflammation exacerbation (IE). *J Control Release* 344:50–61. doi:10.1016/j.jconrel.2021.12.027.

74 Li, Fujita, and Boraschi, Endotoxin contamination in nanomaterials leads to the misinterpretation of immunosafety results.
75 USP-NF. (2023) Analytical procedures for mRNA vaccine quality (Draft Guidelines)—2nd Edition. United States Pharmacopoeia-National Formular. Retrieved from www.uspnf.com/notices/analytical-procedures-mrna-vaccines-20230428.
76 Palmer, M., Gilthorpe, J. (2023) COVID-19 mRNA vaccines contain excessive quantities of bacterial DNA: Evidence and implications. Doctors for COVID Ethics. Retrieved from doctors4covidethics.org/covid-19-mrna-vaccines-contain-excessive-quantities-of-bacterial-dna-evidence-and-implications/.
77 McKernan, K., Helbert, Y., Kane, L.T., McLaughlin, S. (2023) Sequencing of bivalent Moderna and Pfizer mRNA vaccines reveals nanogram to microgram quantities of expression vector dsDNA peer dose. ResearchGate. doi:10.31219/osf.io/b9t7m Retrieved from www.researchgate.net/publication/369967228_Sequencing_of_bivalent_Moderna_and_Pfizer_mRNA_vaccines_reveals_nanogram_to_microgram_quantities_of_expression_vector_dsDNA_per_dose.
78 Buckhaults, P. (2023) Testimony before South Carolina Senate Medical Affairs Ad-Hoc Committee on DHEC. Retrieved from www.youtube.com/watch?v=IEWHhrHiiTY.
79 World Council for Health. (2023) Urgent expert hearing on reports of cancer-promoting DNA contamination in C-19 mRNA vaccines. Retrieved from worldcouncilforhealth.org/multimedia/urgent-hearing-dna-contamination-mrna-vaccines/.
80 Speicher, D. J., Rose, J., Gutschi, L. M., Wiseman, D. M., McKernan, K. (2023) DNA fragments detected in monovalent and Pfizer/BioNTech and Moderna modRNA COVID-19 vaccines from Ontario, Canada: Exploratory dose response relationship with serious adverse events. OSF Preprints. Retrieved from osf.io/mjc97/.
81 Ibid.
82 Josephson, Rapporteur's Rolling Review assessment report.
83 Sheng-Fowler, L., Lewis, A. M. Jr, Peden, K. (2009) Issues associated with residual cell-substrate DNA in viral vaccines. *Biologicals* 37(3):190–95. doi:10.1016/j.biologicals.2009.02.015.
84 Speicher, Rose, Gutschi, Wiseman, and McKernan, DNA fragments detected in monovalent and Pfizer/BioNTech and Moderna modRNA COVID-19 vaccines from Ontario, Canada.
85 Horwood, M., Chartier, N. (2023) Exclusive: Health Canada not concerned about scientists' finding of plasmid DNA contamination in COVID shots. Epoch Times. Retrieved from www.theepochtimes.com/world/exclusive-health-canada-not-concerned-about-scientists-finding-of-plasmid-dna-contamination-in-covid-shots-5449394.
86 Phillips, J. (2023) FDA responds to reports of DNA contamination in COVID vaccines. Epoch Times. Retrieved from www.theepochtimes.com/article/fda-responds-to-reports-of-dna-contamination-in-covid-vaccines-5496717.
87 Demasi, M. (2023) Exclusive: An interview with Buckhaults about DNA contamination in COVID vaccines . . . and the FDA responds. MaryAnne Demasi Substack. Retrieved from maryannedemasi.substack.com/p/exclusive-an-interview-with-buckhaults.
88 Stieber, Z. (2023) European regulator confirms BioNTech did not highlight DNA sequence in COVID-19 vaccine. Epoch Times. Retrieved from www.theepochtimes.com/health/european-regulator-confirms-pfizer-did-not-highlight-dna-sequence-in-covid-19-vaccine-5519668?utm.

89 Speicher, Rose, Gutschi, Wiseman, and McKernan, DNA fragments detected in monovalent and Pfizer/BioNTech and Moderna modRNA COVID-19 vaccines from Ontario, Canada: Exploratory dose response relationship with serious adverse events.
90 Buckhaults, P. (2023) Testimony before South Carolina Senate Medical Affairs Ad-Hoc.
91 Lim, S., Yocum, R. R., Silver, P. A., Way, J. C. (2023) High spontaneous integration rates of end-modified linear DNAs upon mammalian cell transfection. *Sci Rep* 13:6835. doi:10.1038/s41598–023-33862–0
92 Ledwith, B. J., Manam, S., Troilo, P. J., Barnum, A. B., Pauley, C. J., et al. (2000) Plasmid DNA vaccines: Assay for integration into host genomic DNA. *Dev Biol* (Basel) 104:33–43.
93 Nie, Y., Fu, G., Leng, Y. (2023) Nuclear delivery of nanoparticle-based drug delivery systems by nuclear localization signals. *Cells* 12(12):1637. doi:10.3390/cells12121637.
94 Zhang, M. (2024) COVID vaccine gene could integrate into human cancer cells: Researcher. Epoch Times. Retrieved from www.theepochtimes.com/health/covid-vaccine-gene-could-integrate-into-human-cancer-cells-researcher-5604184?utm.
95 Phillips, FDA responds to reports of DNA contamination in COVID vaccines.
96 Chartier, N. (2023) Here are the four e-mails from Health Canada which underpin our work on DNA plasmid contamination and the undisclosed presence of Simian Virus 40 enhancer-promoter. X. Retrieved from twitter.com/nchartieret/status/1716579403243634922?s=46&t=fHNy04S5p-78vK_ah9g3hw.
97 Horwood, M. (2023) Exclusive: Health Canada confirms undisclosed presence of DNA sequence in Pfizer shot. Epoch Times. Retrieved from www.theepochtimes.com/world/exclusive-health-canada-confirms-undisclosed-presence-of-dna-sequence-in-pfizer-shot-5513277.
98 Bai, H., Lester, G. M. S., Petishnok, L. C., Dean, D. A. (2017) Cytoplasmic transport and nuclear import of plasmid DNA. *Biosci Rep* 37(6):BSR20160616. doi:10.1042/BSR20160616.
99 Institute of Medicine (US) Immunization Safety Review Committee (2002) Immunization Safety Review: SV40 contamination of polio vaccine and cancer. Stratton, K., Almario, D. A., McCormick, M. C., editors. Washington (DC): National Academies Press (US). doi:10.17226/10534.
100 McKernan, Helbert, Kane, and McLaughlin, Sequencing of bivalent Moderna and Pfizer mRNA vaccines reveals nanogram to microgram quantities of expression vector dsDNA peer dose.
101 Zhang, L., Richards, A., Barrasa, M. I., Hughes, S. H., Young, R. A., Jaenisch, R. (2021) Reverse-transcribed SARS-CoV-2 RNA can integrate into the genome of cultured human cells and can be expressed in patient-derived tissues. *Proc Natl Acad Sci USA* 118(21):e2105968118. doi:10.1073/pnas.2105968118.
102 Aldén, M., Olofsson Falla, F., Yang, D., Barghouth, M., Luan, C., et al. (2022) Intracellular reverse transcription of Pfizer BioNTech COVID-19 mRNA vaccine BNT162b2 *in vitro* in human liver cell line. *Curr Issues Mol Biol* 2022 Feb 25;44(3):1115–26. doi:10.3390/cimb44030073.
103 Comirnaty European Public Assessment Report.
104 Wang, Z., Hood, E. D., Nong, J., Ding, J., Marcos-Contreras, O. A., et al. (2022) Combating complement's deleterious effects on nanomedicine by conjugating complement regulatory proteins to nanoparticles. *Adv Mater* 34(8):e2107070. doi:10.1002/adma.202107070.

105 Szebeni, J., Simberg, D., González-Fernández, Á., Barenholz, Y., Dobrovolskaia, M. A. (2018) Roadmap and strategy for overcoming infusion reactions to nanomedicines. *Nat Nanotechnol* 13(12):1100–1108. doi:10.1038/s41565–018-0273–1.

106 Moghimi, S. M. (2021) Allergic reactions and anaphylaxis to LNP-Based COVID-19 vaccines. *Mol Ther* 29(3):898–900. doi:10.1016/j.ymthe.2021.01.030.

107 Paramasivam, P., Franke, C., Stöter, M., Höijer, A., Bartesaghi, S., et al. (2022) Endosomal escape of delivered mRNA from endosomal recycling tubules visualized at the nanoscale. *J Cell Biol* 221(2):e202110137. doi: 10.1083/jcb.202110137.

108 Ndeupen, S., Qin, Z., Jacobsen, S., Bouteau, A., Estanbouli, H., Igyártó, B. Z. (2021) The mRNA-LNP platform's lipid nanoparticle component used in preclinical vaccine studies is highly inflammatory. *iScience* 24(12):103479. doi:10.1016/j.isci.2021.103479.

109 Bitounis, D., Jacquinet, E., Rogers, M. A., Amiji, M. M. (2024) Strategies to reduce the risks of mRNA drug and vaccine toxicity. *Nat Rev Drug Discov* 23(4):281–300. doi:10.1038/s41573–023-00859–3.

110 Council of Europe. (2023) Ph. Eur. Commission kicks off elaboration of three general texts on mRNA vaccines and components. Retrieved from www.edqm.eu/en/-/ph.-eur.-commission-kicks-off-elaboration-of-three-general-texts-on-mrna-vaccines-and-components.

111 USP-NF, Analytical procedures for mRNA vaccine quality (Draft Guidelines).

112 World Health Organization. (2022) Evaluation of the quality, safety and efficacy of messenger RNA vaccines for the prevention of infectious diseases: Regulatory considerations.

113 Li, Z., Malla, S., Shin, B., Li, J. M. (2014) Battle against RNA oxidation: Molecular mechanisms for reducing oxidized RNA to protect cells. *Wiley Interdiscip Rev RNA* 5(3):335–46. doi:10.1002/wrna.1214.

114 Jacobsen, E. (2022) Quality control in mRNA vaccine manufacturing—The critical path. Future Lab, Biocompare. Retrieved from www.biocompare.com/Editorial-Articles/592381-Quality-Control-in-mRNA-Vaccine-Manufacturing-The-Critical-Path/.

115 USP-NF, Analytical procedures for mRNA vaccine quality (Draft Guidelines).

116 Josephson, Rapporteur's Rolling Review assessment report.

117 Segalla, G. (2023) Chemical-physical criticality and toxicological potential of lipid nanomaterials contained in a COVID-19 mRNA vaccine. *Int J Vac Theor Prac Res* 3(1):787–817. doi:10.56098/ijvtpr.v3i1.68.

118 Lewis, L. M., Badkar, A. V., Cirelli, D., Combs, R., Lerch, T. F. (2023) The race to develop the Pfizer-BioNTech COVID-19 vaccine: From the pharmaceutical scientists' perspective. *J Pharm Sci* 112(3):640–47. doi:10.1016/j.xphs.2022.09.014.

119 U.S. Food and Drug Administration. (2021) Emergency Use Authorization (EUA) for an unapproved product review memorandum. Retrieved from www.fda.gov/media/153947/download.

120 Rzymski, P., Fal, A. (2022) To aspirate or not to aspirate? Considerations for the COVID-19 vaccines. *Pharmacol Rep* 74(6):1223–27. doi:10.1007/s43440–022-00361–4.

121 Brail, S. (2022) Marc Girardot's unified theory of vaccine injury. Wholistic Substack. Retrieved from wholistic.substack.com/p/marc-girardots-unified-theory-of-vaccine-injury.

122 Di, J., Du, Z., Wu, K., Jin, S., Wang, X., et al. (2022) Biodistribution and non-linear gene expression of mRNA LNPs affected by delivery route and particle size. *Pharm Res* 39(1):105–14. doi:10.1007/s11095–022-03166–5.

123 Mulroney, T. E., Pöyry, T., Yam-Puc, J., Rust, M., Harvey, R. F., et al. (2023) (N)1-methylpseudouridylation of mRNA causes +1 ribosomal frameshifting. *Nature*. e-publication December 6, 2023. doi: 10.1038/s41586–023-06800–3.

124 Wiseman, D., Gutschi, L. M., Speicher, D. J., Rose, J., McKernan (2023) Ribosomal frameshifting and misreading of mRNA in COVID-19 vaccines produces "off-target" proteins and immune responses eliciting safety concerns: Comment on UK study by Mulroney et al. Retrieved from osf.io/nt8jh. doi:10.31219/osf.io/nt8jh.

125 Takeda Pharmaceuticals. (2021) Moderna COVID-19 vaccine recall investigation report. Retrieved from www.takeda.com/ja-jp/announcements/statement-regarding-moderna-covid-19-vaccine-recall-investigation-report—october-2021.

126 Schmeling, M., Manniche, V., Hansen, P. R. (2023) Batch-dependent safety of the BNT162b2 mRNA COVID-19 vaccine. *Eur J Clin Invest* 53(8):e13998. doi:10.1111/eci.13998.

127 FOI Team (2022) Freedom of Information request on specific batch numbers on the adverse reactions reported following the COVID-19 vaccinations (FOI release 22/661). Medicines and Health Products Regulatory Agency. Retrieved from www.gov.uk/government/publications/freedom-of-information-responses-from-the-mhra-week-commencing-6-june-2022/freedom-of-information-request-on-specific-batch-numbers-on-the-adverse-reactions-reported-following-the-covid-19-vaccinations-foi-22661.

128 Fenton, N. E. (2023) The scandal of the Astrazeneca vaccine from the Emergent Biosolutions plant in Baltimore. Substack. Retrieved from wherearethenumbers.substack.com/p/the-scandal-of-the-astrazeneca-vaccine.

129 Blackwell, T. (2021) More than half Canada's AstraZeneca vaccine came from U.S. plant accused of quality-control problems. *National Post*. Retrieved from nationalpost.com/news/canada/more-than-half-canadas-astrazeneca-vaccine-came-from-u-s-plant-accused-by-fda-of-quality-control-problems.

130 Chooi, W. H., Ng, P. W., Hussain, Z., Ming, L. C., Ibrahim, B., Koh, D. (2022) Vaccine contamination: Causes and control. *Vaccine* 40(12):1699–1701. doi:10.1016/j.vaccine.2022.02.034.

131 Schmeling, Manniche, and Hansen, PBatch-dependent safety of the BNT162b2 mRNA COVID-19 vaccine.

132 WHO guidelines on non-clinical evaluation of vaccines TRS No 927.

133 (2005) Annex 1 WHO guidelines on nonclinical evaluation of vaccines. World Health Organization. Retrieved from www.who.int/biologicals/publications/trs/areas/vaccines/nonclinical_evaluation/ANNEX%201Nonclinical.P31–63.pdf?ua=1.

134 World Health Organization. (2014) Annex 2 Guidelines on the Nonclinical Evaluation of Vaccine Adjuvants and Adjuvanted Vaccines. Retrieved from www.who.int/publications/m/item/nonclinical-evaluation-of-vaccine-adjuvants-and-adjuvanted-vaccines-annex-2-trs-no-987.

135 Ibid.

136 (2020) Evaluation of the quality, safety and efficacy of messenger RNA vaccines for the prevention of infectious diseases: Regulatory considerations. Draft December 20, 2020. World Health Organization. Retrieved from www.who.int/docs/default-source/biologicals/ecbs/reg-considerations-on-rna-vaccines_1st-draft_pc_tz_22122020.pdf?sfvrsn=c13e1e20_.

137 Banoun, mRNA: Vaccine or gene therapy? The safety regulatory issues.

138 Food and Drug Administration Center for Biologics Evaluation and Research. (2020) Human therapy for rare diseases. Guidance for industry. Retrieved from www.fda.gov/media/113807/download.
139 Banoun, mRNA: Vaccine or gene therapy? The safety regulatory issues.
140 Sheng-Fowler, Lewis, and Peden, Issues associated with residual cell-substrate DNA in viral vaccines.
141 Spadafora, C. (2017) Sperm-mediated transgenerational inheritance. *Front Microbiol* 8:2401. doi:10.3389/fmicb.2017.02401
142 USFDA. US Department of Health and Human Services. (2020) Chemistry, manufacturing, and control (CMC) information for human gene therapy investigational new drug applications (INDs). CBER, Ed. Retrieved from www.fda.gov/media/113760/download.
143 Dean, D. A., Dean, B. S., Muller, S., Smith, L. C. (1999) Sequence requirements for plasmid nuclear import. *Exp Cell Res* 253(2):713–22. doi:10.1006/excr.1999.4716.
144 Sencer, D., Millar, J. D. (2006) Reflections on the 1976 swine flu vaccination program. *Emerg Infect Dis* 12(1):29–33. doi:10.3201/eid1201.051007.
145 Evans, D., Cauchemez, S., Hayden, F. G. (2009) "Prepandemic" immunization for novel influenza viruses, "swine flu" vaccine, Guillain-Barré syndrome, and the detection of rare severe adverse events. *J Infect Dis* 200(3):321–28. doi:10.1086/603560.

Chapter 12

1 (2023) Approved COVID-19 vaccines. Retrieved from www.canada.ca/en/health-canada/services/drugs-health-products/covid19-industry/drugs-vaccines-treatments/vaccines.html.
2 (2023) Pfizer/BioNTech Comirnaty COVID-19 vaccine. Retrieved from www.canada.ca/en/health-canada/services/drugs-health-products/covid19-industry/drugs-vaccines-treatments/vaccines/pfizer-biontech.html.
3 Ibid.
4 (2023) Moderna Spikevax COVID-19 vaccines. Health Canada. Retrieved from www.canada.ca/en/health-canada/services/drugs-health-products/covid19-industry/drugs-vaccines-treatments/vaccines/moderna.html.
5 Dolgin, E. (2021) The tangled history of mRNA vaccines. *Nature* 597(7876):318–24. doi:10.1038/d41586–021-02483-w.
6 Gutchi, L., Speicher, D. J., Natsheh, S., Oldfield, P., Britz-McKibbon, P., et al. (2022) An independent analysis of the manufacturing and quality issues of the BNT162b BioNtech/Pfizer quasi-vaccine based on the European Medicines Agency's Public Assessment Report (EPAR). Canadian Covid Care Alliance. Retrieved from www.canadiancovidcarealliance.org/wp-content/uploads/2022/11/22OC29_EMA-Analysis-of-BNT162b-Manufacture.pdf.
7 (2020) Summary of product characteristics: Zabdeno suspension for injection. Retrieved from www.ema.europa.eu/en/documents/product-information/zabdeno-epar-product-information_en.pdf.
8 RECOVERY Collaborative Group; Horby, P., Lim, W. S., Emberson, J. R., Mafham, M., Bell, J. L., et al. (2021) Dexamethasone in hospitalized patients with COVID-19. *N Engl J Med* 384(8):693–704. doi:10.1056/NEJMoa2021436.

9 (2021) Pfizer-BioNTech COVID-19 BNT162b2 Vaccine effectiveness study—Kaiser Permanente Southern California. U.S. National Library of Medicine. Retrieved from clinicaltrials.gov/ct2/show/NCT04848584.

10 (2018) Vaccines and Immunizations. Immunizations: The basics. Retrieved from web.archive.org/web/20200317214611/www.cdc.gov/vaccines/vac-gen/imz-basics.htm.

11 Centers for Disease Control and Prevention, Vaccines and Immunizations. Immunizations: The basics.

12 42 U.S. Code § 300aa-22—Standards of responsibility. LII Legal Information Institute. Cornell Law School. Retrieved from www.law.cornell.edu/uscode/text/42/300aa-22.

13 Buckley, S. (2023) Changes to the drug approval test for COVID-19 vaccines: Permitted vaccines to be approved without objective proof of (1) safety, (2) efficacy, or (3) the benefits outweighing the risks. Natural Health Products Protection Association. Retrieved from nhppa.org/wp-content/uploads/2023/03/NHPPA-Discussion-Paper-COVID-19-Vaccine-Test-March-17–2023.pdf.

14 Ibid.

15 Brown, R. B. (2021) Outcome reporting bias in COVID-19 mRNA vaccine clinical trials. *Medicina* (Mex) 57(3):199. doi:10.3390/medicina57030199.

16 Thomas, S. J., Moreira, E. D., Kitchin, N., Absalon, J., Gurtman, A., et al. (2021) Safety and efficacy of the BNT162b2 mRNA COVID-19 vaccine through 6 months. *N Engl J Med* 385:1761–73. doi:10.1056/NEJMoa2110345.

17 Fischhoff, B., Brewer, N. T., Downs, J. S., eds. (2011) FDA. Communicating risks and benefits: An evidence-based user's guide, 242. Retrieved from www.fda.gov/about-fda/reports/communicating-risks-and-benefits-evidence-based-users-guide.

18 Thomas, Moreira, Kitchin, Absalon, Gurtman, et al., Safety and efficacy of the BNT162b2 mRNA COVID-19 vaccine through 6 months.

19 (2022) Ontario's COVID-19 hospitalizations rise to 1,730, most since mid-February. Retrieved from www.cbc.ca/news/canada/toronto/covid-19-ontario-april-26–2022-hospitalizations-1.6431094.

20 Carrigg, D. (2022) Majority of new COVID-19 hospitalizations in B.C. among people admitted for other reasons. *Vancouver Sun*. Retrieved from vancouversun.com/news/local-news/majority-of-new-covid-19-hospitalizations-among-people-admitted-for-other-reasons.

21 Public Health Scotland (2022) COVID-19 and Winter Statistical Report. As at 14 February 2020. See Figure 16. Retrieved from www.publichealthscotland.scot/media/11916/22–02-16-covid19-winter_publication_report.pdf.

22 (2022) COVID-19 Alberta statistics. Interactive aggregate data on COVID-19 cases in Alberta. Retrieved for January 11, 2022 from web.archive.org/web/20220111010547/www.alberta.ca/stats/covid-19-alberta-statistics.htm#vaccine-outcomes.

23 (2023) Internet Archive WayBack Machine. Retrieved from archive.org/web/.

24 (2022) COVID-19 Alberta statistics. Interactive aggregate data on COVID-19 cases in Alberta. Retrieved for November 29, 2021 from web.archive.org/web/20211111180117/www.alberta.ca/stats/covid-19-alberta-statistics.htm#vaccine-outcomes.

25 Polack, F. P., Thomas, S. J., Kitchin, N., Absalon, J., Gurtman, A., et al. (2020) C4591001 Clinical Trial Group. Safety and efficacy of the BNT162b2 mRNA COVID-19 vaccine. *N Engl J Med* 383(27):2603–15. doi:10.1056/NEJMoa2034577.

26 Ibid.

27 Thomas, S. J., Moreira, E. D., Kitchin, N., Absalon, J., Gurtman, A., et al., Safety and efficacy of the BNT162b2 mRNA COVID-19 vaccine through 6 months.

28 (2021) The Pfizer inoculations for COVID-19: More harm than good. www.canadiancovidcarealliance.org/wp-content/uploads/2021/12/The-COVID-19-Inoculations-More-Harm-Than-Good-REV-Dec-16–2021.pdf.
29 Thaker, P. D. (2021) COVID-19: Researcher blows the whistle on data integrity issues in Pfizer's vaccine trial. *BMJ* 375:n2635. doi:10.1136/bmj.n2635.
30 Ibid.
31 Frenck, R. W., Klein, N. P., Kitchin, N., Curtman, A., Absalon, J., et al.; C4591001 Clinical Trial Group (2021) Safety, immunogenicity, and efficacy of the BNT162b2 COVID-19 vaccine in adolescents. *N Engl J Med* 385(3):239–50. doi:10.1056/NEJMoa2107456.
32 Walter, E. B., Talaat, K. R., Sabharwal, C., Gurtman, A., Lockhart, S., et al.; C4591007 Clinical Trial Group (2022) Evaluation of the BNT162b2 Covid-19 vaccine in children 5 to 11 years of age. *N Engl J Med* 386(1):35–46. doi:10.1056/NEJMoa2116298.
33 Ibid.
34 (2021) Health Canada authorizes use of Comirnaty (the Pfizer-BioNTech COVID-19 vaccine) in children 5 to 11 years of age. Retrieved from www.canada.ca/en/health-canada/news/2021/11/health-canada-authorizes-use-of-comirnaty-the-pfizer-biontech-covid-19-vaccine-in-children-5-to-11-years-of-age.html.
35 (2022) Health Canada authorizes use of Moderna Spikevax (50 mcg) COVID-19 vaccine in children 6 to 11 years of age. Retrieved from www.canada.ca/en/health-canada/news/2022/03/health-canada-authorizes-use-of-the-moderna-spikevax-50-mcg-covid-19-vaccine-in-children-6-to-11-years-of-age.html.
36 (2022) Vaccines and Related Biological Products Advisory Committee June 14–15, 2022 Meeting Announcement—06/14/2022. Retrieved from www.fda.gov/advisory-committees/advisory-committee-calendar/vaccines-and-related-biological-products-advisory-committee-june-14–15-2022-meeting-announcement.
37 (2022) National Advisory Committee on Immunization (NACI): Meetings. June 17, 2022. Retrieved from www.canada.ca/en/public-health/services/immunization/national-advisory-committee-on-immunization-naci/meetings.html.
38 (2023) Drug and vaccine authorizations for COVID-19: List of authorized drugs, vaccines and expanded indications. Retrieved from www.canada.ca/en/health-canada/services/drugs-health-products/covid19-industry/drugs-vaccines-treatments/authorization/list-drugs.html#wb-auto-4.
39 Muñoz, F. M., Sher, L. D., Sabharwal, C., Gurtman, A., Xu, X., et al.; C4591007 Clinical Trial Group. (2023) Evaluation of BNT162b2 COVID-19 vaccine in children younger than 5 years of age. *N Engl J Med.* 388(7):621–34. doi:10.1056/NEJMoa2211031.
40 (2021) Pfizer and BioNTech commence global clinical trial to evaluate COVID-19 vaccine in pregnant women. Press release retrieved from www.pfizer.com/news/press-release/press-release-detail/pfizer-and-biontech-commence-global-clinical-trial-evaluate.
41 Polack, Thomas, Kitchin, Absalon, Gurtman, et al., C4591001 Clinical Trial Group.
42 Almeida, N. D., Schiller, I., Ke, D., Sakr, E., Plesa, M., et al. (2024) The effect of dose-interval on antibody response to mRNA COVID-19 vaccines: a prospective cohort study. *Front Immunol.* doi:10.3389/fimmu.2024.1330549.
43 DeRoy-Olson, I. (2021) Why Indigenous communities are prioritized for the COVID-19 vaccine. Canadian Broadcasting Corporation Kids News. Retrieved from www.cbc.ca/kidsnews/post/watch-why-indigenous-communities-were-prioritized-for-the-covid-19-vaccine.

44 (2021) Joe Biden town hall in Cincinnati: Here's the full CNN transcript. Retrieved from www.cincinnati.com/story/news/politics/2021/07/21/joe-biden-cnn-town-hall-transcript/8051311002/.

45 (2021) Press briefing by White House COVID-19 Response Team and public health officials. Retrieved from www.whitehouse.gov/briefing-room/press-briefings/2021/07/01/press-briefing-by-white-house-covid-19-response-team-and-public-health-officials-43/.

46 (2023) Canada COVID-19 Situation. Retrieved from covid19.who.int/region/amro/country/ca.

47 (2023) COVID-19 vaccination: Vaccination coverage. Retrieved from health-infobase.canada.ca/covid-19/vaccination-coverage/.

48 Mercadé-Besora, N., Li, X., Kolde, R., Trinh, N. T., Sanchez-Santos, M. T., et al. (2024) The role of COVID-19 vaccines in preventing post-COVID-19 thromboembolic and cardiovascular complications. *Heart* 110(9):635–643. doi: 10.1136/heartjnl-2023–323483.

49 Cohn, B. A., Cirillo, P. M., Murphy, C. C., Krigbaum, N., Wallace, A. W. (2022) SARS-CoV-2 vaccine protection and deaths among US veterans during 2021. *Science* 375(6578):331–36. doi:10.1126/science.abm0620.

50 COVID-19 vaccination: Vaccination coverage.

51 Thomas, Moreira, Kitchin, Absalon, Gurtman, et al. Safety and efficacy of the BNT162b2 mRNA COVID-19 vaccine through 6 months.

52 Riemersma, K. K., Haddock, L. A 3rd, Wilson, N. A., Minor, N., Eickhoff, J., et al. (2022) Shedding of infectious SARS-CoV-2 despite vaccination. *PLOS Pathog* 18(9):e1010876. doi:10.1371/journal.ppat.1010876.

53 Franco-Paredes, C. (2022) Transmissibility of SARS-CoV-2 among fully vaccinated individuals. *Lancet Infect Dis* 22(1):16. doi:10.1016/S1473–3099(21)00768–4.

54 (2021) Dr. Fauci on COVID-19 spread: Vaccinated people who have an ... infection are capable of transmitting. Retrieved from www.youtube.com/watch?v=mP9iHyj1uiU.

55 Boucau, J., Marino, C., Regan, J., Uddin, R., Choudhary, M. C., et al. (2022) Duration of shedding of culturable virus in SARS-CoV-2 Omicron (BA.1) infection. *New Engl. J. Med* 387:275–277. doi:10.1056/NEJMc2202092.

56 (2023) BCCDC COVID-19 Regional Surveillance Dashboard—Archived. Retrieved from public.tableau.com/app/profile/bccdc/viz/BCCDCCOVID-19RegionalSurveillanceDashboardArchived/Introduction.

57 Horwood, M. (2024) One-third of doctors, half of nurses in Canada were reluctant to take COVID vaccines: Government survey. Epoch Times. Retrieved from www.theepochtimes.com/world/one-third-of-doctors-half-of-nurses-in-canada-reluctant-to-take-covid-vaccines-government-survey-5590179?utm.

58 (2022) COVID-19 vaccine surveillance report. Week 11. assets.publishing.service.gov.uk/media/623310c88fa8f504a316aa21/Vaccine_surveillance_report_-_week_11.pdf.

59 (2023) UKHSA vaccine efficacy data stopped after new footnote added. Retrieved from twitter.com/Jikkyleaks/status/1675005411014107136.

60 Fenton, N. E. and Neil, M. (2023) Claims the unvaccinated were at higher risk of hospitalisation and death were based on deliberately murky record keeping 2023. Substack. Retrieved from wherearethenumbers.substack.com/p/claims-the-unvaccinated-were-at-higher.

61 (2022) COVID hospitalisation rates. Retrieved from www.gov.wales/atisn16308.

62 Nantel, S., Sheikh-Mohamed, S., Chao, G. Y. C., Kurtesi, A., Hu, Q., et al. (2024) Comparison of Omicron breakthrough infection versus monovalent SARS-CoV-2

intramuscular booster reveals differences in mucosal and systemic humoral immunity. *Mucosal Immunol* 17(2):201–10. doi:10.1016/j.mucimm.2024.01.004.

63 Fleming-Dutra, K. E., Britton, A., Shang, N., Derado, G., Link-Gelles, R., et al. (2022) Association of prior BNT162b2 COVID-19 vaccination with symptomatic SARS-CoV-2 infection in children and adolescents during Omicron predominance. *JAMA* 327(22):2210–19. doi:10.1001/jama.2022.7493.

64 Dorabawila, V., Hoefer, D., Bauer, U. E., Bassett, M.T., Lutterloh, E., Rosenberg, E.S. (2022) Effectiveness of the BNT162b2 vaccine among children 5–11 and 12–17 years in New York after the emergence of the Omicron variant. medRxiv (preprint). doi:10.1101/2022.02.25.22271454.

65 Gagne, M., Moliva, J. I., Foulds, K. E., Andrew, S. F., Flynn, B. J., et al. (2022) mRNA-1273 or mRNA-Omicron boost in vaccinated macaques elicits comparable B cell expansion, neutralizing antibodies and protection against Omicron. bioRxiv (preprint). doi:10.1101/2022.02.03.479037.

66 Ying, B., Scheaffer, S. M., Whitener, B., Liang, C-Y., Dymtrenko, O., et al. (2022) Boosting with Omicron-matched or historical mRNA vaccines increases neutralizing antibody responses and protection against B.1.1.529 infection in mice. bioRxiv (preprint). doi:10.1101/2022.02.07.479419.

67 Hawman, D. W., Meade-White, K., Clancy, C., Archer, J., Hinkley, T., et al. (2022) Replicating RNA platform enables rapid response to the SARS-CoV-2 Omicron variant and elicits enhanced protection in naïve hamsters compared to ancestral vaccine. bioRxiv (preprint). doi:10.1101/2022.01.31.478520.

68 Lee, I.-J., Sun, C.-P., Wu, P.-Y., Lan, Y.-H., Wang, I.-H., et al. (2022) Omicron-specific mRNA vaccine induced potent neutralizing antibody against Omicron but not other SARS-CoV-2 variants. bioRxiv (preprint). doi:10.1101/2022.01.31.478406.

69 Hawman, Meade-White, Clancy, Archer, Hinkley, et al., Replicating RNA platform enables rapid response to the SARS-CoV-2 Omicron variant and elicits enhanced protection in naïve hamsters compared to ancestral vaccine.

70 Lee, Sun, Wu, Lan, Wang, et al. Omicron-specific mRNA vaccine induced potent neutralizing antibody against Omicron but not other SARS-CoV-2 variants.

71 Tseng, H. F., Ackerson, B. K., Bruxvoort, K. J., Sy, L. S., Tubert, J. E., et al. (2023) Effectiveness of mRNA-1273 vaccination against SARS-CoV-2 omicron subvariants BA.1, BA.2, BA.2.12.1, BA.4, and BA.5. *Nat Commun* 14(1):189. doi:10.1038/s41467–023-35815–7.

72 Cherry, N., Adisesh, A., Burstyn, I., Charlton, C., Chen, Y., et al. (2024) Determinants of SARS-CoV-2 IgG response and decay in Canadian healthcare workers: a prospective cohort study. *Vaccine*. doi:10.1016/j.vaccine.2024.01.052.

73 Chalkias, S., Harper, C., Vrbicky, K., Walsh, S. R., Essink, B., et al. (2022) A bivalent omicron-containing booster vaccine against COVID-19. *New Eng. J. Med* 387(14):1279–91. doi:10.1056/NEJMoa2208343.

74 (2022) Coronavirus (COVID-19) update: FDA authorizes Moderna, Pfizer-BioNTech bivalent COVID-19 vaccines for use as booster dose. Retrieved from www.fda.gov/news-events/press-announcements/coronavirus-covid-19-update-fda-authorizes-moderna-pfizer-biontech-bivalent-covid-19-vaccines-use.

75 Vogel, G. (2022) Omicron booster shots are coming—with lots of questions. *Science* 377(6610):1029–30. doi:10.1126/science.ade6580.

76 Rawle, D. J., Le, T. T., Dumenil, T., Yan, K., Tang, B., et al. (2022) ACE2-lentiviral transduction enables mouse SARS-CoV-2 infection and mapping of receptor interactions. *PLOS Pathog* 17(7):e1009723. doi:10.1371/journal.ppat.1009723.

77 Vogel, Omicron booster shots are coming—with lots of questions.

78 Ko, L., Malet, G., Chang, L. L., Nguyen, H., Mayes, R. (2023) COVID-19 infection rates in vaccinated and unvaccinated inmates: A retrospective cohort study. *Cureus* 15(9): e44684. doi:10.7759/cureus.44684.

79 Tamada, Y., Takeuchi, K., Kusama, T., Maeda, M., Murata, F., et al. (2024) Bivalent mRNA vaccine effectiveness against COVID-19 among older adults in Japan: a test-negative study from the VENUS study. *BMC Infect Dis* 24(1):135. doi:10.1186/s12879–024-09035–3.

80 Ibid.

81 Shrestha, N. K., Burke, P. C., Nowacki, A. S., Simon J. F., Hagen, A., Gordon, S. M. (2023) Effectiveness of the coronavirus disease 2019 bivalent vaccine. *Open Forum Infect Dis* 10(6):ofad209. doi:10.1093/ofid/ofad209.

82 Shrestha, N. K., Burke, P. C., Nowacki, A. S., Simon J. F., Hagen, A., Gordon, S. M. (2024) Effectiveness of the 2023–2024 formulation of the Coronavirus Disease 2019 mRNA vaccine against the JN.I variant. MedRxiv (preprint). Retrieved from doi.org/10.1101/2024.04.27.24306378.

83 (2023) 182nd meeting of Vaccines and Related Biological Products Advisory Committee. June 15, 20123. Retrieved from www.youtube.com/watch?v=gBOyPREXGh8.

84 Monk, E. (2023) Is it really true that no healthy under 50s died from COVID-19 in Israel? West Country Voices. Retrieved from www.westcountryvoices.com/is-it-really-true-that-no-healthy-under-50s-died-from-covid-19-in-israel/.

85 Ibid.

86 Espino, A. M., Armina-Rodriguez, A., Alvarez, L., Ocasio-Malavé, C., Ramos-Nieves, R., et al. (2024) The anti-SARS-CoV-2 IgG1 and IgG3 antibody isotypes with limited neutralizing capacity against Omicron elicited in a Latin population a switch toward IgG4 after multiple doses with the mRNA Pfizer-BioNTech Vaccine. *Viruses* 16(2):187. doi:10.3390/v16020187.

87 Uversky, V. N., Redwan, E. M., Makis, W., Rubio-Casillas, A. (2023) IgG4 antibodies induced by repeated vaccination may generate immune tolerance to the SARS-CoV-2 spike protein. *Vaccines* (Basel) 11(5):991. doi:10.3390/vaccines11050991.

88 Irrgang, P., Gerling, J., Kocher, K., Lapuente, D., Steininger, P., et al. (2023) Class switch toward noninflammatory, spike-specific IgG4 antibodies after repeated SARS-CoV-2 mRNA vaccination. *Sci Immunol* 8(79):eade2798. doi:10.1126/sciimmunol.ade2798.

89 Buhre, J. S., Pongracz, T., Künsting, I., Lixenfeld, A. S., Wang, W., et al. (2023) mRNA vaccines against SARS-CoV-2 induce comparably low long-term IgG Fc galactosylation and sialylation levels but increasing long-term IgG4 responses compared to an adenovirus-based vaccine. *Front Immunol* 13:1020844. doi:10.3389/fimmu.2022.1020844.

90 Kiszel, P., Sík, P., Miklós, J., Kajdácsi, E., Sinkovits, G., et al. (2023) Class switch towards spike protein-specific IgG4 antibodies after SARS-CoV-2 mRNA vaccination depends on prior infection history. *Sci Rep* 13(1):13166. doi:10.1038/s41598–023.

91 Uversky, Redwan, Makis, Rubio-Casillas, IgG4 antibodies induced by repeated vaccination may generate immune tolerance to the SARS-CoV-2 spike protein.

92 Valk, A. M., Keijer, J. B. D., van Dam, K. P. J., Stalman, E. W., Wieske, L., et al. (2023) Suppressed IgG4 class switching in dupilumab- and TNF inhibitor-treated patients

after repeated SARS-CoV-2 mRNA vaccination. medRxiv (preprint). doi:10.1101/2023.09.29.23296354.

93 Kalkeri, R., Zhu, M., Cloney-Clark, S., Plested, J. S., Parekh, A., et al. (2024) Altered IgG4 antibody response to repeated mRNA versus protein COVID vaccines. medRxiv [Preprint] 2024.01.17.24301374. doi:10.1101/2024.01.17.24301374.

94 McKinney, E. F., Lee, J. C., Jayne, D. R., Lyons, P. A., Smith, K. G. (2015) T cell exhaustion, co-stimulation and clinical outcome in autoimmunity and infection. *Nature* 523(7562):612–16. doi:10.1038/nature14468.

95 Chevaisrakul, P., Lumjiaktase, P., Kietdumrongwong, P., Chuatrisorn, I., Chatsangjaroen, P., Phanuphak, N. (2023) Hybrid and herd immunity 6 months after SARS-CoV-2 exposure among individuals from a community treatment program. *Sci Rep* 13(1):763. doi:10.1038/s41598–023-28101–5.

96 Shrestha, Burke, Nowacki, Simon Hagen, Gordon. Effectiveness of the coronavirus disease 2019 bivalent vaccine.

97 Shrestha, N. K., Burke, P. C., Nowacki, A. S., Gordon, S. M. (2023) Risk of Coronavirus Disease 2019 (COVID-19) among those up-to-date and not up-to-date on COVID-19 vaccination by US CDC criteria. *PLoS One* 18(11):e0293449. doi:10.1371/journal.pone.0293449.

98 Boretti A. (2024) mRNA vaccine boosters and impaired immune system response in immune compromised individuals: a narrative review. *Clin Exp Med* 24(1):23. doi: 10.1007/s10238–023-01264–1.

99 Vecchio, E., Rotundo, S., Veneziano, C., Abatino, A., Aversa, I., et al. (2024) The spike-specific TCRβ repertoire shows distinct features in unvaccinated or vaccinated patients with SARS-CoV-2 infection. *J Transl Med* 22:33. doi.10.1186/s12967–024-04852–1.

100 Adhikari, B., Bednash, J. S., Horowitz, J. C., Rubinstein, M. P., Vlasova, A. N. (2024) Corrigendum: Brief research report: impact of vaccination on antibody responses and mortality from severe COVID-19. *Front Immunol* 15:1384209. doi:10.3389/fimmu.2024.1384209.

Chapter 13

1 Parry, P. I., Lefringhausen, A., Turni, C., Neil, C. J., Cosford, R., et al. (2023) "Spikeopathy": COVID-19 spike protein is athogenic, from both virus and vaccine mRNA. *Biomedicines* 11(8):2287. doi:10.3390/biomedicines11082287.

2 Said, E. A., Al-Rubkhi, A., Jaju, S., Koh, C. Y., Al-Balushi, M. S., et al. (2024) Association of the magnitude of anti-SARS-CoV-2 vaccine side effects with sex, allergy history, chronic diseases, medication intake, and SARS-CoV-2 Infection. *Vaccines* (Basel) 12(1):104. doi: 10.3390/vaccines12010104.

3 Schädlich, A., Hoffmann, S., Mueller, T., Caysa, H., Rose, C., et al. (2012) Accumulation of nanocarriers in the ovary: A neglected toxicity risk? *J Control Release* 160(1):105–12. doi:10.1016/j.jconrel.2012.02.012.

4 (2021) SARS-CoV-2 mRNA Vaccine (BNT162, PF-07302048) 2.6.4 薬物動態試験の概要文 (translation: "Summary of pharmacokinetic study"). Retrieved from pandemictimeline.com/wp-content/uploads/2021/07/Pfizer-report_Japanese-government.pdf.

5 (2021) Assessment report: Comirnaty. Retrieved from www.ema.europa.eu/en/documents/assessment-report/comirnaty-epar-public-assessment-report_en.pdf.

6 SARS-CoV-2 mRNA Vaccine (BNT162, PF-07302048) 2.6.4.

7 Ibid.

8 Yao, W., Ma, D., Wang, H., Tang, X., Du, C., et al. (2021) Effect of SARS-CoV-2 spike mutations on animal ACE2 usage and *in vitro* neutralization sensitivity. bioRxiv (preprint). 2021.01.27.428353. doi:10.1101/2021.01.27.428353.

9 Zhang, C., Cui, H., Li, E., Guo, Z., Wang, T., et al. (2022) The SARS-CoV-2 B.1.351 variant can transmit in rats but not in mice. *Front Immunol* 13:869809. doi:10.3389/fimmu.2022.869809.

10 Rosenke, K., Meade-White, K., Letko, M., Clancy, C., Hansen, F., et al. (2020) Defining the Syrian hamster as a highly susceptible preclinical model for SARS-CoV-2 infection. *Emerg Microbes Infect* 9(1):2673–84. doi:10.1080/22221751.2020.1858177.

11 Polack, F. P., Thomas, S. J., Kitchin, N., Absalon, J., Gurtman, A., et al.; C4591001 Clinical Trial Group. (2020) Safety and efficacy of the BNT162b2 mRNA COVID-19 Vaccine. *N Engl J Med* 383(27):2603–15. doi:10.1056/NEJMoa2034577.

12 Ibid.

13 Thomas, S. J., Moreira, E. D. Jr., Kitchin, N., Absalon, J., Gurtman, A., et al.; C4591001 Clinical Trial Group. (2021) Safety and efficacy of the BNT162b2 mRNA COVID-19 vaccine through 6 months. *N Engl J Med* 385(19):1761–73. doi:10.1056/NEJMoa2110345.

14 Supplement to: Thomas, S.J., Moreira, E.D. Jr, Kitchin, N., Absalon, J., Gurtman, A., et al.; C4591001 Clinical Trial Group. (2021) Safety and efficacy of the BNT162b2 mRNA COVID-19 vaccine through 6 months. N Engl J Med 385(19):1761–73. doi:10.1056/NEJMoa2110345. Retrieved from www.nejm.org/doi/suppl/10.1056/NEJMoa2110345/suppl_file/nejmoa2110345_appendix.pdf.

15 Michels, C., Perrier, D., Kunadhasan, J., Clark, E., Gehrett, J., et al. (2023) Forensic analysis of the 38 subject deaths in the 6-Month Interim Report of the Pfizer/BioNTech BNT162b2 mRNA Vaccine Clinical Trial. *Int J Vacc Theor Prac Res* 3(1):973–1008. doi:10.56098/ijvtpr.v3i1.85.

16 Ibid.

17 Gulbrandsen, T., Martin, N., Fenton, N. (2023) Anomalous patterns of mortality and morbidity in Pfizer's COVID-19 vaccine trial. Substack. Retrieved from wherearethenumbers.substack.com/p/anomalous-patterns-of-mortality-and.

18 Fraiman, J., Erviti, J., Jones, M., Greenland, S., Whelan, P., et al. (2022) Serious adverse events of special interest following mRNA COVID-19 vaccination in randomized trials in adults. *Vaccine*, ISSN 0264–410X. doi:10.1016/j.vaccine.2022.08.036

19 FDA. (2021) Docket No. FDA-2021-N-1088 for "Vaccines and Related Biological Products; Notice of Meeting." Retrieved from www.regulations.gov/comment/FDA-2021-N-1088–129763.

20 Demasi, M. (2021) Are adverse events in COVID-19 vaccine trials under-reported? Substack. Retrieved from maryannedemasi.com/publications/f/are-adverse-events-in-covid-19-vaccine-trials-under-reported.

21 Frenck R. W. Jr, Klein N. P., Kitchin N., Gurtman A., Absalon J., et al.; C4591001 Clinical Trial Group. (2021) Safety, immunogenicity, and efficacy of the BNT162b2 Covid-19 vaccine in adolescents. *N Engl J Med* 385(3):239–50. doi:10.1056/NEJMoa2107456.

22 (2024) Sharyl Attkisson interview with Stephanie de Garay. Vaccine Trials. Retrieved from web.archive.org/web/20240203222026/https:/fullmeasure.news/newest-videos/vaccine-trials.

23 Pfizer, Inc. (2021) BLA Submission for BNT162b2 Module 2.4. Clinical Overview. Public Health and Medical Professionals for Transparency Documents. [Online] April 30, 2021. Retrieved from phmpt.org/wp-content/uploads/2021/12/STN-125742_0_0Section-2.5-Clinical-Overview.pdf.
24 (2021) 5.3.6 Cumulative analysis of post-authorization adverse event reports of PF-07302048 (BNT162B2) received through 28-FEB-2021. Worldwide Safety. Retrieved from phmpt.org/wp-content/uploads/2021/11/5.3.6-postmarketing-experience.pdf.
25 Ibid.
26 (2022) Appendix 2.2: Cumulative and interval summary tabulations of serious and non-serious adverse reactions from post-marketing data sources: BNT162B2. Page 1. Retrieved from lawyerlisa.substack.com/p/pfizer-data-attached-393-pages-of.
27 Wolf, N. (2023) What's in the Pfizer documents? Address to Hillsdale College on March 6, 2023. Retrieved from www.youtube.com/watch?v=T9Y_W_30hsM.
28 (2023) Pfizer reports. Retrieved from dailyclout.io/category/pfizer-reports/.
29 Raethke, M., van Hunsel, F., Luxi, N., Lieber, T., Bellitto, C., et al. (2024) Frequency and timing of adverse reactions to COVID-19 vaccines; A multi-country cohort event monitoring study. *Vaccine* 42(9):2357–2369. doi:10.1016/j.vaccine.2024.03.001.
30 (2024) VAERS COVID vaccine adverse events report. Retrieved from www.openvaers.com/covid-data.
31 Ibid.
32 Ibid.
33 Lazarus, R., Klompas, M. (2011) Harvard Pilgrim Study—Lazarus Final Report 2011. Adverse Effect. Grant Final Report ID R18 HS 017045. Retrieved from digital.ahrq.gov/sites/default/files/docs/publication/r18hs017045-lazarus-final-report-2011.pdf.
34 Kirsch, S., Rose, J., Crawford, M. (2021) Estimating the number of COVID vaccine deaths in America. October 8, 2021 update. Trialsite News 57. Retrieved from www.datascienceassn.org/sites/default/files/Estimating%20the%20number%20of%20COVID%20vaccine%20deaths%20in%20America%20-%20oct%208%202021.pdf.
35 Centers for Disease Control and Prevention. (2023) COVID data tracker. Retrieved from covid.cdc.gov/covid-data-tracker/#datatracker-home
36 Open VAERS, VAERS COVID vaccine adverse events report.
37 Stieber, Z. (2024) CDC ordered to disclose crucial information from COVID-19 vaccine surveillance system. Epoch Times. Retrieved from www.theepochtimes.com/health/cdc-releases-hidden-covid-19-vaccine-injury-reports-5617872.
38 Centers for Disease Control and Prevention. (2024) V-safe. Retrieved from www.cdc.gov/vaccinesafety/ensuringsafety/monitoring/v-safe/index.html.
39 Centers for Disease Control and Prevention. (2024) V-safe publications. V-safe. Retrieved from www.cdc.gov/vaccinesafety/ensuringsafety/monitoring/v-safe/publications.html.
40 Stieber, CDC ordered to disclose crucial information from COVID-19 vaccine surveillance system.
41 Di Pasquale. A., Bonanni, P., Garçon, N., Stanberry, L.R., El-Hodhod, M., Tavares Da Silva, F. (2016) Vaccine safety evaluation: Practical aspects in assessing benefits and risks. *Vaccine* 34(52):6672–80. doi:10.1016/j.vaccine.2016.10.039
42 World Health Organization. (2024) VigiAccess—WHO collaborating center for international drug monitoring. Retrieved from vigiaccess.org/.
43 Ibid.

44 Public Health Canada. (2024) Reported side effects following COVID-19 vaccination in Canada. Retrieved from health-infobase.canada.ca/covid-19/vaccine-safety/.

45 Ontario Physicians and Surgeons Discipline Tribunal. (2023) College of Physicians and Surgeons of Ontario v. Phillips, 2023 ONPSDT 16. Tribunal File No.: 21–023. Retrieved from doctors.cpso.on.ca/cpso/getdocument.aspx?flash=check&pdfid=nfDo8bWUK0M%3d&id=109364&doctype=PastFinding.

46 Dutta, S., Kaur, R. J., Bhardwaj, P., Sharma, P., Ambwani, S., et al. (2021) Adverse events reported from the COVID-19 vaccines: A descriptive study based on the WHO database (VigiBase®). *J Appl Pharm Sci* 11(8):1–9. doi:10.7324/JAPS.2021.110801.

47 Reported side effects following COVID-19 vaccination in Canada.

48 Ibid.

49 Ibid.

50 Shilhavy, B. (2021) Canadian doctor defies gag order and tells the public how Moderna COVID injections killed and permanently disabled indigenous people in his community. Health Impact News. Retrieved from vaccineimpact.com/2021/canadian-doctor-defies-gag-order-and-tells-the-public-how-the-moderna-covid-injections-killed-and-permanently-disabled-indigenous-people-in-his-community/.

51 Mani, A., Ojha, V. (2022) Thromboembolism after COVID-19 vaccination: A systematic review of such events in 286 patients. *Ann Vasc Surg* 84:12–20.e1. doi:10.1016/j.avsg.2022.05.001.

52 Cochrane, D., Tasker, P. (2021) Suspend AstraZeneca use for people under 55, vaccine committee recommends. Canada Broadcasting Corporation News. Retrieved from www.cbc.ca/news/politics/astrazeneca-under-55–1.5968128.

53 Draaisma, M. (2021) Ontario will no longer give AstraZeneca COVID-19 vaccine as 1st dose due to blood clot risk. Canada Broadcasting Corporation News. Retrieved from www.cbc.ca/news/canada/toronto/ontario-update-astrazeneca-vaccine-1.6022545

54 Public Health Agency of Canada. (2023) COVID-19 vaccines: Canada immunization guide. Retrieved from www.canada.ca/en/public-health/services/publications/healthy-living/canadian-immunization-guide-part-4-active-vaccines/page-26-covid-19-vaccine.html.

55 Kaimori, R., Nishida, H., Uchida, T., Tamura, M., Kuroki, K., et al. (2022) Histopathologically TMA-like distribution of multiple organ thromboses following the initial dose of the BNT162b2 mRNA vaccine (Comirnaty, Pfizer/BioNTech): An autopsy case report. *Thromb J* 20(1):61. doi:10.1186/s12959–022-00418–7.

56 Bekal, S., Husari, G., Okura, M., Huang, C.A., Bukari, M.S. (2023) Thrombosis development after mRNA COVID-19 vaccine administration: A case series. *Cureus* 15(7):e41371. doi:10.7759/cureus.41371.

57 Tan, L. J., Koh, C. P., Lai, S. K., Poh, W. C., Othman, M. S., Hussin, H. (2022) A systemic review and recommendation for an autopsy approach to death followed the COVID 19 vaccination. *Forensic Sci Int* 340:111469. doi:10.1016/j.forsciint.2022.111469.

58 Ibid.

59 Canadian Covid Care Alliance. (2023) Morticians speak with the CCCA about abnormal blood clots in the COVID-19 vaccinated deceased. Rumble. Retrieved from rumble.com/v2au84s-morticians-discuss-abnormal-blood-clots-in-covid-19-vaccinated-patients.html.

60 Horwood, M. (2023) Exclusive: Embalmers speak out on unusual blood clots. The Epoch Times. Retrieved from www.theepochtimes.com/world/exclusive-embalmers-speak-out-on-unusual-parasite-blood-clots-5121795.

61 Ask Dr. Drew. (2022) "Foot-long blood clots" from mRNA, says pathologist Dr. Ryan Cole w/ Dr. Kelly Victory—YouTube. Retrieved from www.youtube.com/watch?v=2SLp6B_kkRI.

62 A Midwestern Doctor. (2023) Do the mysterious fibrous clots really exist? The Forgotten Side of Medicine Substack. Retrieved from www.midwesterndoctor.com/p/do-the-mysterious-fibrous-clots-really.

63 Canadian National Citizens Inquiry into COVID-19. (2023) Funeral director Laura Jeffery on post-vaccine embalming. Retrieved from www.youtube.com/watch?v=kYxUS9YO2rE.

64 Ryu, J. K., Sozmen, E. G., Dixit, K., Montano, M., Matsui, Y., et al. (2021) SARS-CoV-2 spike protein induces abnormal inflammatory blood clots neutralized by fibrin immunotherapy. bioRxiv (preprint). doi:10.1101/2021.10.12.464152.

65 Grobbelaar, L. M., Venter, C., Vlok, M., Ngoepe, M., Laubscher, G. J., et al. (2021) SARS-CoV-2 spike protein S1 induces fibrin(ogen) resistant to fibrinolysis: Implications for microclot formation in COVID-19. *Biosci Rep* 41(8):BSR20210611. doi:10.1042/BSR20210611.

66 Montano, M., Ryu, J. K., Sozmen, E. G., Dixit, K., Matsui, Y., et al. (2022) SARS-CoV-2 spike binds fibrinogen-inducing abnormal inflammatory blood clots. *Topics Antiviral Medicine* 30(1 SUPPL.):9. Retrieved from pesquisa.bvsalud.org/global-literature-on-novel-coronavirus-2019-ncov/resource/pt/covidwho-1880599.

67 Kerr, R., Carroll, H. A. (2023) Long COVID is primarily a spike protein induced thrombotic vasculitis. Research Square. doi:10.21203/rs.3.rs-2939263/v1.

68 Mercola, J. (2022) COVID Jabs impact both male and female fertility. Substack. Retrieved from takecontrol.substack.com/p/covid-vaccine-fertility-issues.

69 My Cycle Story Group. (2023) Retrieved from mycyclestory.com/.

70 Wong, K. K., Heilig, C. M., Hause, A., Myers, T. R., Olson, C. K., et al. (2022) Menstrual irregularities and vaginal bleeding after COVID-19 vaccination reported to v-safe active surveillance, USA in December, 2020–January, 2022: an observational cohort study. *Lancet Digit Health* 4(9):e667-e675. doi: 10.1016/S2589–7500(22)00125-X.

71 Wesselink, A. K., Lovett, S. M., Weinberg, J., Geller, R. J., Wang, T. R., et al. (2023) COVID-19 vaccination and menstrual cycle characteristics: A prospective cohort study. *Vaccine* 41(29):4327–34. doi:10.1016/j.vaccine.2023.06.012.

72 Edelman, A., Boniface, E. R., Benhar, E., Han, L., Matteson, K. A., et al. (2022) Association between menstrual cycle length and Coronavirus Disease 2019 (COVID-19) vaccination: A U.S. cohort. *Obstet Gynecol* 139(4):481–89. doi:10.1097/AOG.0000000000004695.

73 Wang, S., Mortazavi, J., Hart, J. E., Hankins, J. A., Katuska, L. M., et al. (2022) A prospective study of the association between SARS-CoV-2 infection and COVID-19 vaccination with changes in usual menstrual cycle characteristics. *Am J Obstet Gyn*ecol 227(5):739.e1–e11. doi:10.1016/j.ajog.2022.07.003.

74 Alvergne, A., Woon, E. V., Male, V. (2022) Effect of COVID-19 vaccination on the timing and flow of menstrual periods in two cohorts. *Front Reprod Health* 4:952976. doi:10.3389/frph.2022.952976.

75 Trogstad, L., Laake, I., Robertson, A. H., Mjaaland, S., Caspersen, I. H., et al. (2023) Heavy bleeding and other menstrual disturbances in young women after COVID-19 vaccination. *Vaccine* 41(36):5271–82. doi:10.1016/j.vaccine.2023.06.088.

76 Blix, K., Laake, I., Juvet, L., Robertson, A. H., Caspersen, I. H., et al. (2023) Unexpected vaginal bleeding and COVID-19 vaccination in nonmenstruating women. *Science Advances* 9(38):eadg1391. doi:10.1126/sciadv.adg1391.

77 Ibid.

78 Lessans, N., Rottenstreich, A., Stern, S., Saar, T. D., Porat, S., Dior, U. P. (2023) The effect of BNT162b2 SARS-CoV-2 mRNA vaccine on menstrual cycle symptoms in healthy women. *Int J Gynecol Obstet* 160(1):313–18. doi:10.1002/ijgo.14356.

79 Baena-García, L., Aparicio, V. A., Molina-López, A., Aranda, P., Cámara-Roca, L., Ocón-Hernández, O. (2022) Premenstrual and menstrual changes reported after COVID-19 vaccination: The EVA project. *Womens Health* (Lond) 18:17455057221112237. doi:10.1177/17455057221112237.

80 Lee, K. M. N., Eleanor J., Junkins, E. J., Luo, C., Fatima, U. A., et al. (2022) Investigating trends in those who experience menstrual bleeding changes after SARS-CoV-2 vaccination. *Science Advances* 8(28):1–15. doi:10.1126/sciadv.abm7201.

81 Hagai, L., Jørgensen, N., Martino-Andrade, A., Mendiola, J., Weksler-Derri, D., et al. (2017) Temporal trends in sperm count: A systematic review and meta-regression analysis, *Hum Reprod Update* 23(6):646–59. doi:10.1093/humupd/dmx022.

82 (2021) SARS-CoV-2 mRNA Vaccine (BNT162, PF-07302048) 2.6.4 薬物動態試験の概要文 (translation: "Summary of pharmacokinetic study"). Retrieved from pandemictimeline.com/wp-content/uploads/2021/07/Pfizer-report_Japanese-government.pdf.

83 Statistics Canada. (2022) Fewer babies born as Canada's fertility rate hit a record low in 2020. Retrieved from www.statcan.gc.ca/o1/en/plus/960-fewer-babies-born-canadas-fertility-rate-hits-record-low-2020.

84 Statistics Canada. (2023) Fertility indicators, provinces and territories: Interactive dashboard. Retrieved from www150.statcan.gc.ca/n1/pub/71–607-x/71–607-x2022003-eng.htm.

85 Statistics Canada. (2023) Crude birth rate, age-specific fertility rates and total fertility rate (live births). Retrieved from www150.statcan.gc.ca/t1/tbl1/en/tv.action?pid=1310041801.

86 Macrotrends. (2023) U.S. Fertility rate 1950–2023. Retrieved from www.macrotrends.net/countries/USA/united-states/fertility-rate.

87 Database Earth. (2023) Total fertility rate of United States of America. Retrieved from https//database.earth/population/united-states-of-america/fertility-rate.

88 Office for National Statistics. (2023) Births in England and Wales: 2022. Retrieved from www.ons.gov.uk/peoplepopulationandcommunity/birthsdeathsandmarriages/livebirths/bulletins/birthsummarytablesenglandandwales/2022.

89 Statista. (2023) Number of live births in the European Union (EU27) from 2009 to 2022. Retrieved from www.statista.com/statistics/253401/number-of-live-births-in-the-eu/.

90 MacroTrends. (2023) World fertility rate 1950–2023. Retrieved from www.macrotrends.net/countries/wld/world/fertility-rate.

91 Mishra, G. D., Pandeya, N., Dobson, A. J., Chung, H. F., Anderson, D., et al. (2017) Early menarche, nulliparity and the risk for premature and early natural menopause. *Hum Reprod* 32(3):679–686. doi:10.1093/humrep/dew350.

92 Braithwaite, J. (2023) Perimenopause symptoms statistics 2023. Forth with Life. Retrieved from www.forthwithlife.co.uk/blog/perimenopause-symptoms-statistics-2023/.

93 Hopper, T. (2023) First Reading: Canada's birth rate has dropped off a cliff (and it's likely because nobody can afford housing). *National Post.* Retrieved from nationalpost.com/opinion/canadas-birth-rate-has-dropped-off-a-cliff-and-its-because-nobody-can-afford-housing.

94 Gat, I., Kedem, A., Dviri, M., Umanski, A., Levi, M., et al. (2022) COVID-19 vaccination BNT162b2 temporarily impairs semen concentration and total motile count among semen donors. *Andrology* 10:1016–22. doi:10.1111/andr.13209.

95 Abd, Z. H., Muter, S. A., Saeed, R. A. M., Ammar, O. (2022) Effects of COVID-19 vaccination on different semen parameters. *Basic Clin Androl* 32(1):13. doi:10.1186/s12610–022-00163-x.

96 Ma, Y.-C., Chao, C., Chi, Y., Xiang, L.-Y., Wen, J., Xi, J. (2023) The effect of COVID-19 vaccines on sperm parameters: A systematic review and meta-analysis. *Asian J. Andrology* 25(4):468–73. doi:10.4103/aja2022100.

97 Gonzalez, D. C., Nassau, D. E., Khodamoradi, K., Ibrahim, E., Blachman-Braun, R., et al. (2021) Sperm parameters before and after COVID-19 mRNA vaccination. *JAMA* 326(3):273–74. doi:10.1001/jama.2021.9976.

98 Barda, S., Laskov, I., Grisaru, D., Lehavi, O., Kleiman, S., et al. (2022) The impact of COVID-19 vaccine on sperm quality. *Int J Gynaecol Obstet* 158(1):116–20. doi:10.1002/ijgo.14135.

99 Safrai, M., Herzberg, S., Imbar, T., Reubinoff, B., Dior, U., Ben-Meir, A. (2022) The BNT162b2 mRNA COVID-19 vaccine does not impair sperm parameters. *Reprod Biomed Online* 44(4):685–88. doi:10.1016/j.rbmo.2022.01.008.

100 Reschini, M., Pagliardini, L., Boeri, L., Piazzini, F., Bandini, V., et al. (2022) COVID-19 vaccination does not affect reproductive health parameters in men. *Front Public Health* 10:839967. doi:10.3389/fpubh.2022.839967.

101 Olana, S., Mazzilli, R., Salerno, G., Zamponi, V., Tarsitano, M. G., et al. (2022) 4BNT162b2 mRNA COVID-19 vaccine and semen: What do we know? *Andrology* 10(6):1023–29. doi:10.1111/andr.13199.

102 Lifshitz, D., Haas, J., Lebovitz, O., Raviv, G., Orvieto, R., Aizer, A. (2022) Does mRNA SARS-CoV-2 vaccine detrimentally affect male fertility, as reflected by semen analysis? *Reprod Biomed Online* 44(1):145–49. doi:10.1016/j.rbmo.2021.09.021.

103 Xia, W., Zhao, J., Hu, Y., Fang, L., Wu, S. (2022) Investigate the effect of COVID-19 inactivated vaccine on sperm parameters and embryo quality in *in vitro* fertilization. *Andrologia* 54(6):e14483. doi:10.1111/and.14483.

104 Gat, I., Kedem, A., Dviri, M., Umanski, A., Levi, M., et al. (2022) COVID-19 vaccination BNT162b2 temporarily impairs semen concentration and total motile count among semen donors. *Andrology* 10:1016–22. doi:10.1111/andr.13209.

105 Ma, Y.-C., Chao, C., Chi, Y., Xiang, L.-Y., Wen, J., Xi, J. (2023) The effect of COVID-19 vaccines on sperm parameters: A systematic review and meta-analysis. *Asian J. Andrology* 25(4):468–73. doi:10.4103/aja2022100.

106 Pourmasumi, S., Nazari, A., Ahmadi, Z., Kouni, S. N., de Gregorio, C., et al. (2022) The effect of Long COVID-19 infection and vaccination on male fertility: A narrative review. *Vaccines* (Basel) 10(12):1982. doi:10.3390/vaccines10121982.

107 Clinical Trial.gov Archive. (2023) History of changes for study: NCT04754594. To evaluate the safety, tolerability, and immunogenicity of BNT162b2 against COVID-19

in healthy pregnant women of 18 years of age and older. Retrieved from classic.clinicaltrials.gov/ct2/history/NCT04754594?V_21=View#StudyPageTop.

108 Fell, D. B., Dimanlig-Cruz, S., Regan, A. K., Håberg, S. E., Gravel, C. A., et al. (2022) Risk of preterm birth, small for gestational age at birth, and stillbirth after COVID-19 vaccination during pregnancy: Population based retrospective cohort study. *BMJ* 378:e071416. doi:10.1136/bmj-2022–071416.

109 Pfizer. (2021) 5.3.6 Cumulative analysis of post-authorization adverse event reports of PF-07302048 (BNT162B2) received through 28-FEB-2021. Worldwide Safety. Retrieved from phmpt.org/wp-content/uploads/2021/11/5.3.6-postmarketing-experience.pdf.

110 Fell, Dimanlig-Cruz, Regan, Håberg, Gravel, et al., Risk of preterm birth, small for gestational age at birth, and stillbirth after COVID-19 vaccination during pregnancy.

111 Pfizer. 5.3.6 Cumulative analysis of post-authorization adverse event reports of PF-07302048 (BNT162B2) received through 28-FEB-2021.

112 Ibid.

113 Ibid.

114 Ibid.

115 Villines, D. (2021) What are the average miscarriage rates by week? Medical News Today. Retrieved from www.medicalnewstoday/com/articles/322634#miscarriage.

116 Pfizer. 5.3.6 Cumulative analysis of post-authorization adverse event reports of PF-07302048 (BNT162B2) received through 28-FEB-2021.

117 Morgan, J. A., Biggio, J. R., Jr., Martin, J. K, Mussarat N., Chawla, H. K., et al. (2022) Maternal outcomes after Severe Acute Respiratory Syndrome Coronavirus 2 (SARSCoV-2) infection in vaccinated compared with unvaccinated pregnant patients. *Obstet Gynecol* 139(1):107–9. doi:10.1097/AOG.0000000000004621.

118 Ibid.

119 Dagan, N., Biron-Shental, T., Makov-Assif, M., Key, C., Kohane, I. S., et al. (2021) Effectiveness of the BNT162b2 mRNA COVID-19 vaccine in pregnancy. *Nat Med* 27(10):1693–95. doi:10.1038/s41591–021-01490–8.

120 Butt, A. A., Chemaitelly, H., Al Khal, A., Coyle, P. V., Saleh, H., et al. (2021) SARS-CoV-2 vaccine effectiveness in preventing confirmed infection in pregnant women. *J Clin Invest* 131(23):e153662. doi:10.1172/JCI153662.

121 Goldshtein, I., Nevo, D., Steinberg, D.M., Rotem, R.S., Gorfine, M., et al. (2021) Association between BNT162b2 vaccination and incidence of SARS-CoV-2 infection in pregnant women. *JAMA* 326(8):728–735. doi:10.1001/jama.2021.11035.

122 Kadour-Peero, E., Sagi-Dain, L., Sagi, S. (2021) Early exploration of COVID-19 vaccination safety and effectiveness during pregnancy: Interim descriptive data from a prospective observational study. *Vaccine* 39(44):6535–38. doi:10.1016/j.vaccine.2021.09.043.

123 Dagan, Biron-Shental, Makov-Assif, Key, Kohane, et al., Effectiveness of the BNT162b2 mRNA COVID-19 vaccine in pregnancy.

124 Goldshtein, Nevo, Steinberg, Rotem, Gorfine, et al., Association between BNT162b2 vaccination and incidence of SARS-CoV-2 infection in pregnant women.

125 Ibid.

126 Bookstein Peretz, S., Regev, N., Novick, L., Nachshol, M., Goffer, E., et al. (2021) Short-term outcome of pregnant women vaccinated with BNT162b2 mRNA COVID-19 vaccine. *Ultrasound Obstet Gynecol* 58(3):450–56. doi:10.1002/uog.23729.

127 Sutton, D., Fuchs, K., D'Alton, M., Goffman, D. (2020) Universal screening for SARS-CoV-2 in women admitted for delivery. *N Engl J Med* 382(22):2163–64. doi:10.1056/NEJMc2009316.

128 Wardhana, M. P., Maniora, A., Maniora, M. C., Aryananda, R. A., Gumilar, K. E., et al. (2021) Lesson from Indonesia: COVID-19 testing strategy in obstetric emergency cases at low-resource health care setting. *Pakistan J Med Health Sci* 15(2):508–13. ISSN 1996–7195.

129 Yanes-Lane, M., Winters, N., Fregonese, F., Bastos, M., Perlman-Arrow, S., et al. (2020) Proportion of asymptomatic infection among COVID-19 positive persons and their transmission potential: A systematic review and meta-analysis. *PLOS One* 15(11):e0241536. doi:10.1371/journal.pone.0241536.

130 McClymont, E., Atkinson, A., Albert, A., Av-Gay, G., Andrade, J., et al.; COVERED Team. (2023) Reactogenicity, pregnancy outcomes, and SARS-CoV-2 infection following COVID-19 vaccination during pregnancy in Canada: A national prospective cohort study. *Vaccine*. S0264–410X(23)01215-X. doi:10.1016/j.vaccine.2023.10.032.

131 Ibid.

132 Statistics Canada. (2023) Between April and August 2022, 98 percent of Canadians had antibodies against COVID-19 and 54 percent had antibodies from a previous infection. Retrieved from www150.statcan.gc.ca/n1/daily-quotidien/230327/dq230327b-eng.htm.

133 McClymont, E., Atkinson, A., Albert, A., Av-Gay, G., Andrade, J., et al.; COVERED Team. Reactogenicity, pregnancy outcomes, and SARS-CoV-2 infection following COVID-19 vaccination during pregnancy in Canada.

134 Fenton, N., Neil, M. (2023) Why is the MHRA hiding critical safety data on the covid vaccines? Where are the numbers? Substack. Retrieved from wherearethenumbers.substack.com/p/461a5df9–22ec-4cfe-a6f3-b19843a52dc3?utm.

135 Ibid.

136 Kelly, A. (2024) CN gov't database reveals catastrophic reproductive damage to men and women. Daily Clout. Retrieved from dailyclout.io/exclusive-cn-govt-database-reveals-catastrophic-reproductive-damage-to-men-and-women/.

137 Sadarangani, M., Soe, P., Shulha, H.P., Valiquette, L., Vanderkooi, O.G., et al. (2022) Safety of COVID-19 vaccines in pregnancy: A Canadian National Vaccine Safety (CANVAS) network cohort study. *Lancet Infect Dis* 22(11):1553–64. doi:10.1016/S1473–3099(22)00426–1.

138 Marchand, G., Masoud, A. T., Grover, S., King, A., Brazil, G., et al. (2023) Maternal and neonatal outcomes of COVID-19 vaccination during pregnancy, a systematic review and meta-analysis. *NPJ Vaccines* 8(1):103. doi:10.1038/s41541–023-00698–8.

139 Ibid.

140 Dick, A., Rosenbloom, J. I., Karavani, G., Gutman-Ido, E., Lessans, N., Chill, H. H. (2022) Safety of third SARS-CoV-2 vaccine (booster dose) during pregnancy. *Am J Obstet Gynecol MFM* 4(4):100637. doi:10.1016/j.ajogmf.2022.100637.

141 Pratama, N. R., Wafa, I. A., Budi, D. S., Putra, M., Wardhana, M. P., Wungu, C. D. K. (2022) mRNA COVID-19 vaccines in pregnancy: A systematic review. *PLOS One* 17(2):e0261350. doi:10.1371/journal.pone.0261350.

142 Kory, P., Pfeiffer, M.B. (2024) Ask why 429 moms died. Covid deaths in pregnancy rose 300 percent during delta. Rescue Substack. Retrieved from rescue.substack.com/p/ask-why-429-moms-died?utm.

143 Spieker, F. (2024) Maternal deaths across the USA. Spieker Substack. Retrieved from maternal.pervaers.com/mm.xlsx.

144 Kachikis, A., Englund, J.A., Covelli, I., Frank, Y., Haghighi, C., et al. (2022) Analysis of vaccine reactions after COVID-19 vaccine booster doses among pregnant and lactating individuals. *JAMA Netw Open* 5(9):e2230495. doi:10.1001/jamanetwork open.2022.30495.
145 Pfizer. 5.3.6 Cumulative analysis of post-authorization adverse event reports of PF-07302048 (BNT162B2) received through 28-FEB-2021.
146 Fu, W., Sivajohan, B., McClymont, E., Albert, A., Elwood, C., et al. (2022) Systematic review of the safety, immunogenicity, and effectiveness of COVID-19 vaccines in pregnant and lactating individuals and their infants. *Int J Gynaecol Obstet* 156(3):406–17. doi:10.1002/ijgo.14008.
147 Trostle, M. E., Limaye, M. A., Avtushka, V., Lighter, J. L., Penfield, C. A., Roman, A. S. (2021) COVID-19 vaccination in pregnancy: Early experience from a single institution. *Am J Obstet Gynecol MFM* 3(6):100464. doi:10.1016/j.ajogmf.2021.100464.
148 Blakeway, H., Prasad, S., Kalafat, E., Heath, P. T., Ladhani, S. N., et al. (2022) COVID-19 vaccination during pregnancy: Coverage and safety. *Am J Obstet Gynecol* 226(2):236.e1–236.e14. doi:10.1016/j.ajog.2021.08.007.
149 Low, J. M., Gu, Y., Ng, M. S. F., Amin, Z., Lee, L. Y., et al. (2021) Codominant IgG and IgA expression with minimal vaccine mRNA in milk of BNT162b2 vaccinees. *NPJ Vaccines* 6(1):105. doi:10.1038/s41541–021-00370-z
150 Hanna, N., De Mejia, C. M., Heffes-Doon, A., Lin, X., Botros, B., et al. (2023) Biodistribution of mRNA COVID-19 vaccines in human breast milk. *EBioMedicine* 96:104800. doi:10.1016/j.ebiom.2023.104800.
151 Pfizer. 5.3.6 Cumulative analysis of post-authorization adverse event reports of PF-07302048 (BNT162B2) received through 28-FEB-2021.
152 Shaw, C. A. (2021) *Dispatches from the Vaccine Wars: Fighting for human freedom during the Great Reset.* New York: Skyhorse Publishing.
153 Public Health Agency of Canada. (2022) Autism spectrum disorder: Highlights from the 2019 Canadian health survey on children and youth. Retrieved from www.canada.ca/en/public-health/services/publications/diseases-conditions/autism-spectrum-disorder-canadian-health-survey-children-youth-2019.html.
154 Erdogan, M. A., Gurbuz, O., Bozkurt, M. F., Erbas O. (2024) Prenatal exposure to COVID-19 mRNA vaccine BNT162b2 induces autism-like behaviors in male neonatal rats: Insights into WNT and BDNF signaling perturbations. *Neurochem Res* 49(4):1034–48. doi:10.1007/s11064–023-04089–2.
155 Ibid.
156 Jaswa, E. G., Cedars, M. I., Lindquist, K. J., Bishop, S. L., Kim, Y. S., et al. (2024) In utero exposure to maternal COVID-19 vaccination and offspring neurodevelopment at 12 and 18 months. *JAMA Pediatr* 178(3):258–265. doi:10.1001/jamapediatrics.2023.5743.
157 Lin, X., Botros, B., Hanna, M., Gurzenda, E., Manzano De Mejia, C., et al. (2024) Transplacental transmission of the COVID-19 vaccine mRNA: Evidence from placental, maternal and cord blood analyses post-vaccination. *Am J Obst. Gynecology*. S0002–9378(24)00063–2. doi:10.1016/j.ajog.2024.01.022.
158 Drory, Y., Turetz, Y., Hiss, Y., Lev, B., Fisman, E.Z., et al. (1991) Sudden unexpected death in persons less than 40 years of age. *Am J Cardiol* 68(13):1388–92. doi:10.1016/0002–9149(91)90251-f.

159 Castiello, T., Georgiopoulos, G., Finocchiaro, G., Claudia, M., Gianatti, A., et al. (2022) COVID-19 and myocarditis: A systematic review and overview of current challenges. *Heart Fail Rev* 27(1):251–61. doi:10.1007/s10741–021-10087–9.

160 Kang, M. (2022) Viral myocarditis. *An J. Viral Myocarditis*. In: StatPearls [Internet]. Treasure Island (FL): StatPearls Publishing. Retrieved from www.ncbi.nlm.nih.gov/books/NBK459259/.

161 Ozierański, K., Tymińska, A., Kruk, M., Koń, B., Skwarek, A., et al. (2021) Occurrence, trends, management and outcomes of patients hospitalized with clinically suspected myocarditis—ten-year perspectives from the MYO-PL nationwide Database. *J Clin Med* 10(20):4672. doi:10.3390/jcm10204672.

162 Ibid.

163 Magnani, J., Dec, G. (2006) Myocarditis: Current trends in diagnosis and treatment. *Circulation* 113(6):876–90. doi:10.1161/CIRCULATIONAHA.105.584532

164 Wang, T.-W.-Y., Lui, R.-B., Huang, C.-Y., Li, H.-Y., Zhang, Z.-X., et al. (2023) Global, regional, and national burdens of myocarditis, 1990–2019: Systematic analysis from GBD 2019. *BMC Public Health* 23(1):714. doi:10.1186/s12889–023-15539–5.

165 Ibid.

166 Nasreen, S., Calzavara, A., Buchan, S.A., Thampi, N., Johnson, C., et al. (2022) Canadian Immunization Research Network (CIRN) Provincial Collaborative Network (PCN) Ontario investigators. Background incidence rates of adverse events of special interest related to COVID-19 vaccines in Ontario, Canada, 2015 to 2020, to inform COVID-19 vaccine safety surveillance. *Vaccine* 40(24):3305–12. doi:10.1016/j.vaccine.2022.04.065.

167 Ibid.

168 Office of the Chief Medical Officer for Ontario. (2021) COVID-19 vaccination in children aged 5–11. Ontario Ministry of Health. Retrieved from www.ontariofamilyphysicians.ca/tools-resources/covid-19-resources/covid-19-vaccines/covid-19-vaccination-children-2021–11-26-session-slides.pdf.

169 Boehmer, T. K., Kompaniyets, L., Lavery, A. M., Hsu, J., Ko, J. Y., et al. (2021) Association between COVID-19 and myocarditis using hospital-based administrative data—United States, March 2020–January 2021. *MMWR Morb Mortal Wkly Rep* 70(35):1228–32. doi:10.15585/mmwr.mm7035e5.

170 Nasreen, Calzavara, Buchan, Thampi, Johnson, et al., Canadian Immunization Research Network (CIRN) Provincial Collaborative Network (PCN) Ontario investigators. Background incidence rates of adverse events of special interest related to COVID-19 vaccines in Ontario, Canada, 2015 to 2020, to inform COVID-19 vaccine safety surveillance.

171 Singer, M. E., Taub, I. B., Kaelber, D. C. (2021) Risk of myocarditis from COVID-19 infection in people under age 20: A population-based analysis. medRxiv (preprint). doi:10.1101/2021.07.23.21260998.

172 Kamath, S., Gomah, M. T., Stepman, G., DiMartino, P., Adetula, I. (2023) COVID-19-associated acute myocarditis: Risk factors, clinical outcomes, and implications for early detection and management. *Cureus* 15(9):e44617. doi:10.7759/cureus.44617.

173 Pirzada, A., Mokhtar, A. T., Moeller, A. D. (2020) COVID-19 and myocarditis: What do we know so far? *CJC Open* 2(4):278–85. doi:10.1016/j.cjco.2020.05.005.

174 Kamath, Gomah, Stepman, DiMartino, and Adetula, COVID-19-associated acute myocarditis.

175 Guo, T., Fan, Y., Chen, M., Wu, X., Zhang, L., et al. (2020) Cardiovascular implications of fatal outcomes of patients with Coronavirus Disease 2019 (COVID-19). *JAMA Cardiol* 5(7):811–18. doi:10.1001/jamacardio.2020.1017.

176 Daniels, C. J., Rajpal, S., Greenshields, J. T., et al. (2021) Prevalence of clinical and subclinical myocarditis in competitive athletes with recent SARS-CoV-2 infection: Results from the Big Ten COVID-19 Cardiac Registry. *JAMA Cardiol* 6(9):1078–87. doi:10.1001/jamacardio.2021.2065.

177 Buckley, B. J. R., Harrison, S. L., Fazio-Eynullayeva, E., Underhill, P., Lane, D. A., Lip, G. Y. H. (2021) Prevalence and clinical outcomes of myocarditis and pericarditis in 718,365 COVID-19 patients. *Eur J Clin Invest* 51(11): e13679. doi:10.1111/eci.13679.

178 Silk, B. J., Scobie, H. M., Duck, W. M., Palmer, T., Ahmad, F. B., et al. (2023) COVID-19 surveillance after expiration of the Public Health Emergency Declaration—United States, May 11, 2023. *MMWR Morb Mortal Wkly Rep* 72(19):523–28. doi:10.15585/mmwr.mm7219e1.

179 Murphy, T. J., Swail, H., Jain, J., Anderson, M., Awadalla, P., et al. (2023) The evolution of SARS-CoV-2 seroprevalence in Canada: A time-series study, 2020–2023. *CMAJ* 195(31):E1030-E1037. doi:10.1503/cmaj.230949.

180 Rose, J., Hulscher, N., McCullough, P. A. (2024) Determinants of COVID-19 vaccine-induced myocarditis. *Therapeutic Advances in Drug Safety* 15. doi:10.1177/20420986241226566.

181 Barda, N., Dagan, N., Ben-Shlomo, Y., Kepten, E., Waxman, J., et al. (2021) Safety of the BNT162b2 mRNA Covid-19 vaccine in a nationwide setting. *N Engl J Med* 385(12):1078–90. doi:10.1056/NEJMoa2110475.

182 Montag, K., Kampf, G. (2022) Hospitalised myocarditis and pericarditis cases in Germany indicate a higher post-vaccination risk for young people mainly after COVID-19 vaccination. *J Clin Med* 11(20):6073. doi:10.3390/jcm11206073.

183 Ibid.

184 Block, J. P., Boehmer. T. K., Forrest, C. B., Carton, T. W., Lee, G. M., et al. (2022) Cardiac complications after SARS-CoV-2 infection and mRNA COVID-19 vaccination—PCORnet, United States, January 2021–January 2022. *MMWR Morb Mortal Wkly Rep* 71(14):517–23. doi:10.15585/mmwr.mm7114e1.

185 Li, M., Wang, X., Feng, J., Feng, Z., Li, W., Ya, B. (2022) Myocarditis or pericarditis following the COVID-19 vaccination in adolescents: A systematic review. *Vaccines* (Basel) 10(8):1316. doi:10.3390/vaccines10081316.

186 Faksova, K., Walsh, D., Jiang, Y., Griffin, J., Phillips, A., et al. (2024) COVID-19 vaccines and adverse events of special interest: A multinational Global Vaccine Data Network (GVDN) cohort study of 99 million vaccinated individuals. *Vaccine* 42(9):2200–2211. doi:10.1016/j.vaccine.2024.01.100.

187 Klein, N. P. (2021) Myocarditis analyses in the Vaccine Safety Datalink: Rapid cycle analyses and "head-to-head" product comparisons. ACIP meeting COVID-19 Vaccines. Retrieved from stacks.cdc.gov/view/cdc/110921.

188 Karlstad, Ø., Hovi, P., Husby, A., Härkänen, T., Selmer, R. M., et al. (2022) SARS-CoV-2 vaccination and myocarditis in a Nordic cohort study of 23 million residents. *JAMA Cardiol* 7(6):600–612. doi:10.1001/jamacardio.2022.0583.

189 Naveed, Z., Li, J., Spencer, M., Wilton, J., Naus, M., García, H. A. V., et al. (2022) Observed versus expected rates of myocarditis after SARS-CoV-2 vaccination: A population-based cohort study. *CMAJ* 94(45):E1529–36. doi:10.1503/cmaj.220676.

190 Sharff, K. A., Dancoes, D. M., Longueil, J. L., Lewis, P. F., Johnson, E. S. (2022) Myopericarditis after COVID-19 booster dose vaccination. *Am J Cardiol* 172:165–66. doi:10.1016/j.amjcard.2022.02.039.
191 Ibid.
192 Naveed, Li, Spencer, Wilton, Naus, García, et al., Observed versus expected rates of myocarditis after SARS-CoV-2 vaccination.
193 Ibid.
194 Ibid.
195 Ibid.
196 Montgomery, J., Ryan, M., Engler, R., Hoffman, D., McClenathan, B., et al. (2021) Myocarditis following immunization with mRNA COVID-19 vaccines in members of the US Military. *JAMA Cardiol* 6(10):1202–6. doi:10.1001/jamacardio.2021.2833.
197 Ibid.
198 Klein, Myocarditis analyses in the Vaccine Safety Datalink.
199 Ibid.
200 Wong, H. L., Hu, M., Zhou, C. K., Lloyd, P. C., Amend, K. L., et al. (2022) Risk of myocarditis and pericarditis after the COVID-19 mRNA vaccination in the USA: A cohort study in claims databases. *Lancet* 399(10342):2191–99. doi:10.1016/S0140–6736(22)00791–7.
201 Ibid.
202 Patone, M., Mei, X. W., Handunnetthi, L., Dixon, S., Zaccardi, F., et al. (2022) Risk of myocarditis after sequential doses of COVID-19 vaccine and SARS-CoV-2 infection by age and sex. *Circulation* 146(10):743–54. doi:10.1161/CIRCULATIONAHA.122.059970.
203 Ibid.
204 Ibid.
205 Husby, A., Hansen, J. V., Fosbøl, E., Thiesson, E. M., Madsen, M., et al. (2021) SARS-CoV-2 vaccination and myocarditis or myopericarditis: Population based cohort study. *BMJ* 375:e068665. doi:10.1136/bmj-2021–068665.
206 Ibid.
207 Nygaard, U., Holm, M., Bohnstedt, C., Chai, Q., Schmidt, L. S., et al. (2022) Population-based incidence of myopericarditis after COVID-19 vaccination in Danish adolescents. *Pediatr Infect Dis J* 1(1):e25-e28. doi:10.1097/INF.0000000000003389.
208 Karlstad, Ø., Hovi, P., Husby, A., Härkänen, T., Selmer, R. M., et al., SARS-CoV-2 vaccination and myocarditis in a Nordic cohort study of 23 million residents.
209 Ibid.
210 Witberg, G., Magen, O., Hoss, S., Talmor-Barkan, Y., Richter, I., et al. (2022) Myocarditis after BNT162b2 vaccination in Israeli adolescents. *N Engl J Med* 387(19):1816–17. doi:10.1056/NEJMc2207270.
211 Mevorach, D., Anis, E., Cedar, N., Bromberg, M., Haas, E. J., et al. (2021) Myocarditis after BNT162b2 mRNA vaccine against COVID-19 in Israel. *N Engl J Med* 385(23):2140–49. doi:10.1056/NEJMoa2109730.
212 Li, X., Lai, F. T. T., Chua, G. T., Kwan, M. Y. W., Lau, Y. L., et al. (2022) Myocarditis following COVID-19 BNT162b2 vaccination among adolescents in Hong Kong. *JAMA Pediatr* 2022 Jun 1;176(6):612–14. doi:10.1001/jamapediatrics.2022.0101.
213 June Choe, Y., Yi, S., Hwang, I., Kim, J., Park, Y. J., et al. (2022) Safety and effectiveness of BNT162b2 mRNA COVID-19 vaccine in adolescents. *Vaccine* 40(5):691–94. doi:10.1016/j.vaccine.2021.12.044.

214 Cronk, T. M. (2020) Pfizer, Moderna produce COVID-19 vaccine. U.S. Department of Defence. Retrieved from www.defense.gov/News/News-Stories/Article/Article/2453288/pfizer-moderna-produce-covid-19-vaccine/.

215 Levi, N., Moravsky, G., Weitsman, T., Amsalem, I., Bar-Sheshet Itach, S., et al. (2023) A prospective study on myocardial injury after BNT162b2 mRNA COVID-19 fourth dose vaccination in healthy persons. *Eur J Heart Fail* 25(2):313–18. doi:10.1002/ejhf.2687.

216 Mansanguan, S., Charunwatthana, P., Piyaphanee, W., Dechkhajorn, W., Poolcharoen, A., Mansanguan, C. (2022) Cardiovascular manifestation of the BNT162b2 mRNA COVID-19 vaccine in adolescents. *Trop. Med. Infect. Dis* 7(8):196. doi:10.3390/tropicalmed7080196.

217 Singer, Taub, and Kaelber, Risk of myocarditis from COVID-19 infection in people under age 20.

218 Kracalik, I., Oster, M. E., Broder, K. R., Cortese, M. M., Glover, M., et al. (2022) Myocarditis outcomes after mRNA COVID-19 vaccination investigators and the CDC COVID-19 Response Team. Outcomes at least 90 days since onset of myocarditis after mRNA COVID-19 vaccination in adolescents and young adults in the USA: A follow-up surveillance study. *Lancet Child Adolesc Health* 6(11):788–98. doi:10.1016/S2352–4642(22)00244–9.

219 Barmada, A., Klein, J., Ramaswamy, A., Brodsky, N. N., Jaycox, J. R., et al. (2023) Cytokinopathy with aberrant cytotoxic lymphocytes and profibrotic myeloid response in SARS-CoV-2 mRNA vaccine-associated myocarditis. *Sci Immunol* 8(83):eadh3455. doi:10.1126/sciimmunol.adh3455.

220 Warren, J., Cheng, D., Crawford, N. W., Jones, B., Lun, R. et al. (2024) Improved diagnosis of COVID-19 vaccine-associated myocarditis with cardiac scarring identified by cardiac magnetic resonance imaging. MedRxiv (preprint). doi:10.1101/2024.03.20.24304640.

221 Patone, Mei, Handunnetthi, Dixon, Zaccardi, et al., Risk of myocarditis after sequential doses of COVID-19 vaccine and SARS-CoV-2 infection by age and sex.

222 Cho, J. Y., Kim, K. H., Lee, N., Cho, S. H., Kim, S. Y., et al. (2023) COVID-19 vaccination-related myocarditis: A Korean nationwide study. *Eur Heart J* 44(24):2234–43. doi:10.1093/eurheartj/ehad339.

223 Kang, M. (2022) Viral myocarditis. *An J. Viral Myocarditis*. In: StatPearls [Internet]. Treasure Island (FL): StatPearls Publishing. Retrieved from www.ncbi.nlm.nih.gov/books/NBK459259/.

224 Hulscher, N., Hodkinson, R., Makis, W., McCullough, P. (2023) Autopsy findings in cases of fatal COVID-19 vaccine-induced myocarditis. *ESC Heart Fail* 2024 Jan 14. doi:10.1002/ehf2.14680.

225 Ibid.

226 Steiber, Z. (2024) Veterans Affairs found safety signal for PfizerCOVID vaccine, Never disclosed it. Epoch Times. www.theepochtimes.com/health/exclusive-veterans-affairs-found-safety-signal-for-pfizer-covid-vaccine-never-disclosed-it-5561709?utm.

227 Steiber, Z. (2024) Email reveals why CDC didn't issue alert on COVID vaccines and myocarditis, CDC officials were worried about causing panic. Epoch Times. www.theepochtimes.com/article/exclusive-email-reveals-why-cdc-didnt-issue-alert-on-covid-vaccines-and-myocarditis-5571675?utm.

228 Sheriff, M. M., Marghalani, R. A., Almana, O. M., et al. (2024) A study on the self-reported physician-diagnosed cardiac complications post mRNA vaccination in Saudi Arabia. *Cureus* 16(1): e52108. doi:10.7759/cureus.52108.

229 Mörz, M. (2022) Case report: Multifocal necrotizing encephalitis and myocarditis after BNT162b2 mRNA vaccination against COVID-19. *Vaccines* (Basel) 10(10):1651. doi:10.3390/vaccines10101651.

230 Burkhardt, A. (2023) The underlying pathology of spike protein biodistribution in people that died post COVID-19 vaccination. Canadian Covid Care Alliance. Retrieved from www.canadiancovidcarealliance.org/all/professor-arne-burkhardt-video.

231 Barmada, Klein, Ramaswamy, Brodsky, Jaycox, et al., Cytokinopathy with aberrant cytotoxic lymphocytes and profibrotic myeloid response in SARS-CoV-2 mRNA vaccine-associated myocarditis.

232 Milano, Gal, Creisson, and Chamorey, Myocarditis and COVID-19 mRNA vaccines.

233 Dousis, A., Ravichandran, K., Hobert, E. M., Moore, M. J., Rabideau, A. E. (2023) An engineered T7 RNA polymerase that produces mRNA free of immunostimulatory byproducts. *Nat Biotechnol* 41(4):560–68. doi:10.1038/s41587–022-01525–6.

234 Paratz, E. D., Nehme, Z., Stub, D., La Gerche, A. (2023) No association between out-of-hospital cardiac arrest and COVID-19 vaccination. *Circulation* 147(17):1309–11. doi:10.1161/CIRCULATIONAHA.122.063753.

235 Ibid.

236 Peterson, D. F., Kucera, K., Thomas, L. C., Maleszewski, J., Siebert, D., et al. (2021) Aetiology and incidence of sudden cardiac arrest and death in young competitive athletes in the USA: A 4-year prospective study. *Br J Sports Med* 55(21):1196–1203. doi:10.1136/bjsports-2020–102666.

237 Bille, K., Figueiras, D., Schamasch, P., Kappenberger, L., Brenner, J.I., et al. (2006) Sudden cardiac death in athletes: The Lausanne Recommendations. *Eur J Cardiovasc Prev Rehabil* 13(6):859–75. doi:10.1097/01.hjr.0000238397.50341.

238 Real Science. (2023) 2024 athlete cardiac arrests or serious issues, 1417 of them dead, since COVID injection. Retrieved from goodsciencing.com/covid/athletes-suffer-cardiac-arrest-die-after-covid-shot/.

239 Binkhorst, M., Goldstein, D. J. (2023) Athlete deaths during the COVID-19 vaccination campaign: Contextualization of online information. medRxiv (preprint). doi:10.1101/2023.02.13.232855851.

240 Peterson, Kucera, Thomas, Maleszewski, Siebert, et al., Aetiology and incidence of sudden cardiac arrest and death in young competitive athletes in the USA.

241 Alonso Castillo, R., Martínez Castrillo, J. C. (2022) Neurological manifestations associated with COVID-19 vaccine. *Neurologia* (Engl Ed) 23:S2173–5808(22)00141–9. doi:10.1016/j.nrleng.2022.09.007.

242 Finsterer, J. (2023) Neurological adverse reactions to SARS-CoV-2 vaccines. *Clin Psychopharmacol Neurosci* 21(2):222–39. doi:10.9758/cpn.2023.21.2.222.

243 Thai-Van, H., Valnet-Rabier, M. B., Anciaux, M., Lambert, A., Maurier, A., et al. (2023) Safety signal generation for sudden sensorineural hearing loss following messenger RNA COVID-19 vaccination: Postmarketing surveillance using the French Pharmacovigilance Spontaneous Reporting Database. *JMIR Public Health Surveill* 9:e45263. doi:10.2196/45263.

244 Finsterer, Neurological adverse reactions to SARS-CoV-2 vaccines 2.

245 Rosca, E. C., Al-Qiami, A., Cornea, A., Simu, M. (2024) Parsonage-Turner Syndrome following COVID-19 vaccination: A systematic review. *Vaccines* (Basel) 12(3):306. doi:10.3390/vaccines12030306.
246 Alonso Castillo and Martínez Castrillo, Neurological manifestations associated with COVID-19 vaccine.
247 Undugodage, C., Dissanayake, U., Kumara, H., Samarasekera, B., Yapa, L., et al. (2021) Reactogenicity to ChAdOx1 nCoV-19 vaccine in health care workers: A multicenter observational study in Sri Lanka. *Ceylon Med J* 66:177–84. doi:10.4038/cmj.v66i4.9508.
248 Salsone, M., Signorelli, C., Oldani, A., Alberti, V. F., Castronovo, et al. (2023) NEURO-COVAX: An Italian population-based study of neurological complications after COVID-19 vaccinations. *Vaccines*. (Basel) 11(10):1621. doi:10.3390/vaccines11101621.
249 Ibid.
250 Hu, M., Shoaibi, A., Feng, Y., Lloyd, P. C., Wong, H. L., et al. (2023) Safety of monovalent BNT162b2 (Pfizer-BioNTech), mRNA-1273 (Moderna), and NVX-CoV2373 (Novavax) COVID-19 vaccines in US children aged 6 months to 17 years. medRxiv (preprint). doi:10.1101/2023.10.13.23296903.
251 Forshee, R. A., Smith, E. R., Wan, Z., Amend, K. L., Secora, A. et al. (2024) Evaluation of febrile seizure risk following ancestral monovalent COVID19 mRNA vaccination among U.S. children aged 2–5 years. MedRxiv preprint. doi:10.1101/2024.03.12.24304127.
252 Mayo Clinic Staff. (2023) Guillain-Barré syndrome. Mayo Clinic. Retrieved from www.mayoclinic.org/diseases-conditions/guillain-barre-syndrome/symptoms-causes/syc-20362793.
253 Yale Medicine. (2023) Guillain-Barré syndrome. Retrieved from www.yalemedicine.org/conditions/guillain-barre-syndrome.
254 Sejvar, J. J., Baughman, A. L., Wise, M., Morgan, O. W. (2011) Population incidence of Guillain-Barré syndrome: A systematic review and meta-analysis. *Neuroepidemiology* 36(2):123–33. doi:10.1159/000324710.
255 Cafasso, J., and Reed-Guy, L. (2021) Guillain-Barré syndrome (GBS). Healthline. Retrieved from www.healthline.com/health/guillain-barre-syndrome.
256 Wikipedia. Guillain-Barrésyndrome. en.wikipedia.org/wiki/Guillain%E2%80%93Barr%C3%A9_syndrome.
257 Ang, C. W., Jacobs, B. C., Laman, J. D. (2004) The Guillain–Barré syndrome: A true case of molecular mimicry. *Trends Immunol* 25(2):61–66. www.sciencedirect.com/science/article/abs/pii/S1471490603003855.
258 Babazadeh, A., Mohseni Afshar, Z., Javanian, M., Mohammadnia-Afrouzi, M., Karkhah, A., et al. (2019) Influenza vaccination and Guillain-Barré Syndrome: Reality or fear. *J Transl Int Med* 7(4):137–42. doi:10.2478/jtim-2019–0028.
259 Wikipedia. Guillain-Barré syndrome.
260 Mayo Clinic Staff. Guillain-Barré syndrome.
261 Wikipedia.Guillain-Barré syndrome.
262 Palaiodimou, L., Stefanou, M. I., Katsanos, A. H., Fragkou, P. C., Papadopoulou, M., et al. (2021) Prevalence, clinical characteristics and outcomes of Guillain-Barré syndrome spectrum associated with COVID-19: A systematic review and meta-analysis. *Eur J Neurol* 28(10):3517–29. doi:10.1111/ene.14860.

263 Keddie, S., Pakpoor, J., Mousele, C., Pipis, M., Machado, P. M., et al. (2021) Epidemiological and cohort study finds no association between COVID-19 and Guillain-Barré syndrome. *Brain* 144(2):682–93. doi:10.1093/brain/awaa433.

264 Ogunjimi, O. B., Tsalamandris, G., Paladini, A., Varrassi, G., Zis, P. (2023) Guillain-Barré Syndrome induced by vaccination against COVID-19: A systematic review and meta-analysis. *Cureus* 15(4):e37578.

265 Zheng, X., Fang, Y., Song, Y., Liu, S., Li, K., et al. (2023) Is there a causal nexus between COVID-19 vaccination and Guillan-Barre syndrome? *Eur J Med Res* 28(1):98. doi:10.1186/s40001–023-01055–0.

266 Mayo Clinic Staff. (2022) Bell's palsy. Mayo Clinic. Retrieved from www.mayoclinic.org/diseases-conditions/bells-palsy/symptoms-causes/syc-20370028.

267 Tiemstra, J. D., Khathate, N. (2007) Bell's palsy: Diagnosis and management. *Am Fam Physician* 76(7): 997–1002.

268 Tamaki, A., Cabrera, C. J., Li, S., Rabbani, C., Thuener, J. E., et al. (2021) Incidence of Bell's palsy in patients with COVID-19. *JAMA Otolaryngol Head Neck Surg* 147(8):767–68. doi:10.1001/jamaoto.2021.1266.

269 Rafati, A., Pasebani, Y., Jameie, M., Yang, Y., Ilkhani, S., et al. (2023) Association of SARS-CoV-2 vaccination or infection with Bell's Palsy: A systematic review and meta-analysis. *JAMA Otolarygology Head Neck Surg* 149(6):493–504. doi:10.1001/jamaoto.2023.0160.

270 Klein, N. P., Lewis, N., Goddard, K., Fireman, B., Zerbo, O., et al. (2021) Surveillance for adverse events after COVID-19 mRNA vaccination. *JAMA* 326(14):1390–99. doi:10.1001/jama.2021.15072.

271 Alonso Castillo and Martínez Castrillo, Neurological manifestations associated with COVID-19 vaccine.

272 Real Science, 2024 athlete cardiac arrests or serious issues, 1417 of them dead, since COVID injection.

273 Makis, W. (2023) Collapsed suddenly—21 videos of collapses on stage and live on air: Greek South African rapper Costa Titch, age 27, collapsed & died; TV reporters collapsing or having strokes live on air. Substack. makismd.substack.com/p/18-videos-of-collapses-on-stage-and?utm_source=substack&utm_medium=email#play.

274 Donato, N. D. (2022) Deaths with unknown causes now Alberta's top killer: Province. Calgary CTV News. Retrieved from calgary.ctvnews.ca/deaths-with-unknown-causes-now-alberta-s-top-killer-province-1.5975536.

275 Statistics Canada. (2023) Table 13–10-0394–01 Leading causes of death, total population, by age group. doi:10.25318/1310039401-eng Retrieved from www150.statcan.gc.ca/n1/en/catalogue/13100394.

276 Rancourt, D. (2023) 2020–06-02: All-cause mortality during COVID-19—No plague and a likely signature of mass homicide by government response. Ontario Civil Liberties Association. Retrieved from denisrancourt.ca/entries.php?id=9&name=2020_06_02_all_cause_mortality_during_covid_19_no_plague_and_a_likely_signature_of_mass_homicide_by_government_response.

277 Rancourt, D.G. (2022) Probable causal association between India's extraordinary April–July 2021 excess-mortality event and the vaccine rollout. Correlation Research in the Public Interest. Retrieved from correlation-canada.org/report-probable-causal-association-between-indias-extraordinary-april-july-2021-excess-mortality-event-and-the-vaccine-rollout/.

278 Rancourt, D. G., Baudin, M., Mercier, J. (2022) Probable causal association between Australia's new regime of high all-cause mortality and its COVID-19 vaccine rollout. Correlation Research in the Public Interest. Retrieved from correlation-canada .org/report-probable-causal-association-between-australias-newregime-of-high-all -cause-mortality-and-its-covid-19-vaccine-rollout/.

279 Rancourt, D. G., Baudin, M., Hickey, J., Mercier, J. (2023) Age-stratified COVID-19 vaccine-dose fatality rate for Israel and Australia. Correlation Research in the Public Interest. Retrieved from correlation-canada.org/report-age-stratified-covid -19-vaccine-dose-fatality-rate-for-israel-and-australia/.

280 Aarstad, J., Kvitastein, O. A. (2023) Is there a link between the 2021 COVID-19 vaccine uptake in Europe and 2022 excess all-cause mortality? *Asian Pacific J Health Sci* 10(1):25–31. doi.10.21276/apjhs.2023.10.1.6.

281 UK Office for National Statistics. (2023) Deaths by vaccination status, England. Deaths occurring between 1 April 2021 and 31 December 2022 edition. Retrieved from www.ons.gov.uk/peoplepopulationandcommunity/birthsdeathsandmarriages/deaths /datasets/deathsbyvaccinationstatusengland.

282 McClelland, R. D., Lin, Y.-C. J., Culp, T. N., Noyce, R., Evans, D., et al. (2023) The domestication of SARS-CoV-2 into a seasonal infection by viral variants. *Front. Microbiol* 14:1289387. doi:10.3389/fmicb.2023.1289387.

283 Pearson-Stuttard, J., Caul, S., McDonald, S., Whamond, E., Newton, J. N. (2023) Excess mortality in England post COVID-19 pandemic: Implications for secondary prevention. *Lancet Reg Health Eur* 36:100802. doi:10.1016/j.lanepe.2023.100802.

284 Alegria, C., Nunes, Y. (2024) UK—Death and disability trends for malignant neoplasms, ages 15–44. Retrieved from www.researchgate.net/publication/378068419_ UK_-_Death_and_Disability_Trends_for_Malignant_Neoplasms_Ages_15–44.

285 Alegria, C., Nunes, Y. (2024) Trends in death rates from neoplasms in the US for all ages and detailed analysis for 75–84. ResearchGate. doi:10.13140/RG.2.2.16221.01760.

286 Kuhbandner, C., Reitzner, M. (2023) Estimation of excess mortality in Germany during 2020–2022. *Cureus* 15(5):e39371. doi:10.7759/cureus.39371.

287 Gibo, M., Kojima, S., Fujisawa, A., Kikuchi, T., Fukushima, M. (2024) Increased age-adjusted cancer mortality after the third mRNA-lipid nanoparticle vaccine dose during the COVID-19 pandemic in Japan. *Cureus* 16(4): e57860. doi:10.7759/ cureus.57860.

288 Alegria and Nunes, UK—Death and disability trends for malignant neoplasms, ages 15–44.

289 Ibid.

290 Alegria and Nunes, Trends in death rates from neoplasms in the US for all ages and detailed analysis for 75–84.

291 Gibo, M., Kojima, S., Fujisawa, A., Kikuchi, T., Fukushima, M. (2024) Increased age-adjusted cancer mortality after the third mRNA-lipid nanoparticle vaccine dose during the COVID-19 pandemic in Japan. *Cureus* 16(4): e57860. doi:10.7759/ cureus.57860.

292 Solis, O., Beccari, A. R., Iaconis, D., Talarico, C., Ruiz-Bedoya, C. A., et al. (2022) The SARS-CoV-2 spike protein binds and modulates estrogen receptors. *Sci Adv* 8(48): eadd4150. doi:10.1126/sciadv.add4150.

293 Rubio-Casillas, A., Cowley, D., Raszek, M., Uversky, V. N., Redwan, E. M. (2024) Review: N1-methyl-pseudouridine (m1Ψ): Friend or foe of cancer? *Int J Biol Macromol* 267(Pt 1):131427. doi:10.1016/j.ijbiomac.2024.131427.

294 Sittplangkoon, C., Alameh, M. G., Weissman, D., Lin, P. J. C., Tam, Y. K., et al. (2022) mRNA vaccine with unmodified uridine induces robust type I interferon-dependent anti-tumor immunity in a melanoma model. *Front Immunol* 13:983000. doi:10.3389/fimmu.2022.983000.

295 Fürst, T., Bazalová, A., Fryčák, T., Janošek, J. (2024) Does the healthy vaccinee bias rule them all? Association of COVID-19 vaccination status and all-cause mortality from an analysis of data from 2.2 million individual health records. *Int J Infect Dis* 142:106976. doi:10.1016/j.ijid.2024.02.019.

296 Alessandria, M., Malatesta, G., Donzelli, A., Berrino, F. (2024) A reanalysis of an Italian study on the effectiveness of COVID-19 vaccination suggests that it might have unintended effects on total mortality. E&P Repository. Retrieved from repo.epiprev.it/2862.

297 Rigs, A. (2023) COVID-19: Quebec drops recommendation that all should get booster vaccine. *Montreal Gazette*. Retrieved from montrealgazette.com/news/local-news/quebec-covid-vaccine-recommendation-hybrid-immunity.

298 Ellyatt, H. (2022) Denmark becomes the first country to halt its COVID vaccination program. CNBC News. Retrieved from www.cnbc.com/2022/04/28/denmark-the-first-country-to-halt-its-covid-vaccination-program.html.

299 Goldenberg, J. (2022) Denmark halts COVID vaccinations for low-risk people under 50. The Suburban. Retrieved from https:/www.thesuburban.com/news/city_news/denmark-halts-covid-vaccinations-for-low-risk-people-under-50/article_1e0264ec-dea3–59e0-bf3e-db59eee4378d.html.

300 France 24. (2021) France advises against Moderna for under-30s over rare heart risk. Retrieved from www.france24.com/en/live-news/20211109-france-advises-against-moderna-for-under-30s-over-rare-heart-risk.

301 Lehto, E. (2021) Finland joins Sweden and Denmark in limiting Moderna's COVID-19 vaccine. Retrieved from www.reuters.com/world/europe/finland-pauses-use-moderna-covid-19-vaccine-young-men2021–10-07/.

302 UK Department of Health and Social Care. (2023) JCVI statement on the COVID-19 vaccination programme for 2023: 8 November 2022. Updated 27 January 2023. Retrieved from www.gov.uk/government/publications/covid-19-vaccination-programme-for-2023-jcvi-interim-advice-8-november-2022/jcvi-statement-on-the-covid-19-vaccination-programme-for-2023–8-november-2022.

303 Federal Office of Public Health. (2023) COVID-19: Vaccination. Retrieved from www.bag.admin.ch/bag/en/home/krankheiten/ausbrueche-epidemien-pandemien/aktuelle-ausbrueche-epidemien/novel-cov/impfen.html#21889874.

304 Australian Government Department of Health and Aged Care. (2023) COVID-19. Australian Immunisation Handbook. Retrieved from www.health.gov.au/our-work/covid-19-vaccines/advice-for-providers/clinical-guidance/clinical-recommendations.

305 Mek, A. (2022) German Hospital Federation demands withdrawal of vaccination mandate after massive side effects revealed. RAIR Foundation USA. Retrieved from rairfoundation.com/german-hospital-federation-demands-withdrawal-of-vaccination-mandate-after-massive-side-effects-revealed/.

306 Joro, V. (2023) European Parliament: How many deaths have been caused by "COVID vaccines"? Question for written answer E-001201/2023. Retrieved from www.europarl.europa.eu/doceo/document/E-9–2023-001201_EN.html.

307 Public Health Ontario. (2023) COVID-19 vaccine uptake in Ontario: December 14, 2020 to November 5, 2023. Retrieved from www.publichealthontario.ca/-/media/documents/ncov/epi/covid-19-vaccine-uptake-ontario-epi-summary.pdf?la=en.

308 Merkowsky, C. M. (2023) Only 3% of Canadians have taken most recent COVID booster: gov't data. LifeSite. Retrieved from www.lifesitenews.com/news/only-3-of-canadians-have-taken-most-recent-covid-booster-govt-data/.

309 Centers for Disease Control and Prevention. (2023) Respiratory viruses. Vaccination trends—Adults. Retrieved from www.cdc.gov/respiratory-viruses/data-research/dashboard/vaccination-trends-adults.html.

310 Ozimek, T. (2024) Moderna posts $1.2 billion loss as sales of COVID-19 vaccine plunge 94 percent. Epoch Times. Retrieved from www.theepochtimes.com/business/moderna-posts-1–2-billion-loss-as-sales-of-covid-19-vaccine-plunge-94-percent-5642322?utm.

Chapter 14

1 Bond, P. (2024) FDA settles lawsuit over ivermectin social media posts. *Newsweek.* Retrieved from www.newsweek.com/fda-settles-lawsuit-over-ivermectin-social-media-posts-1882562.

2 Brinkman, J. E., Toro, F., Sharma, S. (2023) Physiology, Respiratory Drive. In: StatPearls [Internet]. Treasure Island (FL): StatPearls Publishing; Retrieved from www.ncbi.nlm.nih.gov/books/NBK482414/.

3 Beitler, J. R., Malhotra, A., Thompson, B. T. (2016) Ventilator-induced lung injury. *Clin Chest Med* 37(4):633–46. doi:10.1016/j.ccm.2016.07.004.

4 Haribhai, S., Mahboobi, S. K. (2022) Ventilator complications. In: StatPearls [Internet]. Treasure Island (FL): StatPearls Publishing. Retrieved from www.ncbi.nlm.nih.gov/books/NBK560535/.

5 Maslove, D. M., Sibley, S., Boyd, J. G., Goligher, E. C., Munshi, L., et al. (2022) Complications of critical COVID-19: Diagnostic and therapeutic considerations for the mechanically ventilated patient. *Chest* 161(4):989–98. doi:10.1016/j.chest.2021.10.011.

6 Saguil, A., Fargo, M. V. (2020) Acute respiratory distress syndrome: Diagnosis and management. *Am Fam Physician* 101(12):730–38.

7 Ibid.

8 Diamond, M., Peniston, H. L., Sanghavi, D. K., Mahapatra, S. (2023) Acute respiratory distress syndrome. In: StatPearls [Internet]. Treasure Island (FL): StatPearls Publishing. Retrieved from www.ncbi.nlm.nih.gov/books/NBK436002/.

9 Ibid.

10 Powers, K. (2022) Acute respiratory distress syndrome. *JAAPA* 35(4):29–33. doi:10.1097/01.JAA.0000823164.50706.27.

11 Saguil and Fargo, Acute respiratory distress syndrome.

12 Diamond, Peniston, Sanghavi, and Mahapatra, Acute respiratory distress syndrome.

13 Powers, Acute respiratory distress syndrome.

14 Papazian, L., Aubron, C., Brochard, L., Chiche, J. D., Combes, A., et al. (2019) Formal guidelines: Management of acute respiratory distress syndrome. *Ann Intensive Care* 9(1):69. doi:10.1186/s13613–019-0540–9.

15 Powers, Acute respiratory distress syndrome.

16 Fernando, S. M., Ferreyro, B. L., Urner, M., Munshi, L., Fan, E. (2021) Diagnosis and management of acute respiratory distress syndrome. *CMAJ* 193(21):E761–68. doi:10.1503/cmaj.202661.

17 Ibid.

18 Khan, W., Safi, A., Muneeb, M., Mooghal, M., Aftab, A., Ahmed, J. (2022) Complications of invasive mechanical ventilation in critically ill COVID-19 patients—A narrative review. *Ann Med Surg* (Lond) 80:104201. doi:10.1016/j.amsu.2022.104201.

19 Diamond, Peniston, Sanghavi, and Mahapatra, Acute respiratory distress syndrome.

20 Barbeta, E., Motos, A., Torres, A., Ceccato, A., Ferrer, M., et al. (2020) Covid Clinic Critical Care Group: SARS-CoV-2-induced acute respiratory distress syndrome: Pulmonary mechanics and gas-exchange abnormalities. *Ann Am Thorac Soc* 17(9):1164–68. doi:10.1513/AnnalsATS.202005–462RL.

21 Grasselli, G., Tonetti, T., Protti, A., Langer, T., Girardis, M., et al. (2020) Pathophysiology of COVID-19-associated acute respiratory distress syndrome: A multicentre prospective observational study. *Lancet Respir Med* 8(12):1201–8. doi:10.1016/S2213–2600(20)30370–2.

22 Ziehr, D. R., Alladina, J., Petri, C. R., Maley, J. H., Moskowitz, A., et al. (2020) Respiratory pathophysiology of mechanically ventilated patients with COVID-19: A cohort study. *Am J Respir Crit Care Med* 201(12):1560–64. doi:10.1164/rccm.202004–1163LE.

23 Grieco, D. L., Bongiovanni, F., Chen, L., Menga, L. S., Cutuli, S. L., et al. (2020) Respiratory physiology of COVID-19-induced respiratory failure compared to ARDS of other etiologies. *Crit Care* 24(1):529. doi:10.1186/s13054–020-03253–2.

24 Ferrando, C., Suarez-Sipmann, F., Mellado-Artigas, R., Hernández, M., Gea, A., et al. (2020) COVID-19 Spanish ICU Network. Clinical features, ventilatory management, and outcome of ARDS caused by COVID-19 are similar to other causes of ARDS. *Intensive Care Med* 46(12):2200–2211. doi:10.1007/s00134–020-06192–2.

25 Haudebourg, A. F., Perier, F., Tuffet, S., de Prost, N., Razazi, K., et al. (2020) Respiratory mechanics of COVID-19- versus non-COVID-19-associated acute respiratory distress syndrome. *Am J Respir Crit Care Med* 202(2):287–90. doi:10.1164/rccm.202004–1226LE.

26 Kyle-Sidell, C. (2020) From NYC: Does COVID-19 really cause ARDS??!! YouTube. Retrieved from youtu.be/k9GYTc53r2o.

27 Haudebourg, Perier, Tuffet, de Prost, Razazi, et al. Respiratory mechanics of COVID-19- versus non-COVID-19-associated acute respiratory distress syndrome.

28 Haouzi, P., Zamir, A., Villarreal-Fernandez, E., Stauffer, D., Ventola, L., et al. (2020) Mechanics of breathing and gas exchange in mechanically ventilated patients with COVID-19-associated respiratory failure. *Am J Respir Crit Care Med* 202(4):626–28. doi:10.1164/rccm.202004–1041LE.

29 Gattinoni, L., Coppola, S., Cressoni, M., Busana, M., Rossi, S., Chiumello, D. (2020) COVID-19 does not lead to a "typical" acute respiratory distress syndrome. *Am J Res Crit Care Med* 201(10):1299–1300. doi:10.1164/rccm.202003–0817LE.

30 Gattinoni, L., Chiumello, D., Caironi, P., Busana, M., Romitti, F., et al. (2020) COVID-19 pneumonia: Different respiratory treatments for different phenotypes? *Intensive Care Med* 46(6):1099–1102. doi:10.1007/s00134–020-06033–2.

31 Halilton, J. (2020) Ventilators are no panacea for critically ill COVID-19 patients. National Public Radio. Retrieved from www.npr.org/sections/health-shots/2020/04/02/826105278/ventilators-are-no-panacea-for-critically-ill-covid-19-patients.

32 Tsolaki, V., Siempos, I., Magira, E., Kokkoris, S., Zakynthinos, G. E., Zakynthinos, S. (2020) PEEP levels in COVID-19 pneumonia. *Crit Care* 24(1):303. doi:10.1186/s13054–020-03049–4.

33 Ibrahim, G. S., Alkandari, B. M., Shady, I. A. A., Gupta, V. K., Abdelmohsen, M. A. (2021) Invasive mechanical ventilation complications in COVID-19 patients. *Egypt J Radiol Nucl Med* 2021;52(1):226. doi:10.1186/s43055–021-00609–8.

34 Wu, C. P., Adhi, F., Highland, K. (2020) Recognition and management of respiratory co-infection and secondary bacterial pneumonia in patients with COVID-19. *Cleve Clin J Med* 87(11):659–63. doi:10.3949/ccjm.87a.ccc015.

35 Kory, P., Kanne, J. P. (2020) SARS-CoV-2 organising pneumonia: "Has there been a widespread failure to identify and treat this prevalent condition in COVID-19?" *BMJ Open Respir Res* 7(1):e000724. doi:10.1136/bmjresp-2020–000724.

36 Xiang, M., Wu, X., Jing, H., Novakovic, V. A., Shi, J. (2023) The intersection of obesity and (long) COVID-19: Hypoxia, thrombotic inflammation, and vascular endothelial injury. *Front Cardiovasc Med* 10:1062491. doi:10.3389/fcvm.2023.1062491.

37 Herrmann, J., Mori, V., Bates, J. H. T., Suki, B. (2020) Modeling lung perfusion abnormalities to explain early COVID-19 hypoxemia. *Nat Commun* 11:4883. doi:10.1038/s41467–020-18672–6.

38 Bhatia, P., Mohammed, S. (2020) Severe hypoxemia in early COVID-19 pneumonia. *Am J Respir Crit Care Med* 202(4):621–22. doi:10.1164/rccm.202004–1313LE.

39 Scheim D. E. (2022) A deadly embrace: Hemagglutination mediated by SARS-CoV-2 spike protein at its 22 N-Glycosylation sites, red blood cell surface sialoglycoproteins, and antibody. *Int J Mol Sci* 23(5):2558. doi:10.3390/ijms23052558.

40 Boschi, C., Scheim, D. E., Bancod, A., Militello, M., Bideau, M. L., et al. (2022) SARS-CoV-2 spike protein induces hemagglutination: Implications for COVID-19 morbidities and therapeutics and for vaccine adverse effects. *Int J Mol Sci* 23(24):15480. doi:10.3390/ijms232415480.

41 Cavezzi, A., Troiani, E., Corrao, S. (2020) COVID-19: Hemoglobin, iron, and hypoxia beyond inflammation. A narrative review. *Clin Pract* 10(2):1271. doi:10.4081/cp.2020.1271.

42 Russo, A., Tellone, E., Barreca, D., Ficarra, S., Laganà, G. (2022) Implication of COVID-19 on erythrocytes functionality: Red blood cell biochemical implications and morpho-functional aspects. *Int J Mol Sci* 23(4):2171. doi:10.3390/ijms23042171.

43 Thomas, T., Stefanoni, D., Dzieciatkowska, M., Issaian, A., Nemkov, T., et al. (2020) Evidence of structural protein damage and membrane lipid remodeling in red blood cells from COVID-19 patients. *J Proteome Res* 19(11):4455–69. doi:10.1021/acs.jproteome.

44 Harutyunyan, G., Harutyunyan, G., Mkhoyan, G., Harutyunyan, V., Soghomonyan, S. (2020) Haemoglobin oxygen affinity in patients with severe COVID-19 infection: Still unclear. *Br J Haematol* 190(5):725–26. doi:10.1111/bjh.17051.

45 Kronstein-Wiedemann, R., Stadtmüller, M., Traikov, S., Georgi, M., Teichert, M., et al. (2022) SARS-CoV-2 infects red blood cell progenitors and dysregulates hemoglobin and iron metabolism. *Stem Cell Rev Rep* 18(5):1809–21. doi:10.1007/s12015–021-10322–8.

46 Shahbaz, S., Xu, L., Osman, M., Sligl, W., Shields, J., et al. (2021) Erythroid precursors and progenitors suppress adaptive immunity and get invaded by SARS-CoV-2. *Stem Cell Reports* 16(5):1165–81. doi:10.1016/j.stemcr.2021.04.001.

47 Cleveland Clinic. (2023) Mechanical ventilation. Retrieved from my.clevelandclinic.org/health/treatments/15368-mechanical-ventilation.

48 Garcia, A. (2020) Why some doctors are moving away from ventilators for virus patients. National Broadcasting Corporation News. Retrieved from www.nbcnews.com/health/health-news/why-some-doctors-are-moving-away-ventilators-virus-patients-n1179986.

49 Nishikimi, M., Jafari, D., Singh, N., Shinozaki, K., Sison, C. P., et al.; Northwell Health COVID-19 Research Consortium. (2022) Mortality of mechanically ventilated COVID-19 patients in traditional versus expanded intensive care units in New York. *Ann Am Thorac Soc* 19(8):1346–54. doi:10.1513/AnnalsATS.202106–705OC.

50 Gao, C. A., Markov, N. S., Stoeger, T., Pawlowski, A., Kang, M., et al.; NU SCRIPT Study Investigators (2023) Machine learning links unresolving secondary pneumonia to mortality in patients with severe pneumonia, including COVID-19. *J Clin Invest* 133(12):e170682. doi:10.1172/JCI170682.

51 Nolley, E. P., Sahetya, S. K., Hochberg, C. H. Hossen, S., Hager, D. N., et al. (2023) Outcomes among mechanically ventilated patients with severe pneumonia and acute hypoxemic respiratory failure from SARS-CoV-2 and other etiologies. *JAMA Netw Open* 6(1):e2250401. doi:10.1001/jamanetworkopen.2022.50401.

52 Morens, D. M., Taubenberger, J. K., Fauci, A. S. (2008) Predominant role of bacterial pneumonia as a cause of death in pandemic influenza: Implications for pandemic influenza preparedness. *J Infect Dis* 198(7):962–70. doi:10.1086/591708.

53 Mercola, J. (2023) The COVID hospital death trap. X. Retrieved from twitter.com/mercola/status/1666494508433911816?s=20.

54 Gao, C.A., Markov, N.S., Stoeger, T., Pawlowski, A., Kang, M., et al.; NU SCRIPT Study Investigators. (2023) Machine learning links unresolving secondary pneumonia to mortality in patients with severe pneumonia, including COVID-19. *J Clin Invest* 133(12):e170682. doi:10.1172/JCI170682.

55 World Health Organization. (2023) WHO coronavirus (COVID-19) dashboard. Retrieved from covid19.who.int/.

56 Formiga, F. R., Leblanc, R., de Souza Rebouças, J., Farias, L. P., de Oliveira, R. N., Pena L. (2021) Ivermectin: An award-winning drug with expected antiviral activity against COVID-19. *J Control Release* 329:758–61. doi:10.1016/j.jconrel.2020.10.009.

57 Heidary, F., Gharebaghi, R. (2020) Ivermectin: A systematic review from antiviral effects to COVID-19 complementary regimen. *J Antibiot* 73:593–602. doi:10.1038/s41429–020-0336-z.

58 Caly, L., Druce, J. D., Catton, M. G., Jans, D. A., Wagstaff, K. M. (2020) The FDA-approved drug ivermectin inhibits the replication of SARS-CoV-2 *in vitro*. *Antiviral Res* 178:104787. doi:10.1016/j.antiviral.2020.104787.

59 Wehbe, Z., Wehbe, M., Iratni, R., Pintus, G., Zaraket, H., et al. (2021) Repurposing ivermectin for COVID-19: Molecular aspects and therapeutic possibilities. *Front Immunol* 12:2021. ISSN:1664–3224 doi:www.frontiersin.org/articles/10.3389/fimmu.2021.663586.

60 Bernigaud, C., Guillemot, D., Ahmed-Belkacem, A., Grimaldi-Bensouda, L., Lespine, A., et al. (2021) Oral ivermectin for a scabies outbreak in a long-term care facility: Potential value in preventing COVID-19 and associated mortality. *Br J Dermatol* 184(6):1207–9. doi:10.1111/bjd.19821.

61 (2023) Ivermectin for COVID-19: Real-time meta analysis of 95 studies. Retrieved from ivmmeta.com/.

62 Kory, P., Meduri, G. U., Varon, J., Iglesias, J., Marik, P. E. (2021) Review of the emerging evidence demonstrating the efficacy of ivermectin in the prophylaxis and treatment of COVID-19. *Am J Ther* 28(3):e299. doi:10.1097/MJT.0000000000001377.

63 Bryant, A., Lawrie, T. A., Dowswell, T., Fordham, E.J., Mitchell, S., et al. (2021) Ivermectin for prevention and treatment of COVID-19 infection: A systematic review, meta-analysis, and trial sequential analysis to inform clinical guidelines. *Am J Ther* 28(4):e434–60. doi:10.1097/MJT.0000000000001402.

64 Ibid.

65 Popp, M., Reis, S., Schieber, S., Hausinger, R. I., Stegemann, M., et al. (2022) Ivermectin for preventing and treating COVID-19. doi:10.1002/14651858.CD015017.pub3

66 Fordham, E., Lawrie, T. A., MacGilchrist, K., Bryant, A. (2021) The uses and abuses of systematic reviews. doi:10.31219/osf.io/mp4f2.

67 Naggie, S., Boulware, D. R., Lindsell, C. J., Stewart, T. G., Gentile, N., et al. (2022) Effect of ivermectin vs placebo on time to sustained recovery in outpatients with mild to moderate COVID-19: A randomized clinical trial. *JAMA* 328(16):1595–1603. doi:10.1001/jama.2022.18590.

68 U.S. Food and Drug Administration. (2007) Stromectol (Ivermectin). NDA 50–742/S-022. United States Department of Health and Human Services. Retrieved from www.accessdata.fda.gov/drugsatfda_docs/label/2008/050742s022lbl.pdf.

69 Naggie, S. (2022) NIH Pragmatic Trials Collaboratory. Grand Rounds July 22, 2022: ACTIV-6: 1-year later and trial results for ivermectin-400 and inhaled Fluticasone. Retrieved from rethinkingclinicaltrials.org/news/grand-rounds-july-22–2022-activ-6–1-year-later-and-trial-results-for-ivermectin-400-and-inhaled-fluticasone-susanna-naggie-md-mhs/ (see 47:57 minute mark).

70 Naggie, Boulware, Lindsell, Stewart, Gentile, et al., Effect of ivermectin vs placebo on time to sustained recovery in outpatients with mild to moderate COVID-19.

71 Naggie, NIH Pragmatic Trials Collaboratory.

72 Naggie, Boulware, Lindsell, Stewart, Gentile, et al., Effect of ivermectin vs placebo on time to sustained recovery in outpatients with mild to moderate COVID-19.

73 Ibid.

74 Naggie, S. (2022) Ivermectin for treatment of mild-to-moderate COVID-19 in the outpatient setting: A decentralized, placebo-controlled, randomized, platform clinical trial. Accelerating COVID-19 Therapeutic Interventions and Vaccines (ACTIV)-6 study group. medRxiv (preprint). doi:10.1101/2022.06.10.22276252.

75 Nakatsu, K., personal communication.

76 Reis, G., Silva, E., Silva, D., Thabane, L., Milagres, A., et al. (2022) Effect of early treatment with ivermectin among patients with COVID-19. *N Engl J Med* 386:1721–31. doi:10.1056/NEJMoa2115869.

77 Halgas, O. (2022) Analysis of the TOGETHER trial's ivermectin arm results. Canadian Covid Care Alliance. Retrieved from canadiancovidcarealliance.org/media-resources/analysis-together-ivermectin-trial/.

78 Reis, Silva, Silva, Thabane, Milagres, et al., Effect of early treatment with ivermectin among patients with COVID-19.

79 Hayward, G., Yu, L. M., Little, P., Gbinigie, O., Shanyinde, M., et al.; PRINCIPLE Trial Collaborative Group. (2024) Ivermectin for COVID-19 in adults in the community (PRINCIPLE): An open, randomised, controlled, adaptive platform trial of short- and longer-term outcomes. *J Infect* 88(4):106130. doi:10.1016/j.jinf.2024.106130.

80 Ibid.

81 Chamie J. (2021) The latest results of ivermectin's success in treating outbreaks of COVID-19. Front Line COVID-19 Critical Care Alliance (FLCCC). Retrieved from COVID-19criticalcare.com/ivermectin-in-COVID-19/epidemiologic-analyses-on-COVID-19-and-ivermectin/.

82 Kerr, L., Baldi, F., Lobo, R., Assagra, W. L., Proenca, F. C., et al. (2022) Regular use of ivermectin as prophylaxis for COVID-19 led up to a 92% reduction in COVID-19 mortality rate in a dose-response manner: Results of a prospective observational study of a strictly controlled population of 88,012 Subjects. *Cureus* 14(8): e28624. doi:10.7759/cureus.28624.

83 Business Wire. (2023) MedinCell announces positive results for the SAIVE clinical study in prevention of COVID-19 infection in a contact-based population. www.businesswire.com/news/home/20230105005896/en/MedinCell-Announces-Positive-Results-for-the-SAIVE-Clinical-Study-in-Prevention-of-COVID-19-Infection-in-a-Contact-Based-Population.

84 C19early.org group. (2023) Global adoption of COVID-19 early treatments. Retrieved from c19early.org/adoption.html.

85 C19early.org group. (2023) Ivermectin for COVID-19. Retrieved from c19ivm.org/.

86 British Ivermection Recommendation Development Group. (2023) BIRD International. Retrieved from bird-group.org/.

87 World Council for Health. (2023) Early COVID-19 treatment guidelines: A practical approach to home-based care for healthy families. Retrieved from worldcouncilforhealth.org/resources/early-covid-19-treatment-guide/.

88 World Health Organization. (2023) VigiAccess. Retrieved from vigiaccess.org/.

89 Guzzo, C. A., Furtek, C. I., Porras, A. G., Chen, C., Tipping, R., et al. (2002) Safety, tolerability, and pharmacokinetics of escalating high doses of ivermectin in healthy adult subjects. *J Clin Pharmacol* 42(10):1122–33. doi:10.1177/009127002401382731.

90 Business Wire. (2021) MedinCell publishes an extensive Ivermectin safety expert analysis. Press release. Retrieved from www.businesswire.com/news/home/20210305005353/en/COVID-19-MedinCell-Publishes-an-.

91 Descotes, J. (2021) Expert review report: Medical safety of ivermectin. ImmunoSafe. Retrieved from www.covid-factuel.fr/wp-content/uploads/2022/01/Clinical_Safety_of_Ivermectin-March_2021.pdf.

92 Ibid.

93 (2017) WHO model list of essential medicines, 20th List (April 2017). World Health Organization. Retrieved from www.who.int/publications/i/ item/eml-20.

94 Guzzo, Furtek, Porras, Chen, Tipping, et al., Safety, tolerability, and pharmacokinetics of escalating high doses of ivermectin in healthy adult subjects.

95 De Sole, G., Remme, J., Awadzi, K., Accorsi, S., Alley, E. S., et al. (1989) Adverse reactions after large-scale treatment of onchocerciasis with ivermectin: Combined results from eight community trials. *Bulletin of the World Health Organization* 67(6):707–19. europepmc.org/article/PMC/PMC2491300.

96 Twum-Danso, N. A. (2003) Serious adverse events following treatment with ivermectin for onchocerciasis control: A review of reported cases. *Filaria J* 2 Suppl 1(Suppl 1):S3. doi:10.1186/1475–2883-2-S1-S3.

97 Naggie, Boulware, Lindsell, Stewart, Gentile, et al., Effect of ivermectin vs placebo on time to sustained recovery in outpatients with mild to moderate COVID-19.

98 Reis, Silva, Silva, Thabane, Milagres, et al., Effect of early treatment with ivermectin among patients with COVID-19.

99 Drug and Health Product Register—Canada. (2022) Stromectal® Monograph. Last accessed October 23, 2022. Retrieved from pdf.hres.ca/dpd_pm/00047237.pdf.

100 Staff at TrialSite (2022) Uttar Pradesh officials set the record straight: Ivermectin used. TrialSite News. Retrieved from www.trialsitenews.com/a/uttar-pradesh-officials-set-the-record-straight-ivermectin-used-successfully-to-combat-covid-19-in-the-northern-indian-state-a04783f3.

101 Bean, M. (2022) 28 states have legislation to promote ivermectin access. Becker's Hospital Review. Retrieved from www.beckershospitalreview.com/pharmacy/28-states-have-legislation-to-promote-ivermectin-access.html.

102 C19early.org group. (2023) Global adoption of COVID-19 early treatments. Retrieved from c19early.org/adoption.html.

103 Bean, 28 states have legislation to promote ivermectin access.

104 Mehra M. R., Desai, S. S., Ruschitzka, F., Patel, A. N. (2020) Hydroxychloroquine or chloroquine with or without a macrolide for treatment of COVID-19: A multinational registry analysis. *Lancet.* doi:10.1016/S0140–6736(20)31180–6.

105 182 signatories. (2020) Concerns regarding the statistical analysis and data integrity. Open letter to M. R. Mehra, S. S. Desai, F. Ruschitzka, and A. N. Patel, authors of "Hydroxychloroquine or chloroquine with or without a macrolide for treatment of COVID19: a multinational registry analysis." *Lancet* 2020 May 22:S0140–6736(20)31180–31186. doi: 10.1016/S0140–6736(20)31180–6. and to Richard Horton (editor of *The Lancet*). Retrieved from statmodeling.stat.columbia.edu/wp-content/uploads/2020/05/Open-Letter-the-statistical-analysis-and-data-integrity-of-Mehra-et-al_Final-1.pdf.

106 Mehra, M. R., Ruschitzka, F., Patel, A. N. (2020) RETRACTION-Hydroxychloroquine or chloroquine with or without a macrolide for treatment of COVID-19: a multinational registry analysis. *Lancet* 395(10240):1820. doi:10.1016/S0140–6736(20)31324–6.

107 Front Line COVID-19 Critical Care Alliance. (2023) Retrieved from covid19critical-care.com.

108 Lee, K. H., Yoon, S., Jeong, G. H., Kim, J. Y., Han, Y. J. (2020) Efficacy of corticosteroids in patients with SARS, MERS and COVID-19: A systematic review and meta-analysis. *J Clin Med* 9(8):2392. doi:10.3390/jcm9082392.

109 Chetty, S. (2020) A KZN doctor's observations and treatment of COVID-19: Reveal a missing element. *Modern Medicine* 5:3. Retrieved from www.modernmedia.co.za/modernmedicine/DigitalEditions/mm2008–2009-august-september-2020/html5/index.html.

110 McCullough, P. A., Kelly, R. J., Ruocco, G., Lerma, E., Tumlin, J., et al. (2021) Pathophysiological basis and rationale for early outpatient treatment of SARS-CoV-2 (COVID-19) infection. *Am J Med* 134(1):16–22. doi:10.1016/j.amjmed.2020.07.003.

111 Horby, P., Lim, W. S., Emberson, J., Mafham, M., Bell, J., et al. (2021) Dexamethasone in hospitalized patients with COVID-19. *N Engl J Med* 384:693–704. doi:10.1056/NEJMoa2021436.

112 The COVID-19 Therapeutics Working Group. (2022) Current guidance for the management of adult hospitalized patients with COVID-19. Alberta Health Services. Retrieved from www.albertahealthservices.ca/assets/info/ppih/if-ppih-covid-19-recommendations.pdf.

113 BC COVID-19 Therapeutics Committee (CTC) and COVID-19 Therapeutics Review and Advisory Working Group (CTRAWG). (2022) Clinical practice guidance for antimicrobial and immunomodulatory therapy in adult patients with COVID-19.

BC Centre for Disease Control. Retrieved from www.bccdc.ca/health-professionals/clinical-resources/covid-19-care/treatments.

114 (2023) MATH+: Hospital treatment protocol for COVID-19. Front Line COVID-19 Critical Care (FLCCC) Alliance. Retrieved from covid19criticalcare.com/protocol/math-covid-hospital-treatment/.

115 Wang, M., Cao, R., Zhang, L., Yang, X., Liu, J., et al. (2020) Remdesivir and chloroquine effectively inhibit the recently emerged novel coronavirus (2019-nCoV) *in vitro*. *Cell Res* 30(3):269–71. doi:10.1038/s41422–020-0282–0.

116 Beigel, J. H., Tomashek, K. M., Dodd, L. E., Mehta, A. K., Zingman, B. S., et al. (2020) Remdesivir for the treatment of COVID-19—Final report. *New Engl. J Med* 383:1813–26. doi:10.1056/NEJMoa2007764.

117 National Institutes of Health. (2023) Table 4a. Remdesivir: Selected clinical data. Retrieved from www.covid19treatmentguidelines.nih.gov/tables/remdesivir-data/.

118 Ader, F., Bouscambert-Duchamp, M., Hites, M., Peiffer-Smadja, N., Poissy, J., et al. (2021) Remdesivir plus standard of care verses standard of care alone for the treatment of patients admitted to hospital with COVID-19 (DisCoVeRy): A phase 3, randomised, controlled, open-label trial. *Lancet Infectious Diseases* 22(2):P209–21. doi:10.1016/S1473–3099(21)00485–0.

119 Ali, K., Azher, T., Baqi, M., Binnie, A., Borgiam S., et al. (2022) Remdesivir for the treatment of patients in hospital with COVID-19 in Canada: A randomized controlled trial. *CMAJ* 194(7):E242–E251. doi:10.1503/cmaj.211698.

120 Thomson Reuters. (2020) WHO advises against the treating hospitalized COVID-19 patients with remdesivir. Canadian Broadcasting Corporation News. Retrieved from www.cbc.ca/news/health/who-remdesivir-trial-1.5809424.

121 World Health Organization. (2022) Remdesivir for COVID-19. Retrieved from iris.who.int/bitstream/handle/10665/359753/WHO-2019-nCoV-Therapeutics-Remdesivir-Poster-A-2022.1-eng.pdf.

122 Morris, A. M., Juni, P., Odutayo, A., Bobos, P., Andany, N., et al. (2021) Remdesivir for hospitalized patients with COVID-19. Ontario Science Table. Retrieved from covid19-sciencetable.ca/sciencebrief/remdesivir-for-hospitalized-patients-with-covid-19/.

123 Public Services and Procurement Canada. (2022) Government of Canada receives first delivery of COVID-19 oral antiviral treatment. Retrieved from www.canada.ca/en/public-services-procurement/news/2022/01/government-of-canada-receives-first-delivery-of-covid-19-oral-antiviral-treatment.html.

124 Business Wire. (2021) Pfizer announces additional Phase 2/3 study results confirming robust efficacy of novel COVID-19 oral antiviral treatment candidate in reducing risk of hospitalization or death. December 14, 2021. Retrieved from www.businesswire.com/news/home/20211214005548/en/Pfizer-Announces-Additional-Phase-23-Study-Results-Confirming-Robust-Efficacy-of-Novel-COVID-19-Oral-Antiviral-Treatment-Candidate-in-Reducing.

125 Reis, S., Metzendorf, M.-I., Kuehn, R., Popp, M., Gagyor, I., et al. (2022) Nirmatrelvir combined with ritonavir for preventing and treating COVID-19. Cochrane Database of Systematic Reviews 9. Art. No.: CD015395. doi:10.1002/14651858.CD015395.

126 Hammond, J., Fountaine, R. J., Yunis, C., Fleishaker, D., Almas, M., et al. (2024) Nirmatrelvir for vaccinated or unvaccinated adult outpatients with Covid-19. *N Engl J Med* 390(13):1186–95. doi:10.1056/NEJMoa2309003.

127 Wang, L., Berger, N. A., Davis, P. B., Kaelber, D. C., Volkow, N. D., Xu, R. (2022) COVID-19 rebound after Paxlovid and Molnupiravir during January–June 2022. medRxiv (preprint). doi:10.1101/2022.06.21.22276724.

128 Hammond, J., Leister-Tebbe, H., Gardner, A., Abreu, P., Bao, W., et al. (2022) Oral Nirmatrelvir for high-risk, nonhospitalized adults with COVID-19. *N Engl J Med* 386:1397–1408. doi:10.1056/NEJMoa2118542.

129 Ibid.

130 Ontario Science Table. (2022) COVID-19 Advisory for Ontario. Evidence-based recommendations on the use of Nirmatrelvir/Ritonavir (Paxlovid) for adults in Ontario. Retrieved from covid19-sciencetable.ca/sciencebrief/evidence-based-recommendations-on-the-use-of-nirmatrelvir-ritonavir-paxlovid-for-adults-in-ontario/.

131 Hammond, Leister-Tebbe, Gardner, Abreu, Bao, et al., Oral Nirmatrelvir for high-risk, nonhospitalized adults with COVID-19.

132 Pfizer. (2023) Product monograph including patient medical information: Paxlovid. Retrieved from covid-vaccine.canada.ca/info/pdf/paxlovid-pm-en.pdf

133 Chatterjee, S., Bhattacharya, M., Dhama, K., Lee, S. S., Chakraborty, C. (2023) Molnupiravir's mechanism of action drives "error catastrophe" in SARS-CoV-2: A therapeutic strategy that leads to lethal mutagenesis of the virus. *Mol Ther Nucleic Acids* 33:49–52. doi:10.1016/j.omtn.2023.06.006.

134 National Institutes of Health. (2023) Molnupravir. NIH COVID-19 treatment guidelines. Retrieved from www.covid19treatmentguidelines.nih.gov/therapies/antivirals-including-antibody-products/molnupiravir/.

135 Jayk Bernal, A., Gomes da Silva, M. M., Musungaie, D.B., Kovalchuk, E., Gonzalez, A., et al.; MOVe-OUT Study Group. (2022) Molnupiravir for oral treatment of COVID-19 in nonhospitalized patients. *N Engl J Med* 386(6):509–20. doi:10.1056/NEJMoa2116044.

136 Butler, C. C., Hobbs, F. D. R., Gbinigie, O. A., Rahman, N. M., Hayward, G., et al.; PANORAMIC Trial Collaborative Group. (2023) Molnupiravir plus usual care versus usual care alone as early treatment for adults with COVID-19 at increased risk of adverse outcomes (PANORAMIC): An open-label, platform-adaptive randomised controlled trial. *Lancet* 401(10373):281–93. doi:10.1016/S0140–6736(22)02597–1.

137 Wang, L., Berger, N. A., Davis, P. B., Kaelber, D. C., Volkow, N. D., Xu. R. (2022) COVID-19 rebound after Paxlovid and Molnupiravir during January–June 2022. medRxiv (preprint). doi:10.1101/2022.06.21.22276724.

138 (2022) Government of Canada receives first delivery of COVID-19 oral antiviral treatment. Public Services and Procurement Canada. Retrieved from www.canada.ca/en/public-services-procurement/news/2022/01/government-of-canada-receives-first-delivery-of-covid-19-oral-antiviral-treatment.html.

139 Levesque, C. (2022) Thousands of Canadian-made antiviral COVID-19 pills in storage pending Health Canada approval. *National Post.* Retrieved from nationalpost.com/news/canada/thousands-of-canadian-made-antiviral-covid-19-pills-in-storage-pending-health-canada-approval.

140 Health Canada. (2023) Drug and vaccine authorizations for COVID-19: List of applications received. Government of Canada. Retrieved from www.canada.ca/en/health-canada/services/drugs-health-products/covid19-industry/drugs-vaccines-treatments/authorization/applications.html#wb-auto-4.

141 Merck. (2023) Merck and Ridgeback provide update on EU marketing authorization application for Lagevrio™ (molnupiravir). Retrieved from www.merck.com/news

/merck-and-ridgeback-provide-update-on-eu-marketing-authorization-application-for-lagevrio-molnupiravir-2/.

142 Joseph, A. (2022) Officials limit an antibody therapy, says it's ineffective against BA.2 variant of Omicron. STAT. Retrieved from www.statnews.com/2022/03/25/fda-limits-therapy-ineffective-against-ba2-variant-omicron/.

143 Werza, O., Seegers, J., Schaible, A. M., Weinigel, C., Barz, D., et al. (2014) Cannflavins from hemp sprouts, a novel cannabinoid-free hemp food product, target microsomal prostaglandin E_2 synthase-1 and 5-lipoxygenase. *PharmaNutrition* 2(3)53–60. doi: 10.1016/j.phanu.2014.05.001.

144 Bautista, J. L., Yu, S., Tian, L. (2021) Flavonoids in *Cannabis sativa*: Biosynthesis, bioactivities, and biotechnology. *ACS Omega* 6(8):5119–23. doi:10.1021/acsomega.1c00318.

145 Russo, E. B. (2011) Taming THC: Potential cannabis synergy and phytocannabinoid-terpenoid entourage effects. *Br J Pharmacol* 163(7):1344–64. doi:10.1111/j.1476–5381.2011.01238.x.

146 Maresz, K., Pryce, G., Ponomarev, E. D., Marsicano, G., Croxford, J. L., et al. (2007) Direct suppression of CNS autoimmune inflammation via the cannabinoid receptor CB1 on neurons and CB2 on autoreactive T cells. *Nat Med* 13(4):492–97. doi:10.1038/nm1561.

147 Kendall, D. A., Yudowski, G. A. (2017) Cannabinoid receptors in the central nervous system: Their signaling and roles in disease. *Front Cell Neurosci* 10:294. doi:10.3389/fncel.2016.00294.

148 O'Sullivan, S. E. (2016) An update on PPAR activation by cannabinoids. *Br J Pharmacol* 173(12):1899–1910. doi:10.1111/bph.13497.

149 Lei, Y., Zhang, J., Schiavon, C. R., He, M., Chen, L., et al. (2021) SARS-CoV-2 spike protein impairs endothelial function via downregulation of ACE 2. *Circ Res* 128(9):1323–26. doi:10.1161/CIRCRESAHA.

150 Robles, J. P., Zamora, M., Adan-Castro, E., Siqueiros-Marquez, L., Martinez de la Escalera, G., Clapp, C. (2022) The spike protein of SARS-CoV-2 induces endothelial inflammation through integrin α5β1 and NF-κB signaling. *J Biol Chem* 298(3):101695. doi:10.1016/j.jbc.2022.101695.

151 Lei, Zhang, Schiavon, He, Chen, et al., SARS-CoV-2 spike protein impairs endothelial function via downregulation of ACE 2.

152 Ni, W., Yang, X., Yang, D., Bao, J., Li, R., et al. (2020) Role of angiotensin-converting enzyme 2 (ACE2) in COVID-19. *Crit Care* 24(1):422. doi:10.1186/s13054–020-03120–0.

153 Ryu, J. K., Sozmen, E. G., Dixit, K., Montano, M., Matsui Y., et al. (2021) SARS-CoV-2 spike protein induces abnormal inflammatory blood clots neutralized by fibrin immunotherapy. bioRxiv [Preprint] 13:2021.10.12.464152. doi:10.1101/2021.10.12.464152.

154 Van Breemen, R. B., Muchiri, R. N., Bates, T. A., Weinstein, J. B., Leier, H. C., et al. (2022) Cannabinoids block cellular entry of SARS-CoV-2 and the emerging variants. *J Nat Prod* 85(1):176–84. doi:10.1021/acs.jnatprod.1c00946.

155 Ibid.

156 González-Maldonado, P., Alvarenga, N., Burgos-Edwards, A., Flores-Giubi, M. E., Barúa, J. E., et al. (2022) Screening of natural products inhibitors of SARS-CoV-2 entry. *Molecules* 27(5):1743. doi:10.3390/molecules27051743.

157 Bansal, S., Perincheri, S., Fleming, T., Poulson, C., Tiffany, B., et al. (2021) Cutting edge: Circulating exosomes with COVID spike protein are induced by BNT162b2

(Pfizer–BioNTech) vaccination prior to development of antibodies: A novel mechanism for immune activation by mRNA Vaccines. *J Immunol 2*07(10):2405–10. doi:10.4049/jimmunol.2100637.

158 Mishra, R., Banerjea, A. C. (2021) SARS-CoV-2 spike targets USP33-IRF9 Axis *via* exosomal miR-148a to activate human microglia. *Front in Immunol* 12:656700. doi:10.3389/fimmu.2021.656700.

159 DeMarino, C., Cowen, M., Khatkar, P., Cotto, B., Branscome, H., et al. (2022) Cannabinoids reduce extracellular vesicle release from HIV-1 infected myeloid cells and inhibit viral transcription. *Cells* 11(4):723. doi:10.3390/cells11040723.

160 Bansal, S., Perincheri, S., Fleming, T., Poulson, C., Tiffany, B., et al. (2021) Cutting edge: Circulating exosomes with COVID spike protein are induced by BNT162b2 (Pfizer–BioNTech) vaccination prior to development of antibodies: A novel mechanism for immune activation by mRNA vaccines. *J Immunol 2*07(10):2405–10. doi:10.4049/jimmunol.2100637.

161 DeMarino, Cowen, Khatkar, Cotto, Branscome, et al., Cannabinoids reduce extracellular vesicle release from HIV-1 infected myeloid cells and inhibit viral transcription.

162 Vrechi, T. A. M., Leao, A. H. F. F., Morais, I. B. M., Abílio, V. C., Zuardi, A. W., et al. (2021) Cannabidiol induces autophagy via ERK1/2 activation in neural cells. *Sci Rep* 11(1):5434. doi:10.1038/s41598–021-84879–2.

163 Wang, Z., Zheng, P., Chen, X., Xie, Y., Weston-Green, K., Solowij, N., et al. (2022) Cannabidiol induces autophagy and improves neuronal health associated with SIRT1 mediated longevity. *GeroScience* 44(3): 1505–24. doi:10.1007/s11357–022-00559–7.

164 Park, H., Kang, J.-H., Lee, S. (2020) Autophagy in neurodegenerative diseases: A hunter for aggregates. *Int J Mol Sci 21(9):3369.* doi:/10.3390/ijms21093369.

165 Li, F., Li, J., Wang, P. H., Yang, N., Huang, J., et al. (2021) SARS-CoV-2 spike promotes inflammation and apoptosis through autophagy by ROS-suppressed PI3K/AKT/mTOR signaling. *Biochim Biophys Acta Mol Basis Dis* 867(12):166260. doi:10.1016/j.bbadis.2021.166260.

166 Nguyen, V., Zhang, Y., Gao, C., Cao, X., Tian, Y., et al. (2022) The spike protein of SARS-CoV-2 impairs lipid metabolism and increases susceptibility to lipotoxicity: Implication for a role of Nrf2. *Cells 1*1(12):1916. doi:10.3390/cells11121916.

167 Salazar, M., Carracedo, A., Salanueva, I. J., Hernández-Tiedra, S., Lorente, M., et al. (2009) Cannabinoid action induces autophagy-mediated cell death through stimulation of ER stress in human glioma cells. *J Clin Invest* 119(5):1359–72. doi:10.1172/jci37948.

168 Vara, D., Salazar, M., Olea-Herrero, N., Guzmán, M., Velasco, G., and Díaz-Laviada, I. (2011) Anti-tumoral action of cannabinoids on hepatocellular carcinoma: Role of AMPK-dependent activation of autophagy. *Cell Death Differ* 18(7):1099–1111. doi:10.1038/cdd.2011.32.

169 Armstrong, J. L., Hill, D. S., McKee, C. S., Hernandez-Tiedra, S., Lorente, M., et al. (2015) Exploiting cannabinoid-induced cytotoxic autophagy to drive melanoma cell death. *J Invest Dermatol* 135(6):1629–37. doi:10.1038/jid.2015.45.

170 Lee, X. C., Werner, E., Falasca M. (2021) Molecular mechanism of autophagy and its regulation by cannabinoids in cancer. *Cancers* (Basel) 13(6):1211. doi.10.3390/cancers13061211.

171 Hao, F., Feng Y. (2021) Cannabidiol (CBD) enhanced the hippocampal immune response and autophagy of APP/PS1 Alzheimer's mice uncovered by RNA-seq. *Life Sci* 264:118624. doi:10.1016/j.lfs.2020.118624.

172 Xiong, Y., Lim C. S. (2021) Understanding the modulatory effects of cannabidiol on Alzheimer's disease. *Brain Sci* 11(9):1211. doi:10.3390/brainsci11091211.

173 Kang, S., Li, J., Yao, Z., Liu, J. (2021) Cannabidiol induces autophagy to protects neural cells from mitochondrial dysfunction by upregulating SIRT1 to inhibits NF-κB and NOTCH pathways. *Frontiers in Cellular Neuroscience* 15:654340. doi:10.3389/fncel.2021.654340.

174 Muhammad, F., Liu, Y., Wang, N., Zhao, L., Zhou, Y., et al. (2022) Neuroprotective effects of cannabidiol on dopaminergic neurodegeneration and α-synuclein accumulation in *C. elegans* models of Parkinson's disease. *Neurotoxicology* 93:128–39. doi:10.1016/j.neuro.2022.09.001.

175 Vrechi, Leao, Morais, Abílio, Zuardi, et al., Cannabidiol induces autophagy via ERK1/2 activation in neural cells.

176 Wang, Zheng, Chen, Xie, Weston-Green, Solowij, et al., Cannabidiol induces autophagy and improves neuronal health associated with SIRT1 mediated longevity.

177 Jiang, F., Xia, M., Zhang, Y., Chang, J., Cao, J., et al. (2022) Cannabinoid receptor-2 attenuates neuroinflammation by promoting autophagy-mediated degradation of the NLRP3 inflammasome post spinal cord injury. (2022) *Front Immunol* 13:993168. doi:10.3389/fimmu.2022.993168.

178 Shao, B. Z., Wei, W., Ke, P., Xu, Z. Q., Zhou, J. X, Liu, C. (2014) Activating cannabinoid receptor 2 alleviates pathogenesis of experimental autoimmune encephalomyelitis via activation of autophagy and inhibiting NLRP3 inflammasome. *CNS Neurosci Ther* 20(12):1021–28. doi:10.1111/cns.12349.

179 Hiebel, C., Kromm, T., Stark, M., Behl, C. (2014) Cannabinoid receptor 1 modulates the autophagic flux independent of mTOR- and BECLIN1-complex. *J Neurochem* 131(4):484–97. doi:10.1111/jnc.12839.

180 Yan, S., Yang, X., Chen, T., Xi, Z., Jiang, X. (2014) The PPARγ agonist Troglitazone induces autophagy, apoptosis and necroptosis in bladder cancer cells. *Cancer Gene Ther* 21(5):188–93. doi:10.1038/cgt.2014.16.

181 Luo, R., Su, L.Y., Li, G., Yang, J., Liu, Q., et al. (2020) Activation of PPARA-mediated autophagy reduces Alzheimer disease–like pathology and cognitive decline in a murine model. *Autophagy* 16(1):52–69. doi:10.1080/15548627.2019.1596488.

182 Barhoumi, T., Alghanem, B., Shaibah, H., Mansour, F.A., Alamri, H.S., et al. (2021) SARS-CoV-2 coronavirus spike protein-induced apoptosis, inflammatory, and oxidative stress responses in THP-1-like-macrophages: Potential role of angiotensin-converting enzyme inhibitor (Perindopril). *Front Immunol* 20(12):728896. doi:10.3389/fimmu.2021.728896.

183 Khan, S., Shafiei, M. S., Longoria, C., Schoggins, J. W., Savani, R. C., Zaki H. (2021) SARS-CoV-2 spike protein induces inflammation via TLR2-dependent activation of the NF-κB pathway. *Elife* 10:e68563. doi:10.7554/eLife.68563.

184 Li, Li, Wang, Yang, Huang, et al., SARS-CoV-2 spike promotes inflammation and apoptosis through autophagy.

185 Barhoumi, Alghanem, Shaibah, Mansour, Alamri, et al., SARS-CoV-2 coronavirus spike protein-induced apoptosis, inflammatory, and oxidative stress responses in THP-1 -like-macrophages.

186 Nagarkatti, P., Pandey, R., Rieder, S. A., Hegde, V. L., Nagarkatti, M. (2009) Cannabinoids as novel anti-inflammatory drugs. *Future Med Chem* 1(7):1333–49. doi.: 10.4155/fmc.09.93.

187 Anil, S. M., Peeri, H., Koltai, H. (2022) Medical cannabis activity against inflammation: Active compounds and modes of action. *Front Pharmacol* 13:908198. doi:10.3389/fphar.2022.908198.

188 Robles, J. P., Zamora, M., Adan-Castro, E., Siqueiros-Marquez, L., Martinez de la Escalera, G., Clapp, C. (2022) The spike protein of SARS-CoV-2 induces endothelial inflammation through integrin α5β1 and NF-κB signaling. *J Biol Chem* 298(3):101695. doi:10.1016/j.jbc.2022.101695.

189 Khan, Shafiei, Longoria, Schoggins, Savani, and Zaki, SARS-CoV-2 spike protein induces inflammation via TLR2-dependent activation of the NF-κB pathway.

190 Albornoz, E. A., Amarilla, A.A., Modhiran, N., Parker, S., Li, X. X., et al. (2022) SARS-CoV-2 drives NLRP3 inflammasome activation in human microglia through spike protein. *Mol Psychiatry*. doi:10.1038/s41380–022-01831–0.

191 Nagarkatti, Pandey, Rieder, Hegde, and Nagarkatti, Cannabinoids as novel anti-inflammatory drugs.

192 Anil, S. M., Shalev, N., Vinayaka, A. C., Nadarajan, S., Namdar, D., et al. (2021) Cannabis compounds exhibit anti-inflammatory activity *in vitro* in COVID-19-related inflammation in lung epithelial cells and pro-inflammatory activity in macrophages. *Scientific Reports* 11(1):1462. doi:10.1038/s41598–021-81049–2.

193 Kovalchuk, A., Want, B., Li, D., Rodriguez-Juarez, R., Ilnytskyy, S., et al. (2021) Fighting the storm: Could novel anti-TNFα and anti-IL-6 *C. Sativa* cultivars tame cytokine storm in COVID-19? Aging 13(2):1571–90. doi:10.18632/aging.202500.

194 Corpetti, C., Del Re, A., Seguella, L., Palenca, I., Rurgo, S., et al. (2021) Cannabidiol inhibits SARS-Cov-2 spike (S) protein-induced cytotoxicity and inflammation through a PPARγ-dependent TLR4/NLRP3/Caspase-1 signaling suppression in Caco-2 cell line. *Phytother Rese* 35(12):6893–6903. doi:10.1002/ptr.7302.

195 Nagarkatti, Pandey, Rieder, Hegde, and Nagarkatti, Cannabinoids as novel anti-inflammatory drugs.

196 Anil, Shalev, Vinayaka, Nadarajan, Namdar, et al., Cannabis compounds exhibit anti-inflammatory activity *in vitro* in COVID-19-related inflammation in lung epithelial cells and pro-inflammatory activity in macrophages.

197 Nagarkatti, Pandey, Rieder, Hegde, and Nagarkatti, Cannabinoids as novel anti-inflammatory drugs.

198 Jha, N. K., Sharma, C., Hashiesh, H. M., Arunachalam, S., Meeran, M. N., et al. (2021) β-Caryophyllene, a natural dietary CB2 receptor selective cannabinoid can be a candidate to target the trinity of infection, immunity, and inflammation in COVID-19. *Front Pharmacol* 12:590201. doi:10.3389/fphar.2021.590201.

199 Ibid.

200 Gaylis, N. B., Kreychman, I., Sagliani, J., Mograbi, J., Gabet, Y. (2022) The results of a unique dietary supplement (nutraceutical formulation) used to treat the symptoms of long-haul COVID. *Front Nutr* 9:1034169. doi:10.3389/fnut.2022.

201 Rhea, E. M., Logsdon, A. F., Hansen, K. M., Williams, L. M., Reed, et al. (2021) The S1 protein of SARS-CoV-2 crosses the blood-brain barrier in mice. *Nature Neurosci* 24(3):368–78. doi:10.1038/s41593–020-00771–8.

202 Rong, Z., Mai, H., Kapoor, S., Puelles, V. G, Czogalla, J., et al. (2023) SARS-CoV-2 spike protein accumulation in the skull-meninges-brain axis: Potential implications for long-term neurological complications in post-COVID-19. bioRxiv (preprint). doi:10.1101/2023.04.04.535604.

203 Kim, E. S., Jeon, M. T., Kim, K. S., Lee, S., Kim, S., Kim, D. G. (2021) Spike proteins of SARS-CoV-2 induce pathological changes in molecular delivery and metabolic function in the brain endothelial cells. *Viruses* 13(10):2021. doi:10.3390/v13102021.

204 Albornoz, Amarilla, Modhiran, Parker, Li, et al., SARS-CoV-2 drives NLRP3 inflammasome activation in human microglia through spike protein.

205 Frank, M. G., Nguyen, K. H., Ball, J. B., Hopkins, S., Kelley, T., et al. (2022) SARS-CoV-2 spike S1 subunit induces neuroinflammatory, microglial and behavioral sickness responses: Evidence of PAMP-like properties. *Brain Behav Immun* 100:267–77. doi:10.1016/j.bbi.2021.12.007.

206 Chesney, A. D., Maiti, B., Hansmann, U.H.E. (2023) SARS-COV-2 spike protein fragment eases amyloidogenesis of α-Synuclein. bioRxiv [Preprint]. doi:10.1101/2023.05.06.539715.

207 Kendall, D. A., and Yudowski, G. A. (2017) Cannabinoid receptors in the central nervous system: Their signaling and roles in disease. *Front Cell Neurosci* 10:294. doi:10.3389/fncel.2016.00294.

208 Rog, D. J. (2010) Cannabis-based medicines in multiple sclerosis—a review of clinical studies. *Immunobiology* 215(8):658–72. doi:10.1016/j.imbio.2010.03.009.

209 Bhunia, S., Kolishetti, N., Arias, A. Y., Vashist, A., Nair, M. (2022) Cannabidiol for neurodegenerative disorders: A comprehensive review. *Front Pharmacol* 13:989717. doi:10.3389/fphar.2022.989717.

210 Martin-Moreno, A. M., Reigada, D., Ramirez, B. G., Mechoulam, R., Innamorato, N., et al. (2011) Cannabidiol and other cannabinoids reduce microglial activation *in vitro* and *in vivo*: Relevance to Alzheimer's disease. *Mol Pharmacol* 79(6):964–73. doi:10.1124/mol.111.071290.

211 Casarejos, M. J., Perucho, J., Gomez, A., Muñoz, M. P., Fernandez-Estevez, M., et al. (2013) Natural cannabinoids improve dopamine neurotransmission and tau and amyloid pathology in a mouse model of tauopathy. *J Alzheimer's Dis* 35(3):525–39. doi:10.3233/JAD-130050.

212 Aso, E., Sánchez-Pla, A., Vegas-Lozano, E., Maldonado, R., Ferrer, I. (2015) Cannabis-based medicine reduces multiple pathological processes in AβPP/PS1 mice. *J Alzheimers Dis* 43(3):977–91. doi:10.3233/JAD-141014.

213 Kozela, E., Lev, N., Kaushansky, N., Eilam, R., Rimmerman, N., et al. (2011) Cannabidiol inhibits pathogenic T cells, decreases spinal microglial activation and ameliorates multiple sclerosis-like disease in C57BL/6 mice. *Br J Pharmacol* 163(7), 1507–19. doi:10.1111/j.1476–5381.2011.01379.x.

214 Chagas, M. H., Zuardi, A. W., Tumas, V., Pena-Pereira, M. A., Sobreira, E. T., et al. (2014) Effects of cannabidiol in the treatment of patients with Parkinson's disease: An exploratory double-blind trial. *J Psychopharmacol* 28(11):1088–98. doi:10.1177/0269881114550355.

215 Zuardi, A. W., Crippa, J. A., Hallak, J. E., Pinto, J. P., Chagas, M. H., et al. (2009) Cannabidiol for the treatment of psychosis in Parkinson's disease. *J. Psychopharmacol* 23(8):979–83. doi:10.1177/0269881108096519.

216 Leszko, M., and Meenrajan, S. (2021) Attitudes, beliefs, and changing trends of cannabidiol (CBD) oil use among caregivers of individuals with Alzheimer's disease. *Complement Ther Med* 57:102660. doi:10.1016/j.ctim.2021.102660.

217 Bridgeman, M. B., and Abazia, D. T. (2017) Medicinal cannabis: History, pharmacology, and implications for the acute care setting. *P T* 42(3):180–88.

218 Jones, G. (2022) 100 years of vitamin D: Historical aspects of vitamin D. *Endocr Connect* 11(4):e210594. doi:10.1530/EC-21–0594.

219 Christakos, S., Dhawan, P., Verstuyf, A., Verlinden, L., Carmeliet, G. (2016) Vitamin D: Metabolism, molecular mechanism of action, and pleiotropic effects. *Physiol Rev* 96(1):365–408. doi:10.1152/physrev.00014.2015.

220 Lamberg-Allardt, C. (2006) Vitamin D in foods and as supplements. *Prog Biophys Mol Biol* 92(1):33–38. doi:10.1016/j.pbiomolbio.2006.02.017.

221 Prietl, B. Treiber, G., Pieber, T. R., Amrein, K. (2013) Vitamin D and immune function. *Nutrients* 5(7):2502–21. doi:10.3390/nu5072502.

222 Schwalfenberg, G. K., Genuis, S. J., Hiltz, M. N. (2010) Addressing vitamin D deficiency in Canada: A public health innovation whose time has come. *Public Health* 124(6):350–59. doi:10.1016/j.puhe.2010.03.003.

223 Gröber, U., Spitz, J., Reichrath, J., Kisters, K., Holick, M. F. (2013) Vitamin D: Update 2013: From rickets prophylaxis to general preventive healthcare. *Dermatoendocrinol* 5(3):331–47. doi:10.4161/derm.26738.

224 Hyppönen, E., Läärä, E., Reunanen, A., Järvelin, M. R. (2001) Virtanen SM. Intake of vitamin D and risk of type 1 diabetes: A birth-cohort study. *Lancet* 358(9292):1500–1503. doi:10.1016/S0140–6736(01)06580–1.

225 Ashique, S., Gupta, K., Gupta, G., Mishra, N., Singh, S. K., et al. (2023) Vitamin D—A prominent immunomodulator to prevent COVID-19 infection. *Int J Rheum Dis* 26(1):13–30. doi:10.1111/1756–185X.14477.

226 Prietl, B. Treiber, G., Pieber, T. R., Amrein, K. (2013) Vitamin D and immune function. *Nutrients* 5(7):2502–21. doi:10.3390/nu5072502.

227 Wang, T. T., Nestel, F. P., Bourdeau, V., Nagai, Y., Wang, Q., et al. (2004) Cutting edge: 1,25-dihydroxyvitamin D3 is a direct inducer of antimicrobial peptide gene expression. *J Immunol* 173(5):2909–12. doi:10.4049/jimmunol.173.5.2909.

228 Liu, P. T., Stenger, S., Tang, D. H., Modlin, R. L. (2007) Cutting edge: Vitamin D-mediated human antimicrobial activity against *Mycobacterium tuberculosis* is dependent on the induction of cathelicidin. *J Immunol* 179(4):2060–63. doi:10.4049/jimmunol.179.4.2060.

229 Lowry, M. B., Guo, C., Borregaard, N., Gombart, A. F. (2014) Regulation of the human cathelicidin antimicrobial peptide gene by 1α,25-dihydroxyvitamin D3 in primary immune cells. *J Steroid Biochem Mol Biol* 143:183–91. doi:10.1016/j.jsbmb.2014.02.004.

230 Martens, P. J., Gysemans, C., Verstuyf, A., Mathieu, A. C. (2020) Vitamin D's effect on immune function. *Nutrients* 12(5):1248. doi:10.3390/nu12051248.

231 Baeke, F., Takiishi, T., Korf, H., Gysemans, C., Mathieu, C. (2010) Vitamin D: Modulator of the immune system. *Curr Opin Pharmacol* 10(4):482–96. doi:10.1016/j.coph.2010.04.001.

232 Lemire, J. M., Adams, J. S., Sakai, R., Jordan, S. C. (1984) 1 alpha,25-dihydroxyvitamin D3 suppresses proliferation and immunoglobulin production by normal human peripheral blood mononuclear cells. *J Clin Invest* 74(2):657–61. doi:10.1172/JCI11146.

233 Heine, G., Niesner, U., Chang, H. D., Steinmeyer, A., Zügel, U., et al. (2008) 1,25-dihydroxyvitamin D(3) promotes IL-10 production in human B cells. *Eur J Immunol* 38(8):2210–18. doi:10.1002/eji.200838216.

234 Drozdenko, G., Scheel, T., Heine, G., Baumgrass, R., Worm, M. (2014) Impaired T cell activation and cytokine production by calcitriol-primed human B cells. *Clin Exp Immunol* 178(2):364–72. doi:10.1111/cei.12406.

235 Deluca, H. F., Cantorna, M. T. (2002) Vitamin D: Its role and uses in immunology. *FASEB J* 15(14):2579–85. doi:10.1096/fj.01–0433rev.

236 Tieu, S., Charchoglyan, A., Wagter-Lesperance, L., Karimi, K., Bridle, B.W., et al. (2022) Immunoceuticals: Harnessing their immunomodulatory potential to promote health and wellness. *Nutrients* 14(19):4075. doi:10.3390/nu14194075.

237 Grant, W. B., Lahore, H., McDonnell, S. L., Baggerly, C. A., French, et al. (2020) Evidence that vitamin D supplementation could reduce risk of influenza and COVID-19 infections and deaths. *Nutrients* 12(4):988. doi:10.3390/nu12040988.

238 van Ballegooijen, A. J., Pilz, S, Tomaschitz, A., Grübler, M. R., Verheyen, N. (2017) The synergistic interplay between vitamins D and K for bone and cardiovascular health: A narrative review. *Int J Endocrinol* 2017:7454376. doi:10.1155/2017/7454376.

239 Tieu, S., Charchoglyan, A., Wagter-Lesperance, L., Karimi, K., Bridle, B. W., et al. (2022) Immunoceuticals: Harnessing their immunomodulatory potential to promote health and wellness. *Nutrients* 14(19):4075. doi:10.3390/nu14194075.

240 FLCCC and World Council for Health. (2023) Vitamin D for COVID-19. Retrieved from c19early.org/d.

241 Abdollahi, A., Sarvestani, H. K., Rafat, Z., Ghaderkhani, S., Mahmoudi-Aliabadi, M., et al. (2021) The association between the level of serum 25(OH) vitamin D, obesity, and underlying diseases with the risk of developing COVID-19 infection: A case-control study of hospitalized patients in Tehran, Iran. *J Med Virol* 93:2359–64. doi:10.1002/jmv.26726.

242 Jude, E. B., Ling, S. F., Allcock, S., Yeap, B. X. Y., Pappachan, J. M. (2021) Vitamin D deficiency is associated with higher hospitalization risk from COVID-19: A retrospective case-control study. *J Clin Endocrin Metab*. 06(11):e4708–15. doi:10.1210/clinem/dgab439.

243 Borsche, L., Glauner, B., von Mendel, J. (2021) COVID-19 mortality risk correlates inversely with vitamin D3 status, and a mortality rate close to zero could theoretically be achieved at 50 ng/mL 25(OH)D3: Results of a systematic review and meta-analysis. *Nutrients* 13(10):3596. doi:10.3390/nu13103596.

244 Alcala-Diaz, J. F., Limia-Perez, L., Gomez-Huelgas, R., Martin-Escalante, M. D., Cortes-Rodriguez, B., et al. (2021) Calcifediol treatment and hospital mortality due to COVID-19: A cohort study. *Nutrients* 13(6):1760. doi:10.3390/nu13061760.

245 Entrenas Castillo, M., Entrenas Costa, L. M., Vaquero Barrios, J. M., Alcalá Díaz, J. F., López Miranda, J., et al. (2020) Effect of calcifediol treatment and best available therapy versus best available therapy on intensive care unit admission and mortality among patients hospitalized for COVID-19: A pilot randomized clinical study. *J Steroid Biochem Mol Biol* 203:105751. doi:10.1016/j.jsbmb.2020.105751.

246 Sartini, M., Del Puente, F., Oliva, M., Carbone, A., Bobbio, N., et al. (2024) Preventive vitamin D supplementation and risk for COVID-19 infection: A systematic review and meta-analysis. *Nutrients* 16(5):679. doi:10.3390/nu16050679.

247 Jolliffe, D. A., Holt, H., Greenig, M., Talaei, M., Perdek, N., et al. (2022) Effect of a test-and-treat approach to vitamin D supplementation on risk of all cause acute respiratory tract infection and COVID-19: Phase 3 randomised controlled trial (CORONAVIT). *BMJ* 378:e071230. doi:10.1136/bmj-2022–071230.

248 UK Office for National Statistics. (2020) Coronavirus (COVID-19): 2020 in charts. Retrieved from www.ons.gov.uk/peoplepopulationandcommunity/healthandsocialcare/conditionsanddiseases/articles/coronaviruscovid192020incharts/2020–12-18.

249 Brunvoll, S. H., Nygaard, A. B., Ellingjord-Dale, M., Holland, P., Istre, M. S., et al. (2022) Prevention of COVID-19 and other acute respiratory infections with cod liver oil supplementation, a low dose vitamin D supplement: Quadruple blinded, randomised placebo controlled trial. *BMJ* 378:e071245. doi:10.1136/bmj-2022–071245.

250 Borsche, L., Glauner, B., von Mendel, J. (2021) COVID-19 mortality risk correlates inversely with vitamin D3 status, and a mortality rate close to zero could theoretically be achieved at 50 ng/mL 25(OH)D3: Results of a systematic review and meta-analysis . *Nutrients* 13(10):3596. doi:10.3390/nu13103596.

251 Brenner, H., and Schöttker, B. (2020) Vitamin D insufficiency may account for almost nine of ten COVID-19 deaths: Time to act. Comment on: "Vitamin D deficiency and outcome of COVID-19 Patients." *Nutrients* 12(12):3642. doi:10.3390/nu12123642.

252 Carman, K. (2022) From A to Zinc: Your guide to the top nutrients, vitamins and supplements for better health. FLCCC Alliance. Retrieved from covid19criticalcare.com/wp-content/uploads/2023/05/From-A-to-Zinc-the-FLCCC-Nutrient-Guide.pdf.

253 Yuandani, Jantan, I., Rohani, A. S., Sumantri, I.B. (2021) Immunomodulatory effects and mechanisms of *Curcuma* species and their bioactive compounds: A review. *Front Pharmacol* 12:643119. doi.org/10.3389/fphar.2021.643119.

254 Karimi, K. Sarir, H., Mortaz, E., Smit, J. J., Hosseini, H., et al. (2006) Toll-like receptor-4 mediates cigarette smoke-induced cytokine production by human macrophages. *Respir Res* 7(1):66. doi:10.1186/1465–9921-7–66.

255 Vors, C., Couillard, C., Paradis, M.-B., Gigleux, I., Marin, J., et al. (2018) Supplementation with resveratrol and curcumin does not affect the inflammatory response to a high-fat meal in older adults with abdominal obesity: A randomized, placebo-controlled crossover trial. *J Nutr* 148(3):379–88. doi:10.1093/jn/nxx072.

256 Bereswill, S., Muñoz, M., Fischer, A., Plickert, R., Haag, L. M., et al. (2010) Anti-inflammatory effects of resveratrol, curcumin and simvastatin in acute small intestinal inflammation. *PLOS One* 5(12):e15099. doi:10.1371/journal.pone.0015099.

257 Gan, Z., Wei, W., Li, Y., Wu, J., Zhao, Y., et al. (2019) Curcumin and resveratrol regulate intestinal bacteria and alleviate inflammation in weaned piglets. *Molecules* 24(7):1220. doi10.3390/molecules24071220.

258 Dabeek, W. M., Marra, M. V. (2019) Dietary quercetin and kaempferol: Bioavailability and potential cardiovascular-related bioactivity in humans. *Nutrients* 11(10):2288. doi10.3390/nu11102288.

259 Al-Khayri, J. M., Sahana, G. R., Nagella, P., Joseph, B. V., Alessa, F. M., Al-Mssallem, M. Q. (2022) Flavonoids as potential anti-Inflammatory molecules: A review. *Molecules* 27(9):2901. doi:10.3390/molecules27092901.

260 Hasan, Z. T., Atrakji, M. Q. Y. M. A. A., Mehuaiden, A. K. (2022) The effect of melatonin on thrombosis, sepsis and mortality rate in COVID-19 Patients. *Int J Infect Dis* 114:79–84. doi:10.1016/j.ijid.2021.10.012.

261 Imran, M., Thabet, H. K., Alaqel, S. I., Alzahrani, A. R., Abida, A., et al. (2022) The therapeutic and prophylactic potential of quercetin against COVID-19: An outlook on the clinical studies, inventive compositions, and patent literature. *Antioxidants* (Basel) 11(5):876. doi:10.3390/antiox11050876.

262 Mlcek, J., Jurikova, T., Skrovankova, S., Sochor, J. (2016) Quercetin and its anti-allergic immune response. *Molecules* 21(5):623. doi:10.3390/molecules21050623.

263 Zhou, X., Afzal, S., Zheng, Y. F., Münch, G., Li, C. G. (2021) Synergistic protective effect of curcumin and resveratrol against oxidative stress in endothelial EAhy926 cells. *Evid Based Complement Alternat Med* 2021:2661025. doi:10.1155/2021/2661025.

264 Li, Y. H., Niu, Y. B., Sun, Y., Zhang, F, Liu, C., et al. (2015) Role of phytochemicals in colorectal cancer prevention. *World J Gastroenterol* 21(31):9262–72. doi:10.3748/wjg.v21.i31.9262.

265 Xiao, Z., Ye, Q., Duan, X., Xiang, T. (2021) Network pharmacology reveals that resveratrol can alleviate COVID-19-related hyperinflammation. *Dis Markers* 2021:4129993. doi:10.1155/2021/4129993.

266 Pasquereau, S., Nehme, Z., Haidar Ahmad, S., Daouad, F., Van Assche, J., et al. (2021) Resveratrol inhibits HCoV-229E and SARS-CoV-2 coronavirus replication *in vitro*. *Viruses* 13(2):354. doi:10.3390/v13020354.

267 Derwand, R., Scholz, M., Zelenko, V. (2020) COVID-19 outpatients: Early risk-stratified treatment with zinc plus low-dose hydroxychloroquine and azithromycin: A retrospective case series study. *Int J Antimicrob Agents* 56(6):106214. doi:10.1016/j.ijantimicag.2020.106214.

268 Ibid.

269 Moghaddam, A., Heller, R. A., Sun, Q., Seelig, J., Cherkezov, A., et al. (2020) Selenium deficiency is associated with mortality risk from COVID-19. *Nutrients* 12:2098. doi:10.3390/nu12072098.

270 Guillin, O. M., Vindry, C., Ohlmann, T., Chavatte, L. (2019) Selenium, selenoproteins and viral infection. *Nutrients* 11:2101. doi:10.3390/nu11092101.

271 Izquierdo-Alonso, J. L., Pérez-Rial, S., Rivera, C. G., Peces-Barba, G. (2022) N-acetylcysteine for prevention and treatment of COVID-19: Current state of evidence and future directions. *J Infect Public Health* 15(12):1477–83. doi:10.1016/j.jiph.2022.11.009.

272 Jassey, A., Imtiyaz, Z., Jassey, S., Imtiyaz, M., Rasool, S. (2022) Antiviral effects of black seeds: Effect on COVID-19. Black Seeds (*Nigella Sativa*) 2022:387–404. doi:10.1016/B978–0-12–824462-3.00004–4.

273 Tepasse, P. R., Vollenberg, R., Fobker, M., Kabar, I., Schmidt, H., et al. (2021) Vitamin A plasma levels in COVID-19 patients: A prospective multicenter study and hypothesis. *Nutrients* 13(7):2173. doi:10.3390/nu13072173.

274 Cerullo, G., Negro, M., Parimbelli, M., Pecoraro, M., Perna, S., et al. (2020) The long history of Vitamin C: From prevention of the common cold to potential aid in the treatment of COVID-19. *Front Immunol* 11:574029. doi:10.3389/fimmu.2020.574029.

275 Miranda-Massari, J. R., Toro, A. P., Loh, D., Rodriguez, J. R., Borges, R. M., et al. (2021) The effects of Vitamin C on the multiple pathophysiological stages of COVID-19. *Life* (Basel) 11(12):1341. doi:10.3390/life11121341.

276 Sokary, S., Ouagueni, A., Ganji, V. (2022) Intravenous ascorbic acid and lung function in severely ill COVID-19 patients. *Metabolites* 12(9):865. doi:10.3390/metabo12090865.

277 Grand View Research. (2021) Mushroom market size, share & trends analysis report by product (Button, Shiitake, Oyster), by form, by distribution channel, by application (food, pharmaceuticals, cosmetics), by region, and segment forecasts, 2022–2030. Retrieved from www.grandviewresearch.com/industry-analysis/mushroom-market.

278 Sullivan, R., Smith, J. E., Rowan, N. J. (2006) Medicinal mushrooms and cancer therapy: Translating a traditional practice into Western medicine. *Perspect Biol Med* 49(2):159–70. doi:10.1353/pbm.2006.0034.

279 Brown, G. D., Gordon, S. (2003) Fungal beta-glucans and mammalian immunity. *Immunity* 19(3):311–15. doi:10.1016/s1074-7613(03)00233-4.

280 Ina, K., Kataoka, T., Ando, T. (2013) The use of lentinan for treating gastric cancer. *Anticancer Agents Med Chem* 13(5):681–88. doi:10.2174/1871520611313050002.

281 Tzianabos, A. O. (2000) Polysaccharide immunomodulators as therapeutic agents: Structural aspects and biologic function. *Clin Microbiol Rev* 13(4):523–33. doi:10.1128/CMR.13.4.523.

282 Kato, M., Hirose, K., Hakozaki, M., Ohno, M., Saito, Y., et al. (1995) Induction of gene expression for immunomodulating cytokines in peripheral blood mononuclear cells in response to orally administered PSK, an immunomodulating protein-bound polysaccharide. *Cancer Immunol Immunother* 40(3):152–56. doi:10.1007/BF01517346.

283 Liu, F., Fung, M. C., Ooi, V. E., Chang, S. T. (1996) Induction in the mouse of gene expression of immunomodulating cytokines by mushroom polysaccharide-protein complexes. *Life Sci* 58(21):1795–1803. doi:10.1016/0024-3205(96)00163-4.

284 Smith, J. E., Sullivan, R., Rowan, N. J. (2005) Mushrooms and cancer therapy. *Biologist* (London, England) 52(6):328–36.

285 Tan, P., Li, X., Shen, J., Feng, Q. (2020) Fecal microbiota transplantation for the treatment of inflammatory bowel disease: An update. *Front Pharmacol* 11:574533. doi:10.3389/fphar.2020.574533.

286 Tieu, S., Charchoglyan, A., Wagter-Lesperance, L., Karimi, K., Bridle, B. W., et al. (2022) Immunoceuticals: Harnessing their immunomodulatory potential to promote health and wellness. *Nutrients* 14(19):4075. doi:10.3390/nu14194075.

287 Campbell, J. (2023) New safe form of immunization. Retrieved from www.youtube.com/watch?v=elBkEJpvuG8.

288 Nakatsu, K. (2021) Stress proteins in COVID-19: Is carbon monoxide formed by heme oxygenase important in drug therapy? Canadian Covid Care Alliance. Retrieved from www.canadiancovidcarealliance.org/all/stress-proteins-in-covid-19-is-carbon-monoxide-formed-by-heme-oxygenase-important-in-drug-therapy/.

289 Kunnumakkara, A. B., Rana, V., Parama, D., Banik, K., Girisa S., et al. (2021) COVID-19, cytokines, inflammation, and spices: How are they related. *Life Sci* 284:1–35. doi:10.1016/j.lfs.2021.119201.

290 FLCCC Alliance. (2023) I-Prevent. COVID, flu and RSV protection. Retrieved from covid19criticalcare.com/wp-content/uploads/2022/12/I-PREVENT-Summary-1.pdf.

291 Winchester, S., John, S., Jabbar, K., John, I. (2021) Clinical efficacy of nitric oxide nasal spray (NONS) for the treatment of mild COVID-19 infection. *J Infect* 83(2):237–79. doi:10.1016/j.jinf.2021.05.009.

292 Tandon, M., Wu, W., Moore, K., Winchester, S., Tu, Y. P., et al.; Study Group. (2022) SARS-CoV-2 accelerated clearance using a novel nitric oxide nasal spray (NONS) treatment: A randomized trial. *Lancet Reg Health Southeast Asia* 3:100036. doi:10.1016/j.lansea.2022.100036.

293 Miller, C., and Moore, K. (2023) Epidemiological analysis of nitric oxide nasal spray (VirX) use in students exposed to COVID-19 infected individuals. J. *Pulmonary Technique* 18(2):38–40. Retrieved from www.respiratorytherapy.ca/pdf/RT-18-2-Spring-2023-R17-web.pdf.

294 C19 Early Treatment Group. (2023) COVID-19 treatment cost effectiveness. Retrieved on October 12, 2023 from c19early.org/cost.html.

Chapter 15

1 (1947) "Permissible medical experiments." Trials of War Criminals before the Nuremberg Military Tribunals under Control Council Law No 10. Nuremberg October 1946–April 1949, Washington. U.S. Government Printing Office (n.d.), vol 2., 181–82.

2 Palmer, M., Bhakdi, S., DesBois, M., Hooker, B., Rasnick, D., et al. (2023) mRNA vaccine toxicity. D4CE.org. Retrieved from doctors4covidethics.org/mRNA-vaccine-toxicity.

3 Mansanguan, S., Charunwatthana, P., Piyaphanee, W., Dechkhajorn, W., Poolcharoen, A., Mansanguan, C. (2022) Cardiovascular manifestation of the BNT162b2 mRNA COVID-19 vaccine in adolescents. *Trop Med Infect Dis* 7(8):196. doi:10.3390/tropicalmed7080196.

4 Feldstein, S. (2023) Population decline will change the world for the better. *Sci Am*. Retrieved from www.scientificamerican.com/article/population-decline-will-change-the-world-for-the-better/.

5 Dettmers, S. (2022) The great people shortage is coming—and it's going to cause global economic chaos. *Insider*. Retrieved from www.businessinsider.com/great-labor-shortage-looming-population-decline-disaster-global-economy-2022–10.

Photo Insert

1 Tali, S. H. S., LeBlanc, J. J., Sadiq, Z., Oyewunmi, O. D., Camargo, C., et al. (2021) Tools and techniques for severe acute respiratory syndrome coronavirus 2 (SARS-CoV-2)/COVID-19 detection. *Clinical Microbiol* 34(3):1–63. doi:10.1128/CMR.00228-20.

2 Yadav, R., Chaudhary, J. K., Jain, N., Chaudhary, P. K., Khanra, S., et al. (2021) Role of structural and non-structural proteins and therapeutic targets of SARS-CoV-2 for COVID-19. *Cells* 10(4):821. doi:10.3390/cells10040821.

3 Huang, Y., Yang, C., Xu, X.F., Xu, W., Liu, S.W. (2020) Structural and functional properties of SARS-CoV-2 spike protein: Potential antivirus drug development for COVID-19. *Acta Pharmacol Sin* 41(9):1141–49. doi:10.1038/s41401-020-0485-4.

4 Zhao, X., Chen, H., Wang, H. (2021) Glycans of SARS-CoV-2 spike protein in virus infection and antibody production. *Front Mol. Biosci* 8:629873. doi:10.3389/fmolb.2021.629873.

5 Huang et al., Structural and functional properties of SARS-CoV-2 spike protein.

6 Zhao et al., Glycans of SARS-CoV-2 spike protein in virus infection and antibody production.

7 Lamers, M.M., Haagmans, B.L. (2022) SARS-CoV-2 pathogenesis. *Nat Rev Microbiol.* 20(5):270–284. doi:10.1038/s41579-022-00713-0.

8 Wikipedia. (2023) Influenza. Retrieved from en.wikipedia.org/wiki/Influenza#Research.

9 Kim, Sekhon, Shin, Ahn, Cho, et al. Modifications of mRNA vaccine structural elements for improving mRNA stability and translation efficiency.

10 Josephson, F. (2020) Rapporteur's Rolling Review assessment report. Committee for Medicinal Products for Human Use. EMEA/H/C/005735/RR. Retrieved from covidvaccinereactions.com/ema-pfizer-leak/.

11 Shrestha, N.K., Burke, P.C., Nowacki, A.S., Simon J.F., Hagen, A., Gordon, S.M. (2023) Effectiveness of the coronavirus disease 2019 bivalent vaccine. Open Forum Infect Dis. 10(6):ofad209. doi:10.1093/ofid/ofad209
12 UK Office for National Statistics, Deaths by vaccination status, England.
13 C19early.org. (2023) COVID-19 early treatment: Real-time analysis of 3,363 studies. Retrieved August 18, 2023 from c19early.org/; reproduced under Creative Commons license.
14 NIH National Library of Medicine. (2023) PubChem: Explore chemistry. Retrieved from pubchem.ncbi.nlm.nih.gov/.